Molecular Pharmacology and Pathology of Strokes

Molecular Pharmacology and Pathology of Strokes

Special Issue Editor

Joen-Rong Sheu

MDPI • Basel • Beijing • Wuhan • Barcelona • Belgrade

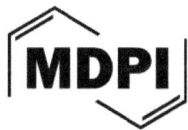

Special Issue Editor
Joen-Rong Sheu
Taipei Medical University
Taiwan

Editorial Office
MDPI
St. Alban-Anlage 66
4052 Basel, Switzerland

This is a reprint of articles from the Special Issue published online in the open access journal *International Journal of Molecular Sciences* (ISSN 1422-0067) from 2017 to 2018 (available at: https://www.mdpi.com/journal/ijms/special_issues/strokes)

For citation purposes, cite each article independently as indicated on the article page online and as indicated below:

LastName, A.A.; LastName, B.B.; LastName, C.C. Article Title. *Journal Name* **Year**, *Article Number*, Page Range.

ISBN 978-3-03897-541-0 (Pbk)
ISBN 978-3-03897-542-7 (PDF)

© 2019 by the authors. Articles in this book are Open Access and distributed under the Creative Commons Attribution (CC BY) license, which allows users to download, copy and build upon published articles, as long as the author and publisher are properly credited, which ensures maximum dissemination and a wider impact of our publications.

The book as a whole is distributed by MDPI under the terms and conditions of the Creative Commons license CC BY-NC-ND.

Contents

About the Special Issue Editor vii

Joen-Rong Sheu
Molecular Pharmacology and Pathology of Strokes
Reprinted from: *Int. J. Mol. Sci.* **2018**, *19*, 4103, doi:10.3390/ijms19124103 1

Li-Ming Lien, Kuan-Hung Lin, Li-Ting Huang, Mei-Fang Tseng, Hou-Chang Chiu, Ray-Jade Chen and Wan-Jung Lu
Licochalcone A Prevents Platelet Activation and Thrombus Formation through the Inhibition of PLCγ2-PKC, Akt, and MAPK Pathways
Reprinted from: *Int. J. Mol. Sci.* **2017**, *18*, 1500, doi:10.3390/ijms18071500 5

Chih-Wei Hsia, Marappan Velusamy, Jeng-Ting Tsao, Chih-Hsuan Hsia, Duen-Suey Chou, Thanasekaran Jayakumar, Lin-Wen Lee, Jiun-Yi Li and Joen-Rong Sheu
New Therapeutic Agent against Arterial Thrombosis: An Iridium(III)-Derived Organometallic Compound
Reprinted from: *Int. J. Mol. Sci.* **2017**, *18*, 2616, doi:10.3390/ijms18122616 21

Piotr K. Janicki, Ceren Eyileten, Victor Ruiz-Velasco, Khaled Anwar Sedeek, Justyna Pordzik, Anna Czlonkowska, Iwona Kurkowska-Jastrzebska, Shigekazu Sugino, Yuka Imamura-Kawasawa, Dagmara Mirowska-Guzel and Marek Postula
Population-Specific Associations of Deleterious Rare Variants in Coding Region of P2RY1–P2RY12 Purinergic Receptor Genes in Large-Vessel Ischemic Stroke Patients
Reprinted from: *Int. J. Mol. Sci.* **2017**, *18*, 2678, doi:10.3390/ijms18122678 37

Ting-Lin Yen, Chao-Chien Chang, Chi-Li Chung, Wen-Chin Ko, Chih-Hao Yang and Cheng-Ying Hsieh
Neuroprotective Effects of Platonin, a Therapeutic Immunomodulating Medicine, on Traumatic Brain Injury in Mice after Controlled Cortical Impact
Reprinted from: *Int. J. Mol. Sci.* **2018**, *19*, 1100, doi:10.3390/ijms19041100 49

A Ra Kho, Bo Young Choi, Song Hee Lee, Dae Ki Hong, Sang Hwon Lee, Jeong Hyun Jeong, Kyoung-Ha Park, Hong Ki Song, Hui Chul Choi and Sang Won Suh
Effects of Protocatechuic Acid (PCA) on Global Cerebral Ischemia-Induced Hippocampal Neuronal Death
Reprinted from: *Int. J. Mol. Sci.* **2018**, *19*, 1420, doi:10.3390/ijms19051420 63

Thanasekaran Jayakumar, Chia-Yuan Hsu, Themmila Khamrang, Chih-Hsuan Hsia, Chih-Wei Hsia, Manjunath Manubolu and Joen-Rong Sheu
Possible Molecular Targets of Novel Ruthenium Complexes in Antiplatelet Therapy
Reprinted from: *Int. J. Mol. Sci.* **2018**, *19*, 1818, doi:10.3390/ijms19061818 82

In-Ae Choi, Cheol Soon Lee, Hahn Young Kim, Dong-Hee Choi and Jongmin Lee
Effect of Inhibition of DNA Methylation Combined with Task-Specific Training on Chronic Stroke Recovery
Reprinted from: *Int. J. Mol. Sci.* **2018**, *19*, 2019, doi:10.3390/ijms19072019 94

Ami P. Raval, Marc Schatz, Pallab Bhattacharya, Nathan d'Adesky, Tatjana Rundek, Dalton Dietrich and Helen M. Bramlett
Whole Body Vibration Therapy after Ischemia Reduces Brain Damage in Reproductively Senescent Female Rats
Reprinted from: *Int. J. Mol. Sci.* **2018**, *19*, 2749, doi:10.3390/ijms19092749 113

Chih-Hao Yang, Chih-Wei Hsia, Thanasekaran Jayakumar, Joen-Rong Sheu, Chih-Hsuan Hsia, Themmila Khamrang, Yen-Jen Chen, Manjunath Manubolu and Yi Chang
Structure–Activity Relationship Study of Newly Synthesized Iridium-III Complexes as Potential Series for Treating Thrombotic Diseases
Reprinted from: *Int. J. Mol. Sci.* **2018**, *19*, 3641, doi:10.3390/ijms19113641 . . . . **125**

About the Special Issue Editor

Joen-Rong Sheu, Ph.D., is a Distinguished Professor of Pharmacology in the Graduate Institute of Medical Sciences, Taipei Medical University, Taiwan. Dr. Sheu gained his Ph.D. in Pharmacology in 1992 from the Institute of Pharmacology, College of Medicine, National Taiwan University, Taiwan. Dr. Sheu has held the higher academic and administrative positions of Dean of the Office of Research and Development; Vice-Dean of the College of Medicine; Director of the Graduate Institute of Medical Sciences, and Director of the Department of Pharmacology at Taipei Medical University. Prof. Sheu has over 300 publications including papers in Circulation, Blood, Journal of Biological Chemistry, Haematologica, Arteriosclerosis, Thrombosis, and Vascular Biology (ATVB), Thrombosis and Haemostasis, Journal of Thrombosis and Haemostasis, Free Radical Biology and Medicine, Cardiovascular Research, and the British Journal of Pharmacology, etc. His major research interests are identifying molecular pathways for antithrombotic and neuroprotection therapy. He has also been widely involved in cardiovascular pharmacology, cancer biology, protein bio-chemistry, and signal transduction studies. Prof. Sheu's recent investigations have included metal-based therapeutic strategies in models of antithrombotic and anti-inflammatory diseases. Despite Prof. Sheu's having served as an eminent academician for over 25 years, it is notable that he has been recognized through several awards and honors, which include the "Research Award of National Science Council, Taiwan; the Academic Award of American Huang Chi-Hsing Fundation, USA; the Research Award of Lee Hung-Hsin Fundation, Taiwan; and Outstanding Researcher Awards from the Taiwan Pharmacological Society and Taipei Medical University, Taiwan".

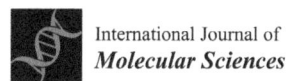 International Journal of
Molecular Sciences

Editorial

Molecular Pharmacology and Pathology of Strokes

Joen-Rong Sheu

Graduate Institute of Medical Sciences, College of Medicine, Taipei Medical University, 250 Wu-Hsing Street, Taipei 110, Taiwan; sheujr@tmu.edu.tw; Tel.: +886-2-2736-1661 (ext. 3199); Fax: +886-2-2739-0450

Received: 13 December 2018; Accepted: 17 December 2018; Published: 18 December 2018

Stroke, an important neurological disease, is becoming an increasingly non-communicable ailment and is the second leading cause of death after coronary heart disease in developed countries [1]. Present treatment options for stroke are adapting lifestyle practice, diabetes treatment, drugs, and other factors management, but no cure is yet available, despite new insights into the molecular and therapeutic targets. Discoveries in explicating the molecular pharmacology in cerebrovascular function and thrombosis have led to significant advancements in the current treatment paradigm for patients with stroke. Hence, this Special Issue invited scientific papers and reviews from researchers to provide solid evidence from a molecular point of view to scrutinize the molecular pharmacology and pathology of strokes. Platelet activation plays a major role in cardio and cerebrovascular diseases. Platelets also play a key role in the hemostatic process and are associated with various pathological events, such as arterial thrombosis and atherosclerosis. While currently used anti-platelet drugs such as aspirin and clopidogrel demonstrate efficacy in many patients, they exert undesirable side effects. Therefore, the development of effective therapeutic strategies for the prevention and treatment of thrombotic diseases is a demanding priority. Recently, precious metal drugs have conquered the subject of metal-based drugs, and several investigators have moved their attention to the synthesis of various ruthenium (Ru) and iridium (Ir) complexes due to their prospective therapeutic values.

In this Special Issue, the authors Hsia et al. [2] found that Ir (III)-derived complex, (Ir-11), showed potent antiplatelet activity by inhibiting platelet activation through the suppression of the phosphorylation of phospholipase Cγ2 (PLCγ2), protein kinase C (PKC) cascade and the subsequent suppression of Akt and mitogen-activated protein kinases (MAPKs) activation, ultimately inhibiting platelet aggregation. A detailed in vitro antiplatelet, in vivo antithrombotic and structure-activity relationship (SAR) study was performed on newly synthesized Ir complexes, Ir-1, Ir-2 and Ir-4, in agonists-induced human platelets [3]. This study found that Ir-1 expressively suppressed collagen-induced Akt, PKC, p38MAPKs and JNK phosphorylation. Interestingly, platelet function analyzer (PFA-100) showed that Ir-1 caused a significant increase in collagen-adenosine diphosphate (C-ADP) induced closure times in mice, but Ir-2 and 4 had no effect on these reactions. Moreover, Ir-1 significantly prolonged the platelet plug formation, increased tail bleeding times and reduced the mortality of adenosine diphosphate (ADP)-induced acute pulmonary thromboembolism in mice. Ir-1 has no substitution on its phenyl group; a water molecule (like cisplatin) can replace its chloride ion and, hence, the rate of hydrolysis might be tuned by the substituent on the ligand system. These features might have played a role for the observed effects of Ir-1. These results indicate that Ir compounds may be a lead compound to design new antiplatelet drugs for the treatment of thromboembolic diseases.

A major review has summarized the antiplatelet activity of newly synthesized ruthenium (Ru)-based compounds (TQ-1, 2, 3, 5 and 6) with their potential molecular mechanisms [4]. This paper condenses the antiplatelet activity of Ru compounds with the major aspects of (i) ruthenium compounds on adenosine triphosphate (ATP) and [Ca^{2+}]i mobilization in antiplatelet therapy, (ii) ruthenium compounds on MAPKs in antiplatelet effects, (iii) ruthenium compounds on cyclic adenosine 3′,5′-monophosphate (cAMP) and cyclic guanosine 3′,5′-cyclic monophosphate (cGMP) signaling in platelets, (iv) molecular targets of ruthenium compounds in antiplatelet property,

(v) antithrombotic effect of ruthenium compounds and (vi) safety and toxicity of ruthenium compounds in platelets. The given information in platelet biology and the functions of ruthenium compounds used for antiplatelet therapy will provide new opportunities to develop therapeutic strategies aimed at promoting cerebro/cardiovascular health.

In addition to the metal complexes, a natural compound, licochalcone A (LA), an active ingredient of licorice, has been studied for its antiplatelet effects. This study demonstrated that LA effectively reduced platelet activation and thrombus formation through the inhibition of PLCγ2-PKC, Akt, and MAPK pathways, without the side effect of bleeding [5]. These results concluded that LA may provide a safe and alternative therapeutic approach for preventing thromboembolic disorders such as stroke.

In the paper by Janicki et al. [6], the population-specific associations of deleterious rare variants in coding region of P2RY1-P2RY12 purinergic receptor genes in large-vessel ischemic stroke patients were studied. In this paper, the authors identified the association between ischemic stroke (IS) and six rare functional and damaging variants in the purinergic genes (P2RY1 and P2RY12 locus). The predicted properties of the most damaging rare variants in P2RY1 and P2RY12 were confirmed by using mouse fibroblast cell cultures transfected with plasmid constructs containing cDNA of mutated variants (FLIPR on FlexStation3). This study recognized a reputed role for rare variants in P2RY1 and P2RY12 genes involved in platelet reactivity on large-vessel IS susceptibility in a Polish population.

Traumatic brain injury (TBI) is one of the leading causes of mortality worldwide and leads to persistent cognitive, sensory, motor dysfunction, and emotional disorders. Yen et al. [7] discovered the neuroprotective effects of platonin, a cyanine photosensitizing dye, against TBI in a controlled cortical impact (CCI) injury model in mice. They found that platonin reduced the neurological severity score, general locomotor activity, and anxiety-related behavior, and improved the rotarod performance of CCI-injured mice, and it reduced lesion volumes, the expression of cleaved caspase-3, and microglial activation in TBI-insulted brains. This natural compound also suppressed mRNA expression of caspase-3, caspase-1, cyclooxygenase-2 (COX-2), tumor necrosis factor-α (TNF-α), interleukin-6 (IL-6), and interleukin-1β (IL-1 β). This study suggested that treatment with platonin exhibited prominent neuroprotective properties against TBI in a CCI mouse model through its anti-inflammatory, anti-apoptotic, and anti-free radical capabilities, and this data indicates that platonin may be a potential therapeutic medicine for use with TBI.

Protocatechuic acid (PCA), a major metabolite of the antioxidant polyphenols, has been found in green tea. Protocatechuic acid had been reported as having antioxidant effects in healthy cells and anti-proliferative effects in tumor cells. Global cerebral ischemia (GCI) is one of the main roots of hippocampal neuronal death. Ischemic damage can be saved by early blood reperfusion. Nevertheless, under some situations reperfusion can activate a cell death process started by the reintroduction of blood, followed by the production of superoxide, a blood brain barrier (BBB) disruption and microglial activation. In the present Special Issue, Kho et al. [8] found that PCA significantly diminishes degenerating neuronal cell death, oxidative stress, microglial activation, astrocyte activation and BBB disruption. Moreover, an ischemia-induced reduction in glutathione concentration in hippocampal neurons is recovered by PCA administration. The obtained results provide evidence supporting the idea that administration of PCA may act as a promising tool for decreasing hippocampal neuronal death after global cerebral ischemia.

The importance of task-specific training (TST) as a neuromotor intervention in neurological restoration has been evidenced [9]. Task-specific training can improve experience-dependent motor skill learning and neural plastic changes in animal and human brains [9]. The effectiveness of TST alone and combined with DNA methyltransferase inhibitor in chronic stroke recovery was investigated. The authors found TST and TST with DNA methyltransferase inhibitor significantly increased the crossing fibers from the contralesional red nucleus, reticular formation in medullar oblongata, and dorsolateral spinal cord. Functional recovery after chronic stroke may involve axonal plasticity and increased mature brain-derived neurotrophic factor (BDNF). These results suggest that combined therapy to enhance axonal plasticity based on TST and DNA methyltransferase inhibitor constitutes a promising approach for promoting the recovery of function in the chronic stage of stroke [10].

Ischemic stroke can cause enhanced frailty. Numerous studies have been proposed in laboratory animals and patients to reduce frailty and subsequent risk of stroke and cognitive decline. Whole body vibration (WBV) improves cerebral function and cognitive ability that deteriorates with increased frailty. A study examined in this Special Issue to test the efficacy of WBV in reducing post-ischemic stroke frailty and brain damage in reproductively senescent female rats. The results establish a noteworthy reduction in inflammatory markers and infarct volume with substantial increases in brain-derived neurotrophic factor and improvement in functional activity after transient middle cerebral artery occlusion (tMCAO) in middle-aged female rats that had been treated with WBV as compared to the no-WBV group. The conclusion of this study may simplify a faster translation of the WBV involvement for improved outcome after stroke, principally among frail women [11].

Overall, we anticipate that readers will find that this Special Issue reports the significant challenges, predictions, and present advances that are currently being faced by stroke research, with the possibility of inspiring the application of novel drug development for enriching the devotion and treatment of patients with cardiovascular diseases.

Funding: Grants from the Ministry of Science and Technology of Taiwan (MOST 104-2622-B-038-003, MOST 104-2320-B-038-045-MY2 and MOST 106-2320-B-038-012).

Conflicts of Interest: The author declares no conflict of interest.

References

1. Shekhar, S.; Cunningham, M.W.; Pabbidi, M.R.; Wang, S.; Booz, G.W.; Fan, F. Targeting vascular inflammation in ischemic stroke: Recent developments on novel immunomodulatory approaches. *Eur. J. Pharmacol.* **2018**, *15*, 531–544. [CrossRef] [PubMed]
2. Hsia, C.W.; Velusamy, M.; Tsao, J.T.; Hsia, C.H.; Chou, D.S.; Jayakumar, T.; Lee, L.W.; Li, J.Y.; Sheu, J.R. New Therapeutic agent against arterial thrombosis: An Iridium(III)-derived organometallic compound. *Int. J. Mol. Sci.* **2017**, *18*, 2616. [CrossRef] [PubMed]
3. Yang, C.H.; Hsia, C.W.; Jayakumar, T.; Sheu, J.R.; Hsia, C.H.; Khamrang, T.; Chen, Y.J.; Manubolu, M.; Chang, Y. Structure–activity relationship study of newly synthesized iridium-III complexes as potential series for treating thrombotic diseases. *Int. J. Mol. Sci.* **2018**, *19*, 3641. [CrossRef] [PubMed]
4. Jayakumar, T.; Hsu, C.Y.; Khamrang, T.; Hsia, C.H.; Hsia, C.W.; Manubolu, M.; Sheu, J.R. Possible molecular targets of novel ruthenium complexes in antiplatelet therapy. *Int. J. Mol. Sci.* **2018**, *19*, 1818. [CrossRef] [PubMed]
5. Lien, L.M.; Lin, K.H.; Huang, L.T.; Tseng, M.F.; Chiu, H.C.; Chen, R.J.; Lu, W.J. Licochalcone A prevents platelet activation and thrombus formation through the inhibition of PLCγ2-PKC, Akt, and MAPK pathways. *Int. J. Mol. Sci.* **2017**, *18*, 1500. [CrossRef] [PubMed]
6. Janicki, P.; Eyileten, C.; Ruiz-Velasco, V.; Sedeek, K.; Pordzik, J.; Czlonkowska, A.; Kurkowska-Jastrzebska, I.; Sugino, S.; Imamura-Kawasawa, Y.; Mirowska-Guzel, D.; Postula, M. Population-specific associations of deleterious rare variants in coding region of P2RY1–P2RY12 purinergic receptor genes in large-vessel ischemic stroke patients. *Int. J. Mol. Sci.* **2017**, *18*, 2678. [CrossRef] [PubMed]
7. Yen, T.L.; Chang, C.C.; Chung, C.L.; Ko, W.C.; Yang, C.H.; Hsieh, C.Y. Neuroprotective effects of platonin, a therapeutic immunomodulating medicine, on traumatic brain injury in mice after controlled cortical impact. *Int. J. Mol. Sci.* **2018**, *19*, 1100. [CrossRef] [PubMed]
8. Kho, A.; Choi, B.; Lee, S.; Hong, D.; Lee, S.; Jeong, J.; Park, K.H.; Song, H.; Choi, H.; Suh, S. Effects of Protocatechuic acid (PCA) on global cerebral ischemia-induced hippocampal neuronal death. *Int. J. Mol. Sci.* **2018**, *19*, 1420. [CrossRef] [PubMed]
9. Okabe, N.; Himi, N.; Maruyama-Nakamura, E.; Hayashi, N.; Narita, K.; Miyamoto, O. Rehabilitative skilled forelimb training enhances axonal remodeling in the corticospinal pathway but not the brainstem-spinal pathways after photothrombotic stroke in the primary motor cortex. *PLoS ONE* **2017**, *12*, e0187413. [CrossRef] [PubMed]

10. Choi, I.A.; Lee, C.; Kim, H.; Choi, D.H.; Lee, J. Effect of inhibition of DNA methylation combined with Task-Specific Training on chronic stroke recovery. *Int. J. Mol. Sci.* **2018**, *19*, 2019. [CrossRef] [PubMed]
11. Raval, A.; Schatz, M.; Bhattacharya, P.; d'Adesky, N.; Rundek, T.; Dietrich, W.; Bramlett, H. Whole body vibration therapy after ischemia reduces brain damage in reproductively senescent female rats. *Int. J. Mol. Sci.* **2018**, *19*, 2749. [CrossRef] [PubMed]

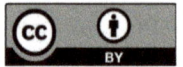

© 2018 by the author. Licensee MDPI, Basel, Switzerland. This article is an open access article distributed under the terms and conditions of the Creative Commons Attribution (CC BY) license (http://creativecommons.org/licenses/by/4.0/).

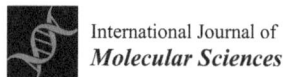

Article

Licochalcone A Prevents Platelet Activation and Thrombus Formation through the Inhibition of PLCγ2-PKC, Akt, and MAPK Pathways

Li-Ming Lien [1,2,†], Kuan-Hung Lin [3,4,†], Li-Ting Huang [5], Mei-Fang Tseng [5], Hou-Chang Chiu [2,6], Ray-Jade Chen [1,5,*] and Wan-Jung Lu [3,5,7,*]

1. School of Medicine, College of Medicine, Taipei Medical University, Taipei 110, Taiwan; M002177@ms.skh.org.tw
2. Department of Neurology, Shin Kong Wu Ho Su Memorial Hospital, Taipei 111, Taiwan; M001012@ms.skh.org.tw
3. Department of Pharmacology and Graduate Institute of Medical Sciences, Taipei Medical University, Taipei 110, Taiwan; d102092002@tmu.edu.tw
4. Central Laboratory, Shin Kong Wu Ho Su Memorial Hospital, Taipei 111, Taiwan
5. Department of Medical Research and Division of General Surgery, Department of Surgery, Taipei Medical University Hospital, Taipei 110, Taiwan; tiffany4441@gmail.com (L.-T.H.); viola0928@hotmail.com (M.-F.T.)
6. College of Medicine, Fu-Jen Catholic University, Taipei 242, Taiwan
7. Graduate Institute of Metabolism and Obesity Sciences, College of Public Health and Nutrition, Taipei Medical University, Taipei 110, Taiwan
* Correspondence: rayjchen@tmu.edu.tw (R.-J.C.); 144106@h.tmu.edu.tw (W.-J.L.); Tel.: +886-2-2737-2181 (ext. 3310) (R.-J.C.); +886-2-2736-1661 (ext. 3201) (W.-J.L.)
† These authors contributed equally to this work.

Received: 5 June 2017; Accepted: 9 July 2017; Published: 12 July 2017

Abstract: Platelet activation is involved in cardiovascular diseases, such as atherosclerosis and ischemic stroke. Licochalcone A (LA), an active ingredient of licorice, exhibits multiple biological activities such as anti-oxidation and anti-inflammation. However, its role in platelet activation remains unclear. Therefore, the study investigated the antiplatelet mechanism of LA. Our data revealed that LA (2–10 µM) concentration dependently inhibited platelet aggregation induced by collagen, but not thrombin and U46619. LA markedly attenuated collagen-stimulated ATP release, P-selectin secretion, calcium mobilization, and GPIIbIIIa activation, but did not interfere with the collagen binding to platelets. Moreover, LA significantly reduced the activation of PLCγ2, PKC, Akt and MAPKs. Thus, LA attenuates platelet activation, possibly by inhibiting collagen receptor downstream signaling but not by blocking the collagen receptors. In addition, LA prevented adenosine diphosphate (ADP)-induced acute pulmonary thrombosis, fluorescein sodium-induced platelet thrombus formation, and middle cerebral artery occlusion/reperfusion-induced brain injury in mice, but did not affect normal hemostasis. This study demonstrated that LA effectively reduced platelet activation and thrombus formation, in part, through the inhibition of PLCγ2–PKC, Akt, and MAPK pathways, without the side effect of bleeding. These findings also indicate that LA may provide a safe and alternative therapeutic approach for preventing thromboembolic disorders such as stroke.

Keywords: Licochalcone A; middle cerebral artery occlusion; platelet activation; PLCγ2–PKC; thrombus formation

---

1. Introduction

Platelet activation is involved in normal hemostasis and in pathological processes such as atherosclerosis and stroke [1,2]. When blood vessels are injured, exposed extracellular matrix proteins (e.g., collagen and von Willebrand factor) activate platelets and further recruit additional platelets from the bloodstream. These platelets form a firm platelet plug at the injury site to stop blood loss; however, under pathological conditions, the platelets are prone to uncontrolled activation and aggregation and may cause vessel occlusion.

Collagen signaling is mediated through the interaction of collagen and its receptor glycoprotein VI (GPVI) and integrin $\alpha 2\beta 1$ [3], which are located on the plasma membrane of platelets; these receptors transmit the activation signals, including those of phospholipase Cγ2 (PLCγ2) and protein kinase C (PKC) activation, and mediate platelet granule release and calcium mobilization [3], all of which finally lead to glycoprotein IIbIIIa (GPIIbIIIa) activation and subsequent platelet aggregation. These processes are crucial for platelet activation and thrombus formation [4]. Moreover, GPVI serves as a promising pharmacological target for the effective and safe treatment of thrombotic and possibly inflammatory diseases [4]. Aspirin and clopidogrel are commonly used to prevent stroke, but account for only a 20% reduction in all recurrent stroke events [5]. Thus, targeting collagen signaling may provide an alternative therapeutic approach to mitigate the recurrence of secondary stroke.

Licochalcone A (LA), a natural chalcone derived from the roots and rhizomes of *Glycyrrhiza* spp., exhibits multiple biological activities such as antibacterial, antioxidant, anti-inflammatory, antimalarial, antiviral, and antitumor effects [6–11]. LA inhibits lipopolysaccharide (LPS)-induced reactive oxygen species (ROS) production and cytokine release in the RAW 264.7 mouse macrophage cell line [12]. LA also alleviates LPS-induced acute lung and kidney injury through NF-κB and p38/ERK mitogen-activated protein kinase (MAPK) signaling and attenuates pertussis toxin-induced autoimmune encephalomyelitis by reducing the production of tumor necrosis factor-α and interferon-γ in vivo [12–14]. In addition, LA induces tumor cell cycle arrest, apoptosis, and autophagy in a various cancer cell lines [10,11]. These observations reveals that LA protects against several pathological processes.

Although, recently, LA was also reported to reduce rabbit and rat platelet activation through the inhibition of cyclooxygenase-1 (COX-1) activity [15,16], its role in platelet activation and thrombosis remains unclear. In the present study, our preliminary data revealed that LA significantly inhibited collagen-induced platelet aggregation through PLCγ2–PKC pathway, suggesting that, in addition to inhibiting COX-1 activity, LA may attenuate platelet activation through other mechanisms. Therefore, we further systemically investigated the mechanism of LA in platelet activation and for the first time determined whether LA has antithrombotic effect in in vivo studies.

2. Results

2.1. Licochalcone A (LA) Inhibited Collagen-Induced Platelet Aggregation

As shown in Figure 1A, LA (2–10 μM) was used to determine its effect on the platelet aggregation induced by collagen (1 μg/mL). The data indicated that LA (at concentrations of 2, 5 and 10 μM) inhibited collagen-induced platelet aggregation by 16.6%, 45.3% and 90.8%, respectively. The IC$_{50}$ was approximately 5.6 μM. In addition, only at a higher concentration of 80 μM did LA affect thrombin (0.01 U/mL)- or U46619 (1 μM)-mediated platelet aggregation (Figure 1B). These results are consistent with that Okuda-Tanino et al. reported [15] and indicate that LA is more sensitive to the inhibition of collagen-mediated platelet activation. Accordingly, in the following experiments, we mainly evaluated the mechanism of LA at concentrations of 2–10 μM in collagen-mediated platelet activation events.

2.2. LA Inhibited Collagen-Mediated ATP Release and P-Selectin Secretion

Platelet granule release plays a crucial role in the amplification of platelet activation and aggregation. Here, two experiments on ATP release and P-selectin secretion, which were assessed by the microplate reader and through flow cytometry, respectively, were performed to determine whether LA interferes with the granule release induced by collagen. As shown in Figure 1C, luciferase/luciferin was used to detect ATP. The data revealed that collagen markedly induced ATP release, which was reversed by LA (2–10 µM) in a concentration-dependent manner. Moreover, LA (5 and 10 µM) significantly reduced collagen-induced P-selectin secretion (Figure 1D), as determined by the intensity of fluorescein isothiocyanate (FITC)–P-selectin. These findings suggest that LA inhibits collagen-mediated platelet activation through the blockade of granule release.

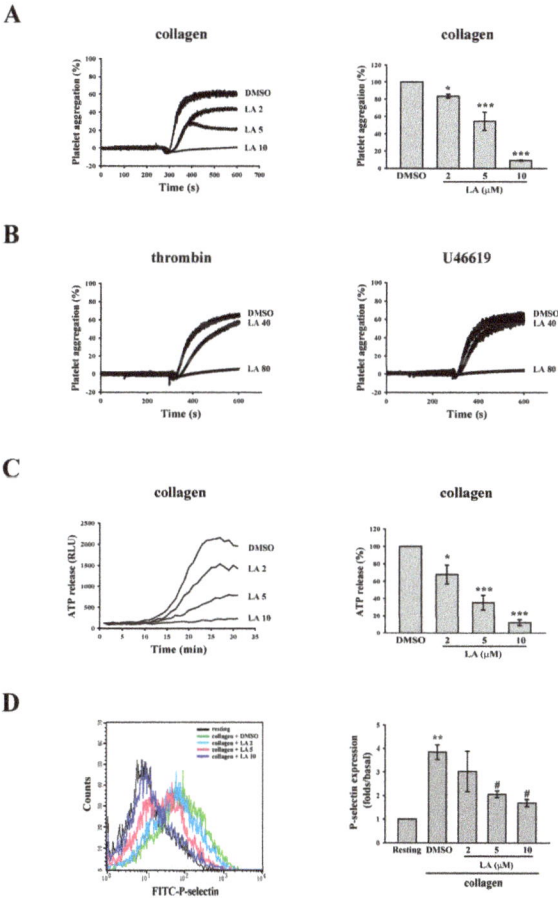

Figure 1. Effects of Licochalcone A (LA) on the collagen-induced platelet aggregation, ATP release, and P-selectin secretion. (**A,B**) Washed platelets (3.6×10^8 cells/mL) were preincubated with DMSO (solvent control) and LA (2–80 µM), and were then stimulated using collagen (1 µg/mL), thrombin (0.01 U/mL), or U46619 (1 µM) to trigger platelet aggregation, as measured by a transmission aggregometer; (**C**) The effect of LA on collagen-induced ATP release was characterized by the detection of chemiluminescent emission from the luciferin–luciferase reaction, which was continually recorded using a microplate reader; (**D**) The effect of LA on collagen-induced P-selectin secretion was detected using FITC–P-selectin antibody. The fluorescence was immediately detected through flow cytometry. The profiles (**B**) are representative examples of five similar experiments. Data (**A,C**) are presented as the mean ± SEM. (**A**, $n = 5$; **C**, $n = 3$). * $p < 0.05$ and *** $p < 0.001$, compared with the DMSO group; Data (**D**) are presented as the mean ± SEM. ($n = 3$). ** $p < 0.01$, compared with the resting group; # $p < 0.05$, compared with the collagen (positive) group.

2.3. LA Inhibited Collagen-Mediated Calcium Mobilization and GPIIbIIIa Activation without Interfering with Collagen Receptors

Calcium signaling is the common platelet activation signaling pathway. Receptor-stimulated PLC catalyzes the hydrolysis of phosphatidylinositol biphosphate to release inositol trisphosphate and diacyglycerol, which activate calcium mobilization and PKC, respectively [17]. The elevation of intracellular Ca^{2+} contributes to several events of platelet activation, such as shape change, granule release, and GPIIbIIIa activaiton [18].

As shown in Figure 2A, fura-2 was used to measure the change in calcium level according to the ratio of F340/F380, which is directly correlated to the amount of intracellular calcium. The data revealed that LA (2–10 µM) markedly inhibited calcium mobilization, as detected using F-4500 Fluorescence Spectrophotometer. Moreover, the FITC–PAC-1 antibody was used to demonstrate that LA (5–10 µM) markedly inhibited GPIIbIIIa activation (Figure 2B), a final step in platelet aggregation, as detected through flow cytometry. These findings indicate that LA blocks calcium mobilization and subsequent GPIIbIIIa activation, thereby inhibiting platelet aggregation. In addition, FITC–collagen was used to determine whether LA directly blocks collagen receptors, leading to the inhibition of its downstream signaling. As shown in Figure 2C, the data obtained from flow cytometry revealed that FITC–collagen markedly binds to platelets. Moreover, pretreated LA did not interfere with the binding of FITC–collagen to platelets. This finding suggests that LA inhibits collagen-induced platelet activation, possibly by inhibiting collagen receptor downstream signaling but not by blocking the collagen receptors. In addition, LA (10–80 µM) did not exhibit cytotoxic effects on platelets, as detected by the LDH assay (Figure 2D), indicating that LA-mediated the inhibition of platelet activation is not due to the cytotoxicity.

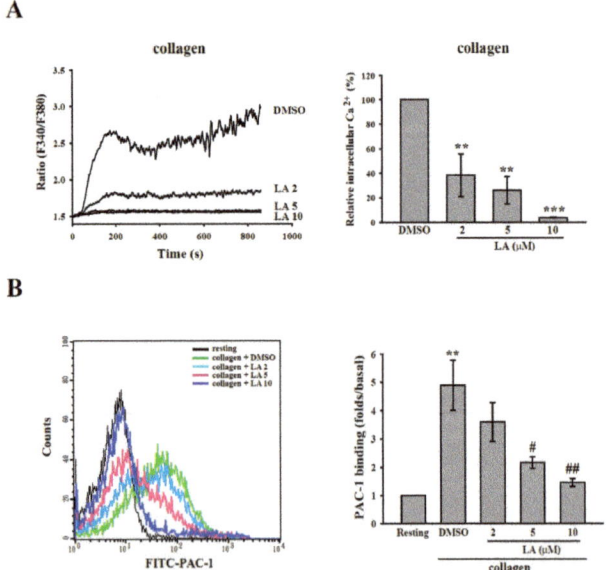

Figure 2. *Cont.*

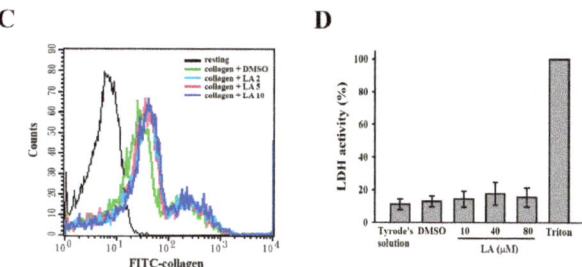

Figure 2. Effects of LA on calcium mobilization, GPIIbIIIa activation, collagen receptors and lactate dehydrogenase (LDH) release. Washed platelets were preincubated with DMSO and LA (2–10 µM), and were then stimulated using 1 µg/mL collagen (**A,B**) or FITC–collagen (**C**). (**A**) The ratio of fura-2 fluorescence (F340/F380) was used to determine calcium mobilization, as measured by a Hitachi F4500 fluorescence spectrophotometer; (**B,C**) GPIIbIIIa activation and the competition with collagen were determined using the FITC–PAC-1 antibody and FITC–collagen, respectively. The fluorescence intensity was measured through flow cytometry; (**D**) The platelets were preincubated with Tyrode's solution, DMSO (solvent control) or various concentrations of LA (10–80 µM) for 10 min at 37 °C, and the supernatant was collected to measure LDH release by the LDH assay kit. LDH activity was expressed as the % of total enzyme activity, which was measured in platelets lysed with 0.5% Triton X-100. Data (**A**) are presented as the means ± SEM (n = 3). ** $p < 0.01$ and *** $p < 0.001$, compared with the DMSO group; Data (**B**) are presented as the means ± SEM (n = 3). ** $p < 0.01$, compared with the resting group # $p < 0.05$ and ## $p < 0.01$, compared with the collagen (positive) group. Profiles (**C,D**) are representative examples of three similar experiments.

2.4. LA Inhibited Collagen-Mediated Platelet Activation Signaling

Collagen mediates platelet activation, mainly by clustering the collagen receptor, GPVI. Therefore, in the present study, we determined the effect of LA on GPVI downstream signaling. As shown in Figure 3A, LA significantly inhibited the collagen-induced PLCγ2 phosphorylation. In addition, the activation of PKC, the downstream of PLCγ2, was also determined. In platelets, the phosphorylation of the major PKC substrate p47 protein (approximately 47 kDa), also known as pleckstrin, has been used to measure PKC activation [19]. Moreover, our data also revealed that the PKC inhibitor Ro318220 (2 µM) markedly inhibited collagen-mediated the phosphorylation of pleckstrin, indicating that this phosphorylation is PKC-dependent (Figure S1). As shown in Figure 3B, LA also inhibited PKC activation (pleckstrin phosphorylation), indicating that LA inhibits platelet activation, in part, through the inhibition of the PLCγ2–PKC pathway. In addition to the common PLCγ2–PKC pathway, the activation of Akt and MAPKs, including Erk, p38 MAPK, and JNK, is involved in collagen-mediated platelet aggregation [20,21]. Hence, we also determined the role of LA in these pathways. As shown in Figure 3C–F, collagen could stimulate the phosphorylation of Akt, p38, JNK, and Erk, and this effect was reversed by LA (2–10 µM). These findings indicate that LA attenuated GPVI downstream signaling, thereby blocking the platelet aggregation induced by collagen.

2.5. LA Alleviated ADP-Induced Pulmonary Thrombosis and Fluorescein Sodium-Induced Platelet Thrombus Formation in the Mesenteric Microvessels of Mice

In the following experiments, we used several animal models to determine the effect of LA on thrombus formation. In the lung thrombosis model of mice, ADP (1.4 g/kg) was used to induce acute pulmonary thrombosis. As shown in Figure 4A (top panel), the lungs of the mice were stained with hematoxylin-eosin. The data revealed that the DMSO group exhibited severe pulmonary thrombosis (arrows), whereas a higher dose of LA (3.6 mg/kg) exerted marked protective effects. In addition, the survival rate of mice was determined at 1 h after ADP was administered (Figure 4A, bottom panel).

The DMSO (solvent control) group had a survival rate of only 12.5% (1/8). Only the higher dose of LA (3.6 mg/kg) effectively increased the survival rate to 75% (6/8, $p < 0.05$).

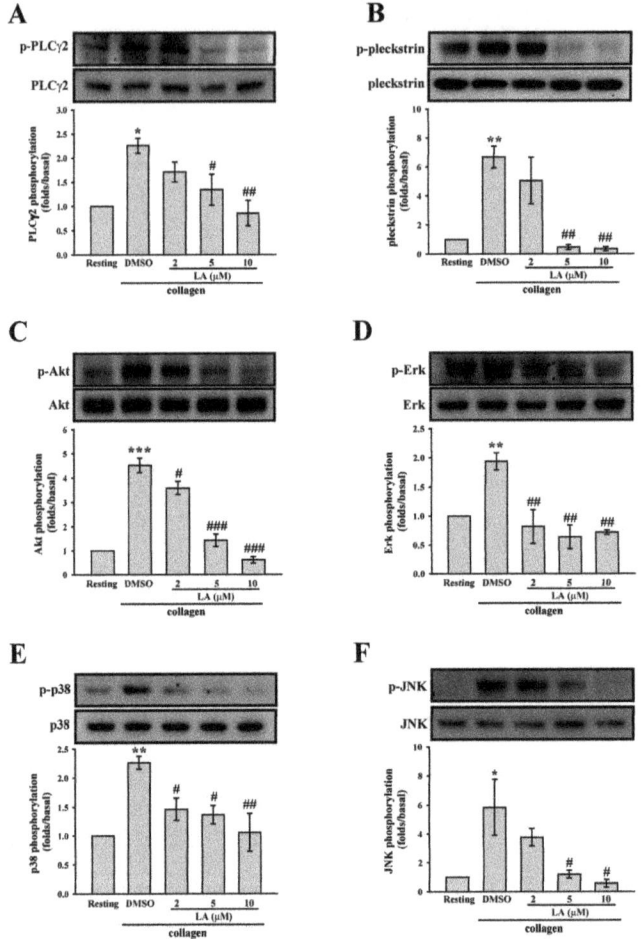

Figure 3. Involvement of LA in the activation of (**A**) PLCγ2; (**B**) PKC; (**C**) Akt; (**D**) Erk; (**E**) p38 mitogen-activated protein kinase (MAPK) and (**F**) JNK. Washed platelets (3.6×10^8 cells/mL) were preincubated with DMSO and LA (2–10 µM), and collagen (1 µg/mL) was then added to trigger platelet activation. Cells were then collected, and subcellular extracts were analyzed through Western blotting. Specific antibodies were used to detect the phosphorylation of PLCγ2, the PKC substrate pleckstrin, Akt, Erk, p38 MAPK, and JNK. Data (**A**–**F**) are presented as the mean ± SEM ($n = 3$). * $p < 0.05$, ** $p < 0.01$ and *** $p < 0.001$, compared with the resting group; # $p < 0.05$, ## $p < 0.01$ and ### $p < 0.001$, compared with the collagen (positive) group.

Fluorescein sodium was used in another model of platelet thrombus formation in mesenteric microvessels; this model was exposed to UV irradiation, which damaged endothelium and subsequently caused vascular occlusion. The occlusion time was recorded using a real-time monitor. As shown in Figure 4B, the data revealed that the DMSO group had an occlusion time of approximately 117.2 s. Compared with the DMSO group, LA (1.8 and 3.6 mg/kg) treatment dose-dependently prolonged the occlusion time by 34.0 and 111.5 s (both $p < 0.01$, $n = 8$), respectively. The findings obtained from these two animal models indicate that LA exerts anti-thrombotic effects.

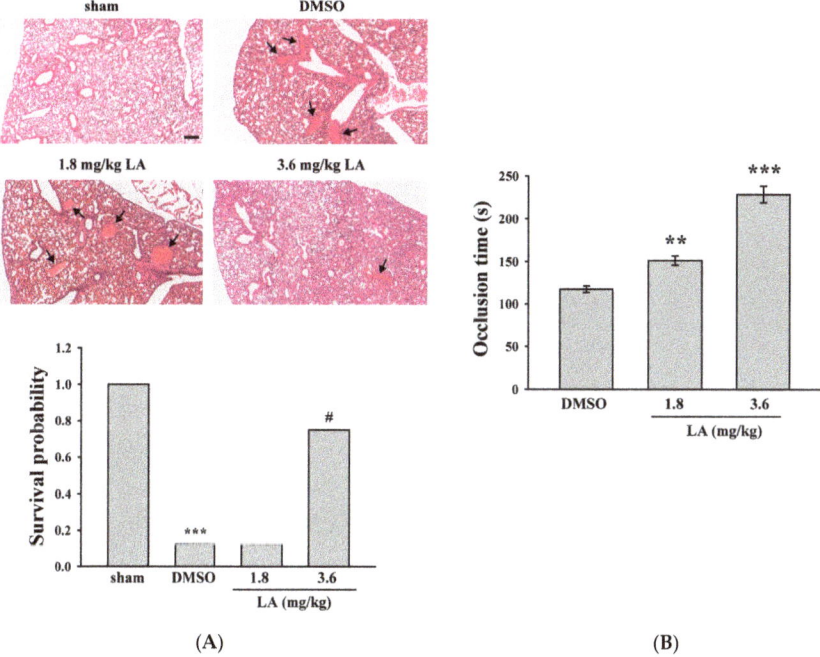

(A)   (B)

Figure 4. Effects of LA on pulmonary thrombosis and fluorescein sodium-induced platelet thrombus formation in the mesenteric microvessels of mice. (**A**) Mice (male, 5–6 weeks old) were intraperitoneally administered with DMSO (solvent control) or LA (1.8 and 3.6 mg/kg) for 30 min. ADP (1.4 g/kg) was injected in the tail vein to induce acute pulmonary thrombosis. The survival rate (bottom panel) was determined at 1 and 24 h after ADP administration, and pulmonary thrombosis (top panel, arrows) was observed by staining lung tissue sections with hematoxylin-eosin. Scale bar: 200 µm. The survival rate was evaluated using the Kaplan–Meier survival method ($n = 8$). *** $p < 0.001$, compared with the sham-operated group. # $p < 0.05$, compared with the DMSO group; (**B**) Mice received an intravenous bolus of DMSO or LA (1.8 and 3.6 mg/kg), and the mesenteric venules were irradiated to induce microthrombus formation. Data are presented as the mean ± SEM ($n = 8$). ** $p < 0.01$ and *** $p < 0.001$, compared with the DMSO group.

2.6. LA Protected against Middle Cerebral Artery Occlusion/Reperfusion-Induced Brain Injury without Affecting Normal Hemostasis

In clinical settings, anti-platelet drugs have been used to prevent secondary stroke. Moreover, previous studies on experimental stroke have revealed the crucial role of platelet activation, in addition to inflammatory responses [22–25]. Hence, we investigated whether LA has a protective effect on middle cerebral artery occlusion (MCAO)-induced brain injury. As shown in Figure 5A, the data described a marked edema (12.6%) and infarct size (61.6%) in the DMSO group. However, the LA treated groups showed a dose-dependent reduction in edema (1.8 mg/kg, 6.0%; 3.6 mg/kg, 4.7%) and infarct size (1.8 mg/kg, 27.7%; 3.6 mg/kg, 8.4%), compared with the DMSO group. This finding indicates that LA protects against MCAO-induced brain injury, at least in part, through the inhibition of platelet activation.

As previously described, LA can reduce thrombus formation and protect against stroke-mediated brain injury. However, in clinical settings, the side effect of bleeding caused by antiplatelet drugs remains a challenge. Hence, we performed an experiment on tail-bleeding time to evaluate whether LA interferes with normal hemostasis. As shown in Figure 5B, the data indicated that the average tail-bleeding time was approximately 92.6 and 99.4 s in the control (saline) and DMSO groups, respectively. There is no significant difference between these two groups ($p > 0.05$, $n = 8$). In addition, the LA-treated groups did not prolong the tail-bleeding time, compared with the DMSO group, indicating that LA is a safer antithrombotic agent.

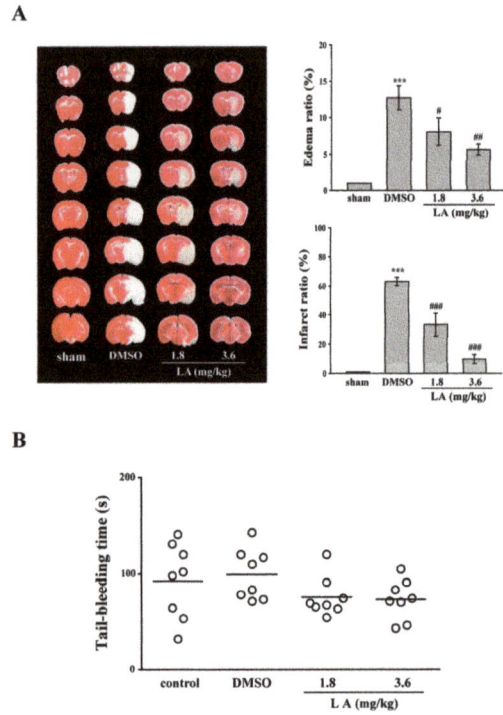

Figure 5. Influence of LA on middle cerebral artery occlusion (MCAO)/reperfusion-induced brain injury and tail bleeding time in mice. Mice (male, 5–6 weeks old) were intraperitoneally administrated with DMSO (solvent control) or LA (1.8 and 3.6 mg/kg) for 30 min. (**A**) Mice were subjected to MCAO for 30 min followed by 24-h reperfusion. Immediately after sacrifice, coronal sections were cut and stained using 2,3,5-triphenyltetrazolium chloride; white areas indicate infarction, and red areas indicate normal tissues (left panel). Edema and infarct ratios (right panel) were calculated through image analysis and are reported as a ratio of the non-ischemic hemisphere. Infarct ratio was corrected for edema. Data are presented as the mean ± SEM. ($n = 8$). *** $p < 0.001$, compared with the sham-operated group; # $p < 0.05$, ## $p < 0.01$ and ### $p < 0.001$, compared with the DMSO group; (**B**) Bleeding was induced by severing the tail at 3 mm from the tail tip, and the bleeding tail stump was immersed in saline. Subsequently, the bleeding time was continually recorded until no sign of bleeding was observed for at least 10 s. Each point in the scatter plots graph represents a mouse ($n = 8$). The bars represent the median bleeding time of each group.

3. Discussion

Medicinal herbs, including those used in traditional medicine are becoming increasingly popular and important in Western countries [26,27]. In China and other countries, traditional medicine has long used medicinal herbs to treat or relieve the symptoms of many human diseases [26,27]. Moreover, the active ingredients of herbs or natural products are among the most crucial resources for developing new lead compounds and scaffolds for treating human diseases [26,27]. Therefore, research on herbs or natural products is a key field for developing new drugs for treating human diseases.

LA is an active ingredient derived from the roots and rhizomes of *Glycyrrhiza* spp.; it possesses multiple biological activities, such as anti-inflammation, antioxidation, antibacteria, and antitumor effects [7,9–11]. Although, LA was recently reported to block rabbit and rat platelet aggregation through the inhibition of COX-1 activity [15,16], the role of LA on platelet activation and thrombosis remains unclear. Therefore, we further systemically investigated its antiplatelet mechanism and for the first time determined whether LA prevents thrombus formation in in vivo studies. Our data reveal that LA is more sensitive to the inhibition of collagen-induced platelet aggregation in human platelets, as well as that which Okuda-Tanino et al. reported [15]. Moreover, LA also inhibits collagen-mediated several activation events, such as granule release, calcium mobilization, and GPIIbIIIa activation. In addition, we further determined the possible antiplatelet mechanisms of LA. Several GPVI-mediated signaling pathways were examined in this study. LA could inhibit the conventional PLCγ2–PKC pathway as well as Akt and MAPK pathways. GPVI-mediated Akt activation in platelets is majorly dependent on PI3K and, in part, on Gi protein stimulation by secreted ADP, indicating that PI3K/Akt is the direct downstream target of GPVI [20]. Moreover, the pharmacological inhibition of PI3K markedly inhibit GPVI-mediated platelet aggregation, secretion, and intracellular calcium mobilization [20]. Similar to the pharmacological inhibitors, the gene deletion of Akt1 impairs collagen-induced platelet activation [28]. These findings indicates that LA inhibits collagen-induced platelet activation, in part, through the inhibition of Akt activation, followed by reducing ADP release.

MAPKs, including Erk, p38 MAPK, and JNK, are also involved in collagen-induced platelet activation [21]. $P2X_1$-mediated Erk2 activation is essential for platelet secretion and aggregation, which is induced by a low dose of collagen ($\leq$1 mg/mL) [21]. Moreover, the Erk upstream MEK1/2 inhibitor prolongs the occlusion time of the arteriolar and venular thrombosis in mice [21]; p38 MAPK activates cytosolic phospholipase A2, leading to subsequent increased thromboxane A_2 formation in collagen-stimulated platelets [21]. Likewise, p38 inhibitors impair platelet aggregation in response to low and medium doses of collagen. Furthermore, p38 MAPK is involved in thrombus formation, as evidenced in $p38^{+/-}$ mice in a model of ferric chloride-induced carotid artery occlusion [21]; the deletion of JNK1 also impairs platelet aggregation and granule release by a low dose of collagen and thrombus formation in an in vivo model of thrombosis induced by photochemical injury to cecum vessels [29]. These observations suggest that LA could reduce collagen-induced platelet activation, including granule release, GPIIbIIIa activation, and platelet aggregation, partly through the inhibition of Erk, p38 MAPK, and JNK activation. In addition, previous studies have demonstrated that LA inhibits COX-1 activity in different species [15,16]. Our data also showed that LA effectively reduced AA-induced human platelet aggregation (Figure S2). This result indirectly implies that LA may has the inhibitory effect on COX-1 activity in human platelets. Collectively, in addition to inhibiting COX-1 activity that Okuda-Tanino et al. and Suo et al. reported [15,16], LA-mediated the inhibition of the PLCγ2-PKC, Akt, and MAPK pathways also contributes to the suppression of platelet activation induced by collagen. Furthermore, the inhibitory effect of LA on platelet activation does not occur through interference with the collagen binding to GPVI, as evidenced by the FITC-collagen binding assay (Figure 2C). Thus, LA may inhibit GPVI downstream signaling, but does act as an antagonist to GPVI.

LA markedly attenuated thrombus formation in two animal models of ADP-induced pulmonary thrombosis and fluorescein sodium-induced platelet thrombus formation in the mesenteric microvessels of mice. Moreover, LA did not affect normal hemostasis. These findings suggest that LA is a relatively safe antithrombotic agent. In our study, our data also showed that LA could inhibit mouse platelet aggregation (Figure S3), which, in part, supports that LA has protective effects in ADP-induced pulmonary thrombosis of mice. However, the influence of LA on ADP-induced platelet aggregation is controversial. LA reportedly inhibited ADP-induced platelet aggregation in rat, but not rabbit, platelets [15,16]. Thus, whether this diversity is attributed to the different species remains to be further clarified. In addition, LA protected against MCAO-induced brain injury. In this ischemia/reperfusion model, several risk factors, including neutrophil infiltration, ROS production, and platelet activation, are involved in the processes of brain injury [22–25]. Actually, previous studies have demonstrated that LA has a potent anti-inflammatory activity in various models, including acute kidney and lung injury, allergic airway inflammation, and endotoxin shock [12,14,30,31]. LA also exhibits anti-oxidant activity; it protects against tert-butyl hydroperoxide-induced oxidative stress by scavenging ROS, and inhibits LPS-induced ROS production, lipid peroxidation, and nitric oxide in RAW 264.7 cells [7,32]. In addition to the antiplatelet effect, these reported biological activities of LA may also contribute to a protective benefit for thrombosis and ischemic stroke.

4. Materials and Methods

4.1. Materials

Licochalcone A (LA, ≥95%) was purchased from Cayman Chemical (Ann Arbor, MI, USA). Collagen, thrombin, and U46619 were purchased from Chrono-Log (Havertown, PA, USA). FITC-conjugated anti-P-selectin and PAC-1 antibodies were purchased from Biolegend (San Diego, CA, USA). FITC-conjugated collagen, phorbol-12, 13-dibutyrate (PDBu), luciferase/luciferin, fluorescein sodium, and 2,3,5-triphenyltetrazolium chloride (TTC) were purchased from Sigma (St. Louis, MO, USA). Fura 2-AM was purchased from Molecular Probe (Eugene, OR, USA). Anti-phospho PLCγ2 (Tyr^{759}), anti-PLCγ2, anti-phospho-(Ser) PKC substrate, anti-phospho-p38 MAPK (Ser^{180}/Tyr^{182}), anti-phospho-p44/42 MAPK (ERK1/2; Thr^{202}/Tyr^{204}), anti-c-Jun N-terminal kinase (JNK), and anti-phospho-Akt (Ser^{473}) polyclonal antibodies and anti-p38 MAPK, anti-p44/42 MAPK, anti-phospho JNK (Thr^{183}/Tyr^{185}), and anti-Akt monoclonal antibodies were purchased from Cell Signaling (Beverly, MA, USA). The pleckstrin (p47) antibody was purchased from GeneTex (Irvine, CA, USA). The Hybond-P polyvinylidene difluoride membrane, an enhanced chemiluminescence (ECL) Western blotting detection reagent and analysis system, horseradish peroxidase (HRP)-conjugated donkey antirabbit IgG, and sheep antimouse IgG were purchased from Amersham (Buckinghamshire, UK). LA was dissolved in dimethyl sulfoxide (DMSO) and stored at 4 °C until use.

4.2. Platelet Aggregation

This study was approved by the Institutional Review Board of Shin Kong Wu Ho-Su Memorial Hospital (Approval No. 20161205R, 9 February 2017) and conformed to the directives of the Helsinki Declaration. All volunteers provided written informed consent before any procedure of experiments. Blood was collected from healthy volunteers who were free from medication during the past 2 weeks, and prepared to human platelet suspensions, as previously described [33,34]. Blood was mixed with an acid-citrate-dextrose solution (9:1, v/v). Following centrifugation, the supernatant platelet-rich plasma (PRP) was collected. Then PRP was supplemented with prostaglandin E1 (0.5 µM) and heparin (6.4 IU/mL) before the second centrifugation. Washed platelets were suspended in Tyrode's solution containing bovine serum albumin (BSA) (3.5 mg/mL). The final concentration of Ca^{2+} in Tyrode's solution was 1 mM.

A turbidimetric method was applied to measure platelet aggregation [33,34] by using a Lumi-Aggregometer (Payton, Scarborough, ON, Canada). Platelet suspensions (3.6 × 10^8 cells/mL) were preincubated with various concentrations of LA (2–80 µM) or an isovolumetric solvent control (0.1% DMSO, final concentration) for 3 min before agonists were added. The reaction was allowed to proceed for 6 min.

4.3. ATP Release Measured Using a Microplate Reader

Platelet suspensions (3.6 × 10^8 cells/mL) were preincubated with luciferase/luciferin and various concentrations of LA or an isovolumetric solvent control (0.1% DMSO, final concentration) for 3 min before collagen was added. The reaction was allowed to proceed for 30 min and the luminescence was continually recorded every minute using a Synergy H1 microplate reader (BioTek, VT, USA).

4.4. P-Selectin Secretion and GPIIbIIIa Activation

This method was previously described by Yacoub et al. [35]. Platelet suspensions (3×10^8 platelets/mL) were preincubated with LA (2–10 µM) or 0.1% DMSO for 3 min, and subsequently, collagen (1 µg/mL) was added for 15 min in glass cuvettes at 37 °C. After the reactions, the platelet suspensions were fixed and stained with FITC–P-selectin or FITC–PAC-1 antibody for 30 min. After centrifugation and washing, platelets were re-suspended with 1 mL phosphate-buffered saline and all samples were immediately measured in a Becton Dickinson flow cytometer (FACScan Syst., San Jose, CA, USA). The number of events was stopped at 10,000 counts. All of the experiments were performed at least three times to ensure reliability.

4.5. Calcium Mobilization

The washed platelets was incubated with Fura 2-AM (5 µM) for 30 min, which allowed Fura 2 to cross the cell membrane and to be trapped within platelets. After centrifugation and washing, platelets were suspended with Tyrode's solution. The final concentration of Ca^{2+} in Tyrode's solution was 1 mM. The real-time change of relative intracellular Ca^{2+} ion ($[Ca^{2+}]i$) concentration was recorded by a fluorescence spectrophotometer (Hitachi F4500, Tokyo, Japan) with excitation wavelengths of 340 and 380 nm and an emission wavelength of 500 nm [36].

4.6. Determination of Lactate Dehydrogenase (LDH)

LDH release was analyzed using a CytoTox 96 non-radioactive cytotoxicity assay kit from Promega (Madison, WI, USA). Washed platelets (3.6×10^8 cells/mL) were pre-incubated with LA (10, 40, and 80 µM) or a solvent control (0.1% DMSO, final concentration) for 10 min at 37 °C. After centrifugation, an aliquot of supernatant was collected to measure the levels of LDH according to manufacturer's protocol (Promega). The levels of LDH were measured at the wavelength of 490 nm using a Synergy H1 microplate reader (BioTek, VT, USA). LDH activity was expressed as the % of total enzyme activity, which was measured in platelets lysed with 0.5% Triton X-100.

4.7. Immunoblotting Study

Washed platelets (3×10^8 cells/mL) were treated with 1 µg/mL collagen to trigger platelet activation for the indicated times in the absence or presence of LA (2–10 µM). After the reaction, all samples was collected and immediately lysed in 200 µL of a lysis buffer for 1 h. The lysates were centrifuged at $5000 \times g$ for 5 min. The amounts of 80 µg of protein lysates were loaded into each well, separated on a 12% SDS-PAGE, and electrotransferred to PVDF membranes through semidry transfer (Bio-Rad, Hercules, CA, USA). PVDF membranes were blocked with 5% BSA in TBST (Tris-base 10 mM, NaCl 100 mM and Tween 20 0.01%) for 1 h at room temperature, and then probed with various specific primary antibodies (diluted at 1:1000 in TBST), followed by incubation with the HRP-linked antimouse IgG or antirabbit IgG (diluted at 1:3000 in TBST) for 1 h. An enhanced chemiluminescence system was used to develop the immunoreactive bands on the membranes. Then the optical density of each band was measured by a videodensitometry software (Bio-Profil; Biolight Windows Application V2000.01, Vilber Lourmat, France); the density of each band was normalized to the corresponding total protein band.

4.8. Competitive Binding Assay of Collagen Receptors through Flow Cytometry

For the flow cytometry, platelet suspensions (1×10^6 platelets/mL) were pre-incubated with LA (2–10 µM) or 0.1% DMSO for 3 min, and subsequently, FITC–collagen (1 µg/mL) was added for

15 min in glass cuvettes at 37 °C. After the reaction, a final volume of 1 mL was used for an immediate analysis through flow cytometry (Becton Dickinson, FACScan Syst., San Jose, CA, USA).

4.9. Animals

ICR and C57BL/6 mice (20–25 g, male, 5–6 weeks old) were obtained from BioLasco (Taipei, Taiwan). All procedures were approved by the Affidavit of Approval of Animal Use Protocol-Shin Kong Wu Ho-Su Memorial Hospital (Approval No. Most1060005, 22 December 2016) and were in accordance with the Guide for the Care and Use of Laboratory Animals (8th edition, 2011). LA (5 and 10 µM) effectively platelet activation in vitro, these two concentrations were chosen and calculated accordingly into mouse doses 1.8 and 3.6 mg/kg, respectively [37].

4.10. ADP-Induced Acute Pulmonary Thrombosis in Mice

This experiment was performed as previously described [38]. Mice were injected with ADP (1.4 g/kg) at the tail vein to induce acute pulmonary thrombosis. The survival rate of the mice in each group was determined at 1 h after injection. Mice that survived the challenge were euthanized in a CO_2 chamber. The lungs were excised and fixed with 4% formalin, and paraffin-embedded sections of the lungs were stained with hematoxylin-eosin. The stained sections were observed and photographed using ScanScope CS (Leica Biosystems, Wetzlar, Germany). The mice were divided into four groups: (1) sham-operated; (2) DMSO (solvent control); (3) LA-treated (1.8 mg/kg, intraperitoneal (i.p.)) and (4) the LA-treated (3.6 mg/kg, i.p.). All treatments were administered 30 min before ADP administration for all the groups except for the sham-operated group.

4.11. Fluorescein Sodium-Induced Platelet Thrombus Formation in Mesenteric Microvessels of Mice

Thrombus formation was assessed as previously described [39]. Mice were anesthetized using a mixture containing 75% air and 3% isoflurane maintained in 25% oxygen, and the external jugular vein was cannulated with a polyethylene 10 (PE-10) tube for intravenously administering the dye and drugs. Venules (30–40 mM) were selected for irradiation at wavelengths of <520 nm to produce a microthrombus. Either 1.8 or 3.6 mg/kg of LA was administered at 10 min after the administration of sodium fluorescein (15 mg/kg), and the time required to occlude the microvessel through thrombus formation (occlusion time) was recorded.

4.12. Middle Cerebral Artery Occlusion/Reperfusion-Induced Brain Injury in Mice

In this experiment of stroke, the intraluminal suture method was used, as described previously [40]. In brief, after mice were anesthetized with a mixture of 75% air and 25% oxygen containing 3% isoflurane, the right common carotid artery was exposed. Then, the right middle cerebral artery (MCA) was occluded by inserting a 6–0 monofilament nylon suture coated with silicon from the external to the internal carotid artery until no longer advanceable. After the closure of the operative site, the mice were allowed to recover from anesthesia. During another brief anesthesia period, the suture was gently withdrawn to restore blood supply after 30 min of MCAO. All groups of mice were euthanized through decapitation after 24 h reperfusion. The brains were cut into 1-mM coronal slices and stained with 2% 2,3,5-triphenyltetrazolium chloride. The infarct areas were calculated using a computerized image analyzer (Image-Pro Plus, Rockville, MD, USA) and then compiled to obtain the infarct volume (in cubic millimeters) per brain. Infarct volumes were expressed as a percentage of the contralateral hemisphere volume by using the formula (area of the intact contralateral (left) hemisphere-area of the intact region of the ipsilateral (right) hemisphere) to compensate for edema formation in the ipsilateral hemisphere. Four groups were designed as follows: (1) sham-operated; (2) DMSO (solvent control); (3) LA-treated (1.8 mg/kg, i.p.) and (4) LA-treated (3.6 mg/kg, i.p.). All treatments were administered 30 min prior to the onset of MCAO in all the groups except for the sham-operated group.

4.13. Tail Bleeding Time

Mice were anesthetized with a mixture containing 75% air and 3% isoflurane maintained in 25% oxygen and were intraperitoneally administered with saline (control), DMSO (solvent control), or LA (1.8 or 3.6 mg/kg) for 30 min. Immediately, bleeding was induced by severing the tail at 3 mm from the tail tip, and the bleeding tail stump was immersed in saline. Subsequently, the bleeding time was continually recorded until no sign of bleeding was observed for at least 10 s.

4.14. Data Analysis

The experimental results are expressed as the mean ± SEM. and are accompanied by the number of observations (n). Values of n refer to the number of experiments, each of which was conducted with different blood donors. All experimental results were assessed using analysis of variance (ANOVA). Significant differences were investigated using the Newman–Keuls method. Survival rates were calculated using the Kaplan–Meier method, and the groups were compared using the log rank test. Results with $p < 0.05$ were considered statistically significant.

5. Conclusions

The major findings of this study revealed that LA prevents platelet activation and thrombus formation partly through the inhibition of PLCγ2–PKC, Akt, and MAPK pathways (Figure 6), without affecting normal hemostasis. These findings indicate the potential of LA as a safe and effective therapy for preventing thromboembolic disorders such as secondary stroke. In addition, LA may serve as a leading compound for the development of novel antithrombotic drugs.

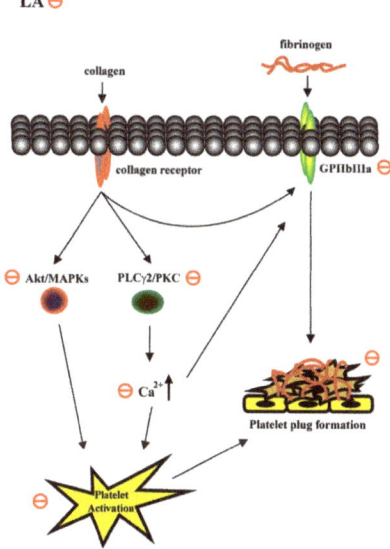

Figure 6. Hypothetical scheme of the involvement of LA in human platelet activation. LA may inhibit PLCγ2–PKC, Akt and MAPK activation and subsequently attenuate granule release and GPIIbIIIa activation, thereby blocking platelet aggregation and thrombus formation. Arrows indicate positive regulation; red circles indicate inhibition.

Supplementary Materials: Supplementary materials can be found at www.mdpi.com/1422-0067/18/7/1500/s1.

Acknowledgments: This work was supported by grants from the Ministry of Science and Technology of Taiwan (MOST105-2314-B-341-004, MOST105-2320-B-341-001, and MOST105-2311-B-038-005-MY3), Taipei Medical University Hospital (105TMU-TMUH-02-01 and 105TMUH-SP-02), Taipei Medical University (TMU105-AE1-B01), and Shin Kong Wu Ho-Su Memorial Hospital (SKH-8302-104-DR-15, SKH-8302-105-NDR-07, SKH-8302-106-NDR-06).

Author Contributions: Li-Ming Lien and Kuan-Hung Lin designed the study, performed research, analyzed the data and wrote the manuscript; Hou-Chang Chiu discussed the in vitro experimental data and reviewed the manuscript; Li-Ting Huang and Mei-Fang Tseng performed the in vitro and in vivo experiments and data analysis; Ray-Jade Chen and Wan-Jung Lu conceived of the study and wrote the manuscript; and Wan-Jung Lu approved the final version of the manuscript. All authors have read and approve the final manuscript.

Conflicts of Interest: The authors declare no conflict of interest.

Abbreviations

GPIIbIIIa	Glycoprotein IIbIIIa
GPVI	Glycoprotein VI
LA	Licochalcone A
MAPK	Mitogen-activated protein kinase
MCAO	Middle cerebral artery occlusion
PKC	Protein kinase C
PLCγ2	Phospholipase Cγ2
ROS	Reactive oxygen species

References

1. Lindemann, S.; Kramer, B.; Seizer, P.; Gawaz, M. Platelets, inflammation and atherosclerosis. *J. Thromb. Haemost.* **2007**, *5*, 203–211. [CrossRef] [PubMed]
2. Nieswandt, B.; Pleines, I.; Bender, M. Platelet adhesion and activation mechanisms in arterial thrombosis and ischaemic stroke. *J. Thromb. Haemost.* **2011**, *9*, 92–104. [CrossRef] [PubMed]
3. Nieswandt, B.; Watson, S.P. Platelet-collagen interaction: Is GPVI the central receptor? *Blood* **2003**, *102*, 449–461. [CrossRef] [PubMed]
4. Dutting, S.; Bender, M.; Nieswandt, B. Platelet GPVI: A target for antithrombotic therapy?! *Trends Pharmacol. Sci.* **2012**, *33*, 583–590. [CrossRef] [PubMed]
5. Baigent, C.; Blackwell, L.; Collins, R.; Emberson, J.; Godwin, J.; Peto, R.; Buring, J.; Hennekens, C.; Kearney, P.; Meade, T.; et al. Aspirin in the primary and secondary prevention of vascular disease: Collaborative meta-analysis of individual participant data from randomised trials. *Lancet* **2009**, *373*, 1849–1860. [PubMed]
6. Adianti, M.; Aoki, C.; Komoto, M.; Deng, L.; Shoji, I.; Wahyuni, T.S.; Lusida, M.I.; Soetjipto; Fuchino, H.; Kawahara, N.; et al. Anti-hepatitis C virus compounds obtained from Glycyrrhiza uralensis and other Glycyrrhiza species. *Microbiol. Immunol.* **2014**, *58*, 180–187. [CrossRef] [PubMed]
7. Fu, Y.; Chen, J.; Li, Y.J.; Zheng, Y.F.; Li, P. Antioxidant and anti-inflammatory activities of six flavonoids separated from licorice. *Food Chem.* **2013**, *141*, 1063–1071. [CrossRef] [PubMed]
8. Hao, H.; Hui, W.; Liu, P.; Lv, Q.; Zeng, X.; Jiang, H.; Wang, Y.; Zheng, X.; Zheng, Y.; Li, J.; et al. Effect of licochalcone A on growth and properties of Streptococcus suis. *PLoS ONE* **2013**, *8*, e67728. [CrossRef]
9. Messier, C.; Grenier, D. Effect of licorice compounds licochalcone A, glabridin and glycyrrhizic acid on growth and virulence properties of Candida albicans. *Mycoses* **2011**, *54*, e801–e806. [CrossRef] [PubMed]
10. Tang, Z.H.; Chen, X.; Wang, Z.Y.; Chai, K.; Wang, Y.F.; Xu, X.H.; Wang, X.W.; Lu, J.H.; Wang, Y.T.; Chen, X.P.; et al. Induction of C/EBP homologous protein-mediated apoptosis and autophagy by licochalcone A in non-small cell lung cancer cells. *Sci. Rep.* **2016**, *6*, 26241. [CrossRef] [PubMed]
11. Xiao, X.Y.; Hao, M.; Yang, X.Y.; Ba, Q.; Li, M.; Ni, S.J.; Wang, L.S.; Du, X. Licochalcone A inhibits growth of gastric cancer cells by arresting cell cycle progression and inducing apoptosis. *Cancer Lett.* **2011**, *302*, 69–75. [CrossRef] [PubMed]
12. Chu, X.; Ci, X.; Wei, M.; Yang, X.; Cao, Q.; Guan, M.; Li, H.; Deng, Y.; Feng, H.; Deng, X. Licochalcone a inhibits lipopolysaccharide-induced inflammatory response in vitro and in vivo. *J. Agric. Food Chem.* **2012**, *60*, 3947–3954. [CrossRef] [PubMed]

13. Fontes, L.B.; Dos Santos Dias, D.; de Carvalho, L.S.; Mesquita, H.L.; da Silva Reis, L.; Dias, A.T.; Da Silva Filho, A.A.; do Amaral Correa, J.O. Immunomodulatory effects of licochalcone A on experimental autoimmune encephalomyelitis. *J. Pharm. Pharmacol.* **2014**, *66*, 886–894. [CrossRef] [PubMed]
14. Hu, J.; Liu, J. Licochalcone a attenuates lipopolysaccharide-induced acute kidney injury by inhibiting nf-κ activation. *Inflammation* **2016**, *39*, 569–574. [CrossRef] [PubMed]
15. Okuda-Tanino, A.; Sugawara, D.; Tashiro, T.; Iwashita, M.; Obara, Y.; Moriya, T.; Tsushima, C.; Saigusa, D.; Tomioka, Y.; Ishii, K.; et al. Licochalcones extracted from Glycyrrhiza inflata inhibit platelet aggregation accompanied by inhibition of COX-1 activity. *PLoS ONE* **2017**, *12*, e0173628. [CrossRef] [PubMed]
16. Suo, T.; Liu, J.; Chen, X.; Yu, H.; Wang, T.; Li, C.; Wang, Y.; Wang, C.; Li, Z. Combining chemical profiling and network analysis to investigate the pharmacology of complex prescriptions in traditional chinese medicine. *Sci. Rep.* **2017**, *13*, 40529. [CrossRef] [PubMed]
17. Li, Z.; Delaney, M.K.; O'Brien, K.A.; Du, X. Signaling during platelet adhesion and activation. *Arterioscler. Thromb. Vasc. Biol.* **2010**, *30*, 2341–2349. [CrossRef] [PubMed]
18. Varga-Szabo, D.; Braun, A.; Nieswandt, B. Calcium signaling in platelets. *J. Thromb. Haemost.* **2009**, *7*, 1057–1066. [CrossRef] [PubMed]
19. Toker, A.; Bachelot, C.; Chen, C.S.; Falck, J.R.; Hartwig, J.H.; Cantley, L.C.; Kovacsovics, T.J. Phosphorylation of the platelet p47 phosphoprotein is mediated by the lipid products of phosphoinositide 3-kinase. *J. Biol. Chem.* **1995**, *270*, 29525–29531. [CrossRef] [PubMed]
20. Kim, S.; Mangin, P.; Dangelmaier, C.; Lillian, R.; Jackson, S.P.; Daniel, J.L.; Kunapuli, S.P. Role of phosphoinositide 3-kinase β in glycoprotein VI-mediated Akt activation in platelets. *J. Biol. Chem.* **2009**, *284*, 33763–33772. [CrossRef] [PubMed]
21. Adam, F.; Kauskot, A.; Rosa, J.P.; Bryckaert, M. Mitogen-activated protein kinases in hemostasis and thrombosis. *J. Thromb. Haemost.* **2008**, *6*, 2007–2016. [CrossRef] [PubMed]
22. Jin, R.; Yang, G.; Li, G. Inflammatory mechanisms in ischemic stroke: Role of inflammatory cells. *J. Leukoc. Biol.* **2010**, *87*, 779–789. [CrossRef] [PubMed]
23. Mao, Y.; Zhang, M.; Tuma, R.F.; Kunapuli, S.P. Deficiency of PAR4 attenuates cerebral ischemia/reperfusion injury in mice. *J. Cereb. Blood Flow Metab.* **2010**, *30*, 1044–1052. [CrossRef] [PubMed]
24. Vital, S.A.; Becker, F.; Holloway, P.M.; Russell, J.; Perretti, M.; Granger, D.N.; Gavins, F.N. Formyl-peptide receptor 2/3/lipoxin a4 receptor regulates neutrophil-platelet aggregation and attenuates cerebral inflammation: Impact for therapy in cardiovascular disease. *Circulation* **2016**, *133*, 2169–2179. [CrossRef] [PubMed]
25. Ishikawa, M.; Cooper, D.; Arumugam, T.V.; Zhang, J.H.; Nanda, A.; Granger, D.N. Platelet-leukocyte-endothelial cell interactions after middle cerebral artery occlusion and reperfusion. *J. Cereb. Blood Flow Metab.* **2004**, *24*, 907–915. [CrossRef] [PubMed]
26. Lee, K.H. Research and future trends in the pharmaceutical development of medicinal herbs from Chinese medicine. *Public Health Nutr.* **2000**, *3*, 515–522. [CrossRef] [PubMed]
27. Yuan, H.; Ma, Q.; Ye, L.; Piao, G. The traditional medicine and modern medicine from natural products. *Molecules* **2016**, *21*, E559. [CrossRef] [PubMed]
28. Chen, J.; De, S.; Damron, D.S.; Chen, W.S.; Hay, N.; Byzova, T.V. Impaired platelet responses to thrombin and collagen in AKT-1-deficient mice. *Blood* **2004**, *104*, 1703–1710. [CrossRef] [PubMed]
29. Adam, F.; Kauskot, A.; Nurden, P.; Sulpice, E.; Hoylaerts, M.F.; Davis, R.J.; Rosa, J.P.; Bryckaert, M. Platelet JNK1 is involved in secretion and thrombus formation. *Blood* **2010**, *115*, 4083–4092. [CrossRef] [PubMed]
30. Chu, X.; Jiang, L.; Wei, M.; Yang, X.; Guan, M.; Xie, X.; Wei, J.; Liu, D.; Wang, D. Attenuation of allergic airway inflammation in a murine model of asthma by Licochalcone A. *Immunopharmacol. Immunotoxicol.* **2013**, *35*, 653–661. [CrossRef] [PubMed]
31. Kwon, H.S.; Park, J.H.; Kim, D.H.; Kim, Y.H.; Shin, H.K.; Kim, J.K. Licochalcone A isolated from licorice suppresses lipopolysaccharide-stimulated inflammatory reactions in RAW264.7 cells and endotoxin shock in mice. *J. Mol. Med.* **2008**, *86*, 1287–1295. [CrossRef] [PubMed]
32. Lv, H.; Ren, H.; Wang, L.; Chen, W.; Ci, X. Lico a enhances nrf2-mediated defense mechanisms against t-bhp-induced oxidative stress and cell death via akt and erk activation in raw 264.7 cells. *Oxid. Med. Cell. Longev.* **2015**, *2015*, 709845. [CrossRef] [PubMed]
33. Lin, K.H.; Hsiao, G.; Shih, C.M.; Chou, D.S.; Sheu, J.R. Mechanisms of resveratrol-induced platelet apoptosis. *Cardiovasc. Res.* **2009**, *83*, 575–585. [CrossRef] [PubMed]

34. Shen, M.Y.; Chen, F.Y.; Hsu, J.F.; Fu, R.H.; Chang, C.M.; Chang, C.T.; Liu, C.H.; Wu, J.R.; Lee, A.S.; Chan, H.C.; et al. Plasma L5 levels are elevated in ischemic stroke patients and enhance platelet aggregation. *Blood* **2016**, *127*, 1336–1345. [CrossRef] [PubMed]
35. Yacoub, D.; Theoret, J.F.; Villeneuve, L.; Abou-Saleh, H.; Mourad, W.; Allen, B.G.; Merhi, Y. Essential role of protein kinase C delta in platelet signaling, α IIb β 3 activation, and thromboxane A2 release. *J. Biol. Chem.* **2006**, *281*, 30024–30035. [CrossRef] [PubMed]
36. Lu, W.J.; Lin, K.H.; Hsu, M.J.; Chou, D.S.; Hsiao, G.; Sheu, J.R. Suppression of NF-κB signaling by andrographolide with a novel mechanism in human platelets: Regulatory roles of the p38 MAPK-hydroxyl radical-ERK2 cascade. *Biochem. Pharmacol.* **2012**, *84*, 914–924. [CrossRef] [PubMed]
37. Reagan-Shaw, S.; Nihal, M.; Ahmad, N. Dose translation from animal to human studies revisited. *FASEB J.* **2008**, *22*, 659–661. [CrossRef] [PubMed]
38. Lu, W.J.; Lee, J.J.; Chou, D.S.; Jayakumar, T.; Fong, T.H.; Hsiao, G.; Sheu, J.R. A novel role of andrographolide, an NF-κB inhibitor, on inhibition of platelet activation: The pivotal mechanisms of endothelial nitric oxide synthase/cyclic GMP. *J. Mol. Med.* **2011**, *89*, 1261–1273. [CrossRef] [PubMed]
39. Lin, K.H.; Kuo, J.R.; Lu, W.J.; Chung, C.L.; Chou, D.S.; Huang, S.Y.; Lee, H.C.; Sheu, J.R. Hinokitiol inhibits platelet activation ex vivo and thrombus formation in vivo. *Biochem. Pharmacol.* **2013**, *85*, 1478–1485. [CrossRef] [PubMed]
40. Yen, T.L.; Chen, R.J.; Jayakumar, T.; Lu, W.J.; Hsieh, C.Y.; Hsu, M.J.; Yang, C.H.; Chang, C.C.; Lin, Y.K.; Lin, K.H.; et al. Andrographolide stimulates p38 mitogen-activated protein kinase-nuclear factor erythroid-2-related factor 2-heme oxygenase 1 signaling in primary cerebral endothelial cells for definite protection against ischemic stroke in rats. *Transl. Res.* **2016**, *170*, 57–72. [CrossRef] [PubMed]

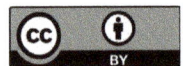

© 2017 by the authors. Licensee MDPI, Basel, Switzerland. This article is an open access article distributed under the terms and conditions of the Creative Commons Attribution (CC BY) license (http://creativecommons.org/licenses/by/4.0/).

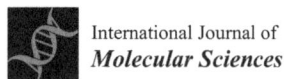

Article

New Therapeutic Agent against Arterial Thrombosis: An Iridium(III)-Derived Organometallic Compound

Chih-Wei Hsia [1,†], Marappan Velusamy [1,2,†], Jeng-Ting Tsao [1,3,†,‡], Chih-Hsuan Hsia [1], Duen-Suey Chou [1], Thanasekaran Jayakumar [1], Lin-Wen Lee [4], Jiun-Yi Li [5] and Joen-Rong Sheu [1,*]

[1] Department of Pharmacology and Graduate Institute of Medical Sciences, College of Medicine, Taipei Medical University, 250 Wu-Hsing Street, Taipei 110, Taiwan; d119106003@tmu.edu.tw (C.-W.H.); mvelusamy@gmail.com (M.V.); p95421019@ntu.edu.tw (J.-T.T.); d119102013@tmu.edu.tw (C.-H.H.); fird@tmu.edu.tw (D.-S.C.); tjaya_2002@yahoo.co.in (T.J.)
[2] Department of Chemistry, North Eastern Hill University, Shillong 793022, India
[3] Division of Allergy and Immunology, Department of Internal Medicine, Cathay General Hospital, Taipei 106, Taiwan
[4] Department of Microbiology and Immunology, Taipei Medical University, Taipei 110, Taiwan; lucie@tmu.edu.tw
[5] Department of Cardiovascular Surgery, Mackay Memorial Hospital, and Mackay Medical College, Taipei 104, Taiwan; jyl5891@gmail.com
* Correspondence: sheujr@tmu.edu.tw; Tel.: +886-2-2736-1661 (ext. 3199); Fax: +886-2-2739-0450
† These authors contributed equally to this work.
‡ Current address: Division of General Internal Medicine, Koo Foundation Sun Yat Sen Cancer Center, Taipei 112, Taiwan.

Received: 12 October 2017; Accepted: 29 November 2017; Published: 5 December 2017

Abstract: Platelet activation plays a major role in cardio and cerebrovascular diseases, and cancer progression. Disruption of platelet activation represents an attractive therapeutic target for reducing the bidirectional cross talk between platelets and tumor cells. Platinum (Pt) compounds have been used for treating cancer. Hence, replacing Pt with iridium (Ir) is considered a potential alternative. We recently developed an Ir(III)-derived complex, [Ir(Cp*)1-(2-pyridyl)-3-(2-hydroxyphenyl)imidazo[1,5-a]pyridine Cl]BF_4 (Ir-11), which exhibited strong antiplatelet activity; hence, we assessed the therapeutic potential of Ir-11 against arterial thrombosis. In collagen-activated platelets, Ir-11 inhibited platelet aggregation, adenosine triphosphate (ATP) release, intracellular Ca^{2+} mobilization, P-selectin expression, and OH· formation, as well as the phosphorylation of phospholipase Cγ2 (PLCγ2), protein kinase C (PKC), mitogen-activated protein kinases (MAPKs), and Akt. Neither the adenylate cyclase inhibitor nor the guanylate cyclase inhibitor reversed the Ir-11-mediated antiplatelet effects. In experimental mice, Ir-11 prolonged the bleeding time and reduced mortality associated with acute pulmonary thromboembolism. Ir-11 plays a crucial role by inhibiting platelet activation through the inhibition of the PLCγ2–PKC cascade, and the subsequent suppression of Akt and MAPK activation, ultimately inhibiting platelet aggregation. Therefore, Ir-11 can be considered a new therapeutic agent against either arterial thrombosis or the bidirectional cross talk between platelets and tumor cells.

Keywords: Ir(III)-derived complex; platelet activation; protein kinases; OH· free radical; bleeding time; pulmonary thromboembolism

---

1. Introduction

Intravascular thrombosis is a cause of various cardiovascular diseases (CVDs). The growth of thrombus inside the stent lumen is the outcome of platelet adhesion, and platelet activation followed by platelet aggregation. Thus, platelets play a crucial role in the pathogenesis of CVDs, including coronary artery disease and stroke [1]. Platelets are also critical for maintaining the integrity of the vascular system, and are the first-line defense against hemorrhage. During platelet activation, the release of several mediators (e.g., adenosine triphosphate (ATP) and thromboxane A$_2$) occurs in conjunction with relative intracellular Ca^{2+} ([Ca^{2+}]i) mobilization; these processes attract additional platelets toward the injured endothelium, and consequently cause thickening of the initial platelet monolayer. Finally, fibrinogen binds to its specific platelet receptor (integrin $\alpha_{IIb}\beta_3$), thus completing the final common pathway for platelet aggregation. Platelet surface membrane contains glycoprotein IIb/IIIa receptors, receptors for thromboxane, adenosine diphosphate (ADP), thrombin, serotonin, epinephrine, histamine, and PAF [2]. Platelets are activated via high-affinity and low-affinity hypersensitivity receptors, which can induce Kounis hypersensitivity-associated thrombotic syndrome.

Platelet activation has also been associated with the key steps of cancer progression. Platelets have been proposed to affect malignancy development through a controlled process that triggers the pathobiology of cancer cells. Cancer cells interact with all the major components of the hemostatic system, including platelets. Platelets are involved in some critical steps of cancer metastasis, including regulation of tumor cell migration, invasion, and arrest within the vasculature [3,4]. The contents of platelets may be released into the peritumoral space following platelet activation, thus enhancing tumor cell extravasation and metastases [5]. Hence, a complex interaction between platelet-induced tumor growth and tumor-stimulated platelet activation occurs with the association of several machineries within the tumor microenvironment that augment metastasis.

Casing polymers, and metals establish an essential class of substances that can act as antigens. Apart from the well-known importance of nickel, chromium, and cobalt in triggering skin hypersensitivity, other metals such as aluminum, beryllium, copper, gold, iridium, mercury, palladium, platinum, rhodium, and titanium are developing as human body sensitizers. Iridium (Ir) is a noble and precious metal belonging to the platinum (Pt) group elements, which also consist of rare metals such as Pt, palladium, rhodium, ruthenium, and osmium. These metals have similar physical and chemical properties [6]. In nature, metallic Ir can be obtained from Pt ores. It is also obtained as a by-product of nickel mining and processing [7]. Various metal complexes have been identified as anticancer therapeutic agents; thus, an increasing amount of related research is available. Metal complexes provide a highly versatile platform for drug design. Metal ions have variable geometries and coordination numbers; hence, their chemical reactivity in terms of both kinetics (ligand exchange rates) and thermodynamics (such as metal–ligand bond strength and redox potentials) can be modified. Metals and their ligands pay crucial roles in biological activity.

Organometallic Ir(III) complexes are particularly promising. Currently, researchers are focusing on Ir(III) compounds because these compounds exhibit potential antitumor activity and low toxicity toward normal tissues [8,9]. Furthermore, Ir complexes exert potent antiangiogenic effects by activating distinct antiangiogenic signaling pathways [8]. Antiangiogenic therapy is considered a promising cancer treatment strategy. On the basis of these observations, we developed a new biologically active Ir(III) derivative, also referred to as Ir-11 (Figure 1). Although in vitro and in vivo pharmacological studies have demonstrated that Ir-based compounds exhibit potent anticancer activity, to date, no study has investigated their effects on platelet activation. Preliminary studies have reported strong activity of Ir-11 toward human platelets. Thus, we further examined the characteristics and functional activity of Ir-11 in platelet activation ex vivo and in vivo. The present study confirms the development of a new class of Ir-based antiplatelet agent.

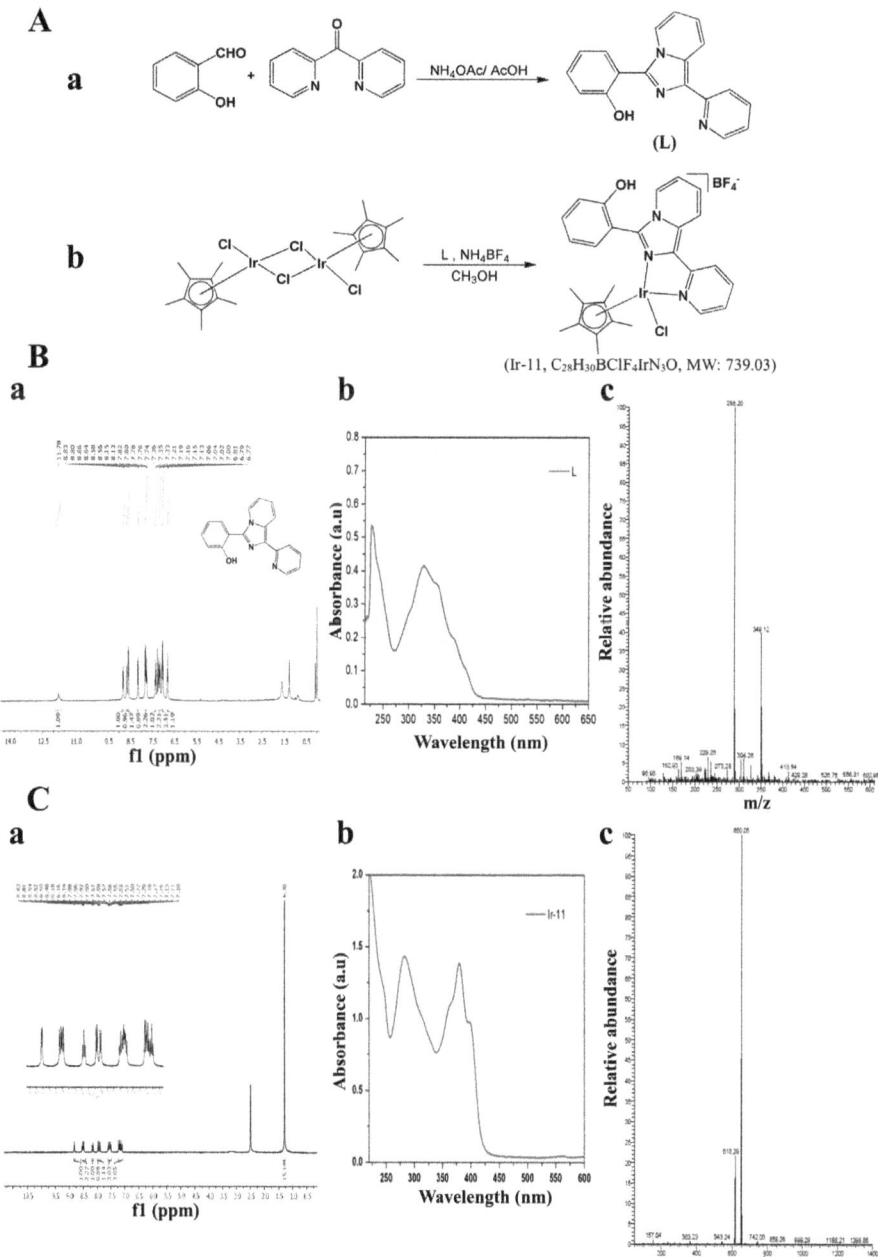

Figure 1. Chemical synthesis of Ir-11 compound. (**A**) Synthesis of (**a**) ligand (L) and (**b**) the complex [Ir(Cp*)(L)Cl]BF$_4$ (Ir-11); (**B**) Spectral image of ligand 2-(1-pyridin-2-yl-imidazo[1,5-a]pyridin-3-yl)-phenol (**a**) nuclear magnetic resonance (NMR) (**b**) UV–vis absorption and (**c**) electrospray ionization mass spectrometry (ESI-MS); (**C**) Spectral image of Ir-11 complex (**a**) NMR (**b**) UV–vis absorption and (**c**) ESI-MS.

2. Results

2.1. Inhibitory Effects of Ir-11 on Aggregation of Washed Human Platelets

Ir-11 (2–10 µM; Figure 2) strongly inhibited aggregation of collagen-stimulated (1 µg/mL) human platelets in a concentration-dependent manner. Furthermore, Ir-11 (20–100 µM) exhibited moderate activity against stimulation by arachidonic acid (AA, 120 µM) or U46619 (1 µM), a prostaglandin endoperoxide; however, Ir-11 (100–500 µM) exhibited relatively low inhibition of platelet aggregation that was stimulated using thrombin (0.01 U/mL) (Figure 2). The 50% inhibitory concentration (IC_{50}) of Ir-11 for collagen-stimulated aggregation was approximately 6 µM. Therefore, in the subsequent experiments, the IC_{50} (6 µM) and maximal concentration (10 µM) of Ir-11 were used for exploring the possible mechanisms of action of Ir-11 on human platelets. In addition, the solvent control (0.1% dimethyl sulfoxide, DMSO) did not significantly affect platelet aggregation (Figure 2A).

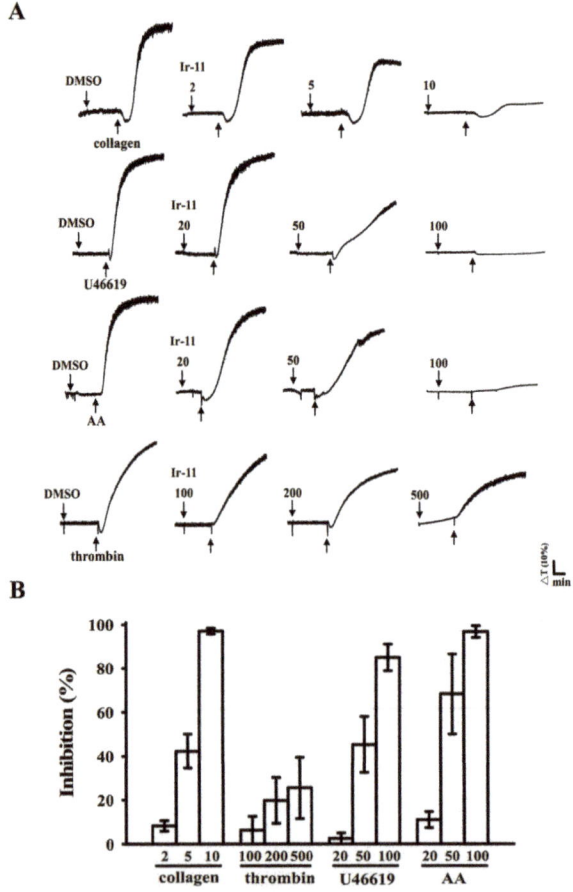

Figure 2. Comparison of the relative inhibitory activity of Ir-11 against platelet aggregation stimulated by various agonists in washed human platelets. (**A**) Washed human platelets (3.6 × 10^8 cells/mL) were preincubated with the solvent control 0.1% DMSO or various concentrations of Ir-11 (2–500 µM) and subsequently treated with collagen (1 µg/mL), thrombin (0.01 U/mL), U46619 (1 µM), and AA (120 µM) to stimulate platelet aggregation; (**B**) Concentration–response histograms of Ir-11 against platelet aggregation stimulated by agonists. Data are presented as means ± standard error of the mean (*n* = 4).

2.2. Regulatory Role of Ir-11 in Adenosine Triphosphate (ATP) Release, Relative [Ca^{2+}]i Mobilization, Surface P-Selectin Expression, Cytotoxicity, and Cyclic Nucleotide Formation in Washed Human Platelets

Platelet activation is associated with the release of granular contents (e.g., ATP and Ca^{2+} from the dense granules, and P-selectin from the α-granules), resulting in substantial platelet activation. In the present study, Ir-11 (6 and 10 µM) markedly reduced both ATP release (Figure 3A) and relative [Ca^{2+}]i mobilization (resting control, 93.0 ± 12.7 nM; collagen-stimulated, 362.3 ± 22.1 nM; 6 µM, 206.9 ± 22.7 nM; and 10 µM, 101.3 ± 14.8 nM; $n = 4$, Figure 3B) in platelets stimulated by collagen (1 µg/mL). In resting platelets, P-selectin is located on the inner wall of the α-granules. Platelet activation exposes the inner walls of the granules to the outside of the cell [10]. Treatment with Ir-11 markedly reduced collagen-induced surface P-selectin expression (resting control, 59.3 ± 8.5; collagen-activated, 641.8 ± 95.7; 6 µM, 200.5 ± 54.1; 10 µM, 170.3 ± 49.2; $n = 4$, Figure 3C). The corresponding statistical data are presented in the right panels of Figure 3A–C.

The aggregation curves of platelets preincubated with Ir-11 (50 µM) for 10 min and subsequently washed two times with Tyrode solution were not significantly different from those of platelets preincubated with the solvent control (0.1% DMSO) under equivalent conditions (Figure 3D); this observation preliminarily indicated that the effects of Ir-11 on platelet aggregation are reversible and noncytotoxic. The lactate dehydrogenase (LDH) detection results revealed that Ir-11 (10, 20, and 50 µM) incubated with platelets for 20 min did not significantly increase LDH activity in the platelets or exert cytotoxic effects on them (Figure 3E), thus demonstrating that Ir-11 does not affect platelet permeability or induce platelet cytolysis. Furthermore, SQ22536 (9-(tetrahydro-2-furanyl)-9H-purin-6-amine, 100 µM), an adenylate cyclase inhibitor, and ODQ (1H-[1,2,4] oxadiazolo [4,3-a]quinoxalin-1-one, 10 µM), a guanylate cyclase inhibitor, significantly reversed the prostaglandin E_1 (PGE_1)-mediated (1 µM) or nitroglycerin (NTG)-mediated (10 µM) inhibition of platelet aggregation stimulated by collagen (Figure 3F). Neither SQ22536 nor ODQ significantly reversed Ir-11-mediated antiplatelet activity stimulated by collagen (Figure 3F).

2.3. Effect of Ir-11 on the Phospholipase Cγ2/Protein Kinase C (PLCγ2/PKC) Cascade and Mitogen-Activated Protein Kinase (MAPK) and Akt Activation

PLCs hydrolyze phosphatidylinositol 4,5-bisphosphate to generate the secondary messengers inositol 1,4,5-trisphosphate (IP_3) and diacylglycerol (DAG). IP_3 triggers relative [Ca^{2+}]i mobilization and DAG activates PKC, yielding an approximately 47 kDa protein that is predominantly phosphorylated (p47 protein; pleckstrin) and causes ATP release [11]. As stated previously, Ir-11 markedly reduced relative [Ca^{2+}]i mobilization (Figure 3B). We further examined the effect of Ir-11 on the phosphorylation of the PLCγ2-PKC signaling cascade. As shown in Figure 4A,B, Ir-11 (10 µM) markedly reduced both PLCγ2 phosphorylation and PKC activation (p47 phosphorylation) in collagen-activated platelets. Nonetheless, Ir-11 (6 and 10 µM) did not significantly affect platelet aggregation stimulated by 150 nM PDBu, a well-known PKC activator (Figure 4C), thus indicating that although Ir-11 did not directly disturb PKC activation, it may have interfered with the upstream regulators of PKC, such as PLCγ2. Additionally, Akt is a serine/threonine-specific protein kinase that plays a key role in multiple cellular processes, such as platelet activation, cell proliferation, apoptosis, and cell migration [12]. Ir-11 (6 and 10 µM) also markedly inhibited collagen-induced Akt phosphorylation (Figure 4D). To further analyze the inhibitory mechanisms of Ir-11, several signaling molecules associated with the mitogen-activated protein kinases (MAPKs) were evaluated. The major MAPK kinase, including p38 MAPK, extracellular signal–regulated kinases (ERKs), and c-Jun N-terminal kinases (JNKs), regulate cellular responses in eukaryotic organisms through cell proliferation, migration, differentiation, and apoptosis. ERK2, JNK1, and p38 MAPK have been identified in platelets [13]. As shown in Figure 5A–C, Ir-11 (6 and 10 µM) inhibited collagen-stimulated phosphorylation of all these proteins in a concentration-dependent manner.

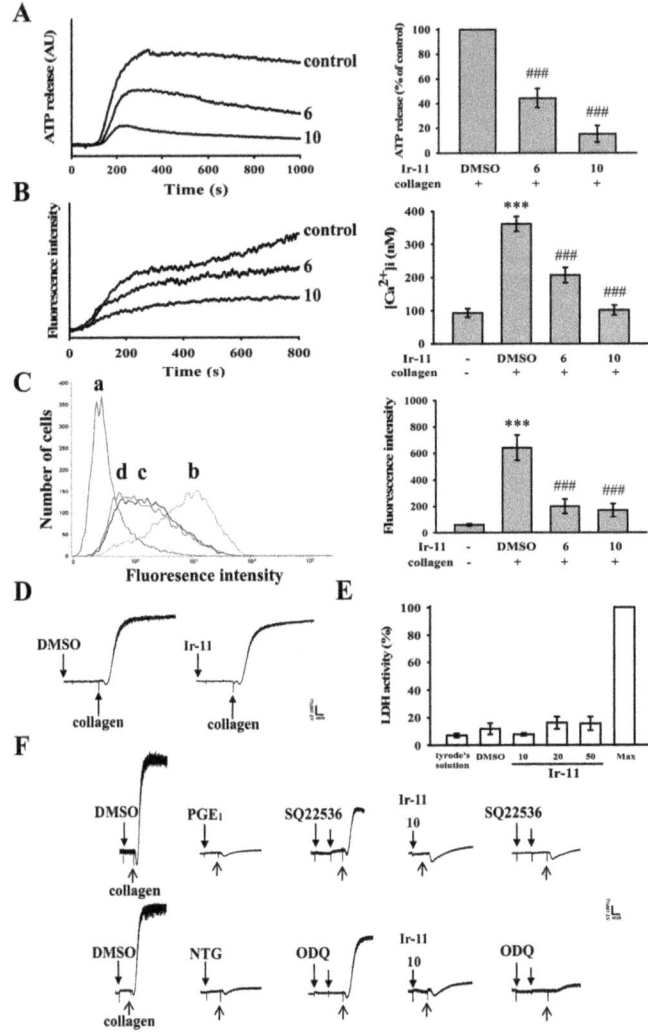

Figure 3. Effect of Ir-11 on ATP release, relative [Ca^{2+}]i mobilization, surface P-selectin expression, cytotoxicity, LDH release, and cyclic nucleotide formation in human platelets. Washed platelets (3.6 × 10^8 cells/mL) were preincubated with the solvent control (0.1% DMSO), Ir-11 (6 and 10 µM), or fluorescein isothiocyanate (FITC)–P-selectin (2 µg/mL), and collagen (1 µg/mL) was then added to trigger either (**A**) ATP release (AU; arbitrary unit), (**B**) relative [Ca^{2+}]i mobilization, or (**C**) surface P-selectin expression (a) Tyrode's solution (resting control), (b) 0.1% DMSO, (c) 6 µM Ir-11, or (d) 10 µM Ir-11. The corresponding statistical data are shown in the right panel of each figure (**A**–**C**); (**D**) Washed platelets were preincubated with the solvent control (0.1% DMSO) or Ir-11 (50 µM) for 10 min and subsequently washed two times with Tyrode solution; collagen (1 µg/mL) was then added to trigger platelet aggregation; (**E**) Washed platelets were preincubated with the solvent control (0.1% DMSO) or Ir-11 (10, 20, and 50 µM) for 20 min, and a 10 µL aliquot of the supernatant was deposited on a Fuji Dri-Chem slide LDH-PIII; (**F**) For other experiments, washed platelets were preincubated with PGE$_1$ (1 µM), NTG (10 µM), or Ir-11 (10 µM) with or without SQ22536 (100 µM) or ODQ (10 µM), and were subsequently treated with collagen (1 µg/mL) to induce platelet aggregation. Data are presented as means ± standard error of the means (n = 4). Profiles in (**D**,**F**) are representative of four independent experiments. *** $p < 0.001$ compared with the resting control; ### $p < 0.001$, compared with the DMSO-treated group.

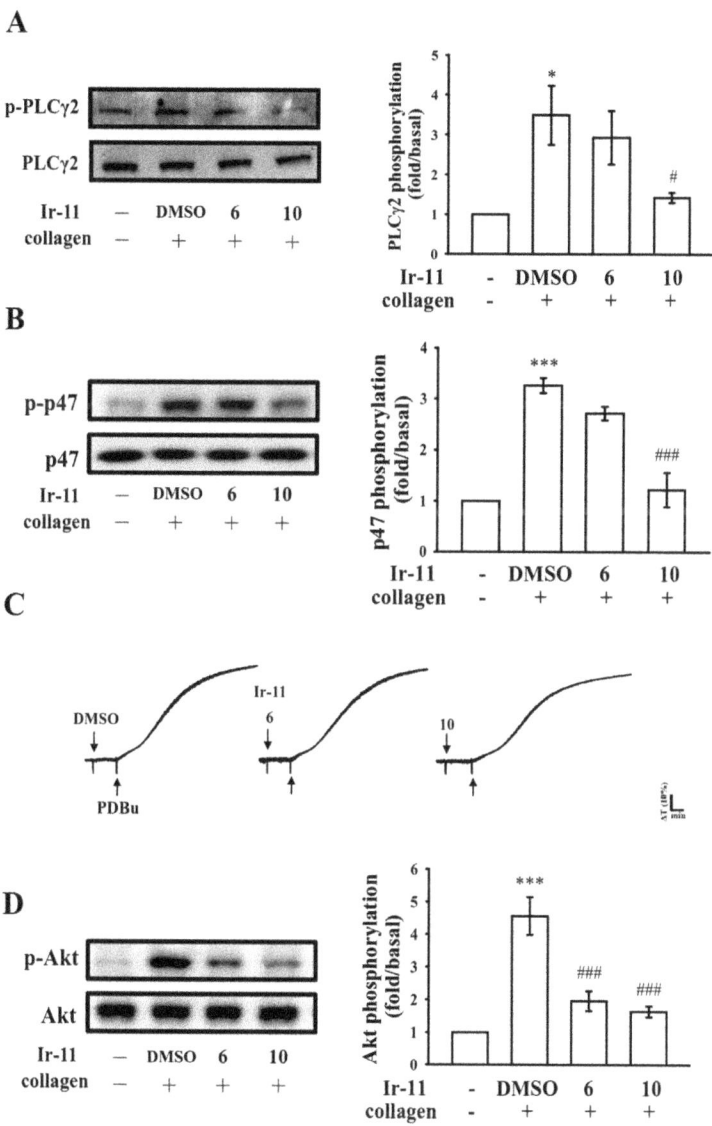

Figure 4. Inhibitory effects of Ir-11 on PLCγ2, PKC, and Akt activation in platelets. Washed platelets were preincubated with the solvent control (0.1% DMSO) or Ir-11 (6 and 10 µM), and subsequently treated with collagen (1 µg/mL) or PDBu (150 nM) to induce (**A**) PLCγ2 and (**B**) PKC activation (p47, pleckstrin phosphorylation); (**C**) platelet aggregation; and (**D**) Akt phosphorylation. Platelets were collected, and their subcellular extracts were analyzed to determine the levels of protein phosphorylation. Data are presented as means ± standard error of the means (n = 4). * $p < 0.05$ and *** $p < 0.001$, compared with the resting control; # $p < 0.05$ and ### $p < 0.001$, compared with the DMSO-treated group. The profiles in (**C**) are representative of four independent experiments.

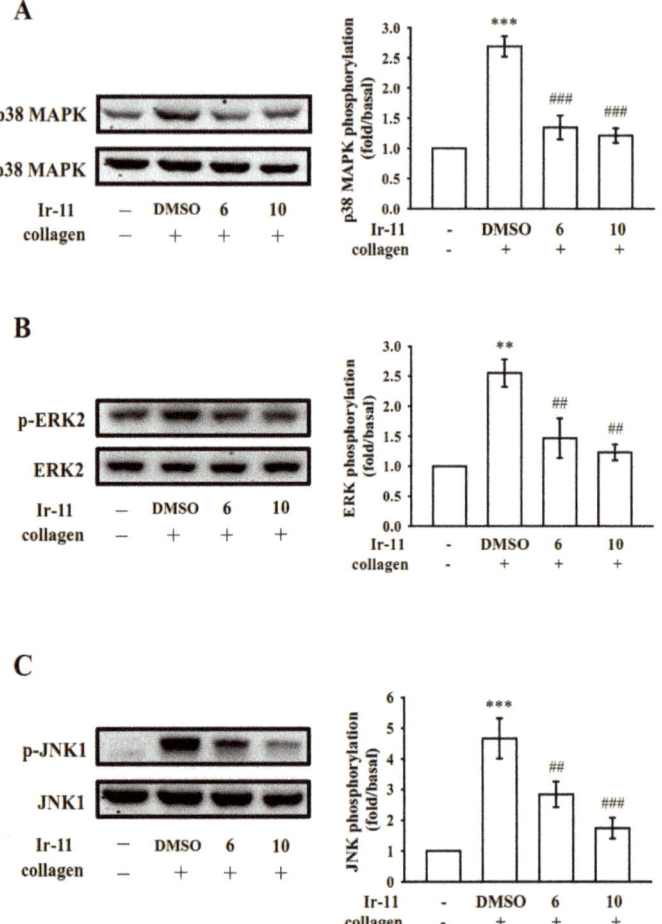

Figure 5. Effects of Ir-11 on p38 MAPK, ERK2, and JNK1 phosphorylation in collagen-activated platelets. Washed platelets were preincubated with the solvent control (0.1% DMSO) or Ir-11 (6 and 10 µM) and subsequently treated with collagen (1 µg/mL) to trigger (**A**) p38 MAPK; (**B**) ERK2; and (**C**) JNK1 activation. Platelets were collected, and their subcellular extracts were analyzed to determine the levels of protein phosphorylation. Data are presented as means ± standard error of the means (n = 4). ** $p < 0.01$ and *** $p < 0.001$, compared with the resting control; ## $p < 0.01$ and ### $p < 0.001$, compared with the DMSO-treated group.

2.4. Assessment of OH·-Scavenging Activity of Ir-11 through ESR Spectrometry

An ESR signal indicative of OH· radical formation was observed in both collagen-stimulated platelet suspensions (Figure 6(Ab)) and the Fenton reaction solution (cell-free system; Figure 6(Bb)) compared with the resting control (Figure 6(Aa,Ba)). Treatment with Ir-11 (6 and 10 µM) considerably reduced the OH· signals in the collagen-stimulated platelet suspensions (Figure 6(Ac,d)) but not in the Fenton reaction solution (Figure 6(Bc,d)), suggesting that Ir-11 reduced intracellular OH· radical formation, but it did not exhibit this effect in a cell-free system.

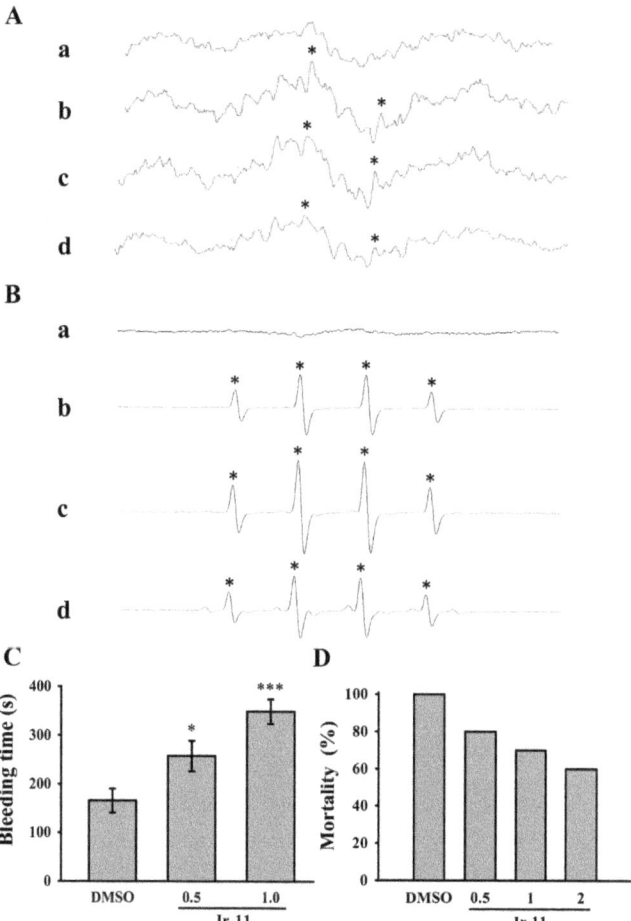

Figure 6. Regulatory activities of Ir-11 on OH· formation in platelet suspensions or the Fenton reaction solution, and bleeding time in the tail vein as well as acute pulmonary thromboembolism in experimental mice. (**A**) Washed platelets or (**B**) the Fenton reaction solution was preincubated with Tyrode solution (**a**, resting control), (**b**) 0.1% DMSO, or Ir-11 at (**c**) 6 µM or (**d**) 10 µM. Collagen (1 µg/mL) was then added for the ESR experiments as described in **Materials and Methods**. Profiles are representative of four independent experiments, and an asterisk (*) indicates OH· formation; (**C**) The bleeding time was measured through transection of the mouse tail after 30 min of administering either 0.1% DMSO, 0.5 mg/kg, or 1.0 mg/kg Ir-11 intraperitoneally (all in 50 µL); (**D**) For acute pulmonary thrombosis study, 0.1% DMSO or Ir-11 in various doses (0.5, 1, and 2 mg/kg) (all in 50 µL) was administered intraperitoneally to the mice, and ADP (0.7 mg/g) was then injected through the tail vein. Data are presented as means ± standard error of the means (C, n = 8; D, n = 10). * $p < 0.05$ and *** $p < 0.001$, compared with the DMSO (0.1%)-treated group.

2.5. Crucial Roles of Ir-11 in Bleeding Time and Adenosine Diphosphate (ADP)-Induced Acute Pulmonary Thromboembolism In Vivo

In the tail transection model of mice, after 30 min of administering 0.5 or 1.0 mg/kg Ir-11 intraperitoneally, the bleeding times recorded were 165.4 ± 24.9 s (0.1% DMSO-treated group; n = 8), 257.4 ± 31.3 s (group treated with Ir-11, 0.5 mg/kg; n = 8), and 348.9 ± 25.1 s (group treated with

Ir-11, 1.0 mg/kg; n = 8) (Figure 6C). Each mouse was monitored for 10 min after the bleeding stopped, for detection of any re-bleeding. We also investigated the therapeutic effects of Ir-11 in preventing acute pulmonary embolism death in mice, as shown in Figure 6D. The results indicated that Ir-11 significantly lowered mortality in mice challenged with ADP (0.7 mg/g), and treatment with Ir-11 at 0.5, 1.0, and 2.0 mg/kg considerably reduced mortality from control (DMSO-treated, 100%) to 80%, 70%, and 60% (n = 10), respectively.

3. Discussion

In addition to the regulation of hemostasis and coagulation, platelets play a crucial role in potentiating tumor cell growth and metastasis [14]. The activation of platelets is associated with the thrombotic events in patients with cancer [15]. Chemotherapeutics may amplify this effect and stimulate vascular thromboembolic events (VTEs) by aggravating endothelial cell damage, augmenting platelet aggregation, aggregating oxidative damage, and consequently leading vascular toxicity [16]. Among the Pt-based chemotherapy agents, cisplatin is associated with a high incidence of treatment-related VTEs [17]. Gemcitabine, combined with a Pt-based agent, is associated with increased thrombotic and vascular side effects [18,19]. Therefore, researchers are focusing on the development of new metal-based agents for inhibiting platelet activation to treat vascular diseases, reduce toxic side effects, and overcome Pt resistance. Notably, this study provides preliminary evidence demonstrating that Ir-11, belonging to a novel class of synthetic Ir(III)-derived compound, exhibits powerful antiplatelet activity ex vivo and in vivo.

Platelets adhere to the subendothelial matrix (i.e., collagen), thus altering their shape and releasing granular contents (e.g., ATP, Ca^{2+}, and P-selectin). P-selectin is an adhesion molecule stored in the α-granules of platelets, and it is expressed on the platelet surface membrane upon activation. Subsequently, it is expressed on the external membrane through membrane flipping. P-selectin mediates the initial formation of platelet aggregates and facilitates the formation of large platelet aggregates [20]. Several agonists, such as collagen, thrombin, and AA, mobilize $[Ca^{2+}]i$ to phosphorylate the Ca^{2+}/calmodulin-dependent myosin light chain (20 kDa), which is involved in the secretion of granule contents, such as serotonin and ATP [21], as well as platelet aggregation. Therefore, the inhibition of relative $[Ca^{2+}]i$ mobilization and ATP production are crucial for evaluating the antiplatelet effects of a compound. In the present study, Ir-11 inhibited platelet aggregation to different degrees, depending on the agonist used, indicating that Ir-11 did not act as the specific individual receptor of these agonists. Therefore, Ir-11 probably exerts its inhibitory effects on stimulated platelets through a common signaling cascade.

Platelet activation by agonists, such as collagen, substantially alters PLC activation. PLC activation results in IP_3 and DAG production, which activates PKC and consequently induces p47 phosphorylation [11]. PKC activation triggers particular responses, facilitating the transmission of specific activating signals in distinct cellular compartments. The PLCγ family consists of the isozymes PLCγ1 and PLCγ2; PLCγ2 is involved in collagen-dependent signaling in human platelets [22]. Ir-11 considerably reduced collagen-induced PLCγ2-PKC activation; however, Ir-11 did not exert direct effects on PKC activation because it did not inhibit PDBu-induced platelet aggregation, suggesting that the Ir-11-mediated inhibition of platelet activation involves PLCγ2 downstream signaling. This result also explains why Ir-11 was more efficacious in inhibiting platelet aggregation induced by collagen, than that induced by thrombin, U46619, and AA.

Human platelet activation is inhibited through intracellular cyclic-AMP- and cyclic-GMP-mediated pathways, and cyclic nucleotides are crucial modulators of platelet activation [23]. At elevated levels, cyclic nucleotides inhibit most platelet responses and reduce the $[Ca^{2+}]i$ level by mediating Ca^{2+} uptake by the dense tubular system; thus, the cyclic nucleotides suppress PLC and PKC activation [22]. Therefore, cyclic AMP and cyclic GMP synergistically inhibit platelet activation. In the present study, neither SQ22536 nor ODQ significantly reversed the

Ir-11-mediated inhibition of collagen-induced platelet aggregation. Therefore, the Ir-11-mediated mechanisms are independent of increasing cyclic nucleotide formation in platelets.

MAPKs are activated by specific MAPK kinases (MEKs); specifically, MEK1/2, MEK3/6, and MEK4/7 activate ERKs, p38 MAPK, and JNKs, respectively [24]. Cytosolic phospholipase A_2 (cPLA$_2$) is a substrate of p38 MAPK activity induced by various agonists, such as von Willebrand factor (vWF) and thrombin [25]. Therefore, p38 MAPK is essential for cPLA$_2$ stimulation and AA release [26]. We observed that SB203580, a p38 MAPK inhibitor, inhibited collagen-induced platelet aggregation substantially [27]. ERK activation is involved in platelet aggregation requiring prior ATP release, which triggers P_2X_1-mediated Ca^{2+} influx and activates ERKs, thereby increasing the phosphorylation of myosin light chain kinase [24]. JNK1 is the most recently identified MAPK in platelets, and therefore, its activation or role is poorly established. It is activated by several agonists such as thrombin, vWF, collagen, and ADP [28]. In addition, a study demonstrated that $JNK^{-/-}$ platelets are associated with an increased bleeding time, decreased integrin $\alpha_{IIb}\beta_3$ activation, and severe granule secretion impairment [25]. In accordance with these findings, the present results demonstrated that Ir-11 markedly inhibits the collagen-induced phosphorylation of these three MAPKs.

Akt is a downstream effector of phosphoinositide 3 (PI3)-kinase. Akt-knockout mice have been reported to exhibit defects in agonist-induced platelet activation, suggesting that Akt regulates platelet activation, and that such regulation potentially has consequences concerning thrombosis [12,13]. Three mammalian Akt isoforms exist, namely Akt 1, 2, and 3. The first two isoforms were detected in human platelets [29]. Studies using Akt inhibitors in human platelet activation have typically reported similar roles for Akt 1 and 2. Consequently, protein kinases involved in Akt activation, chiefly PI3-kinase β, may be suitable targets for the production of antithrombotic therapeutics agents. In our previous study, we found that both PI3-kinase/Akt and MAPKs (e.g., p38 MAPK) are mutually activated as the upstream regulators of PKC in activated platelets [30].

Reactive oxygen species produced through platelet activation (i.e., H_2O_2 and OH·) might affect cells that they contact, such as endothelial cells, thereby enhancing platelet reactivity during thrombus formation. Free radicals upsurge $[Ca^{2+}]i$ levels during the early stage of platelet activation, and PKC plays role in the receptor-mediated production of free radicals in platelets [31]. In addition, H_2O_2 produced by platelets is converted into OH·, because platelet aggregation is inhibited by OH· scavengers [31]. Our ESR spectrometry results provide direct evidence that Ir-11 significantly reduced OH· formation in collagen-stimulated platelet suspensions.

In studies on acute pulmonary thromboembolism, platelet aggregation is intimately involved in experimental thrombosis, and Ir-11 effectively prevented ADP-induced thromboembolic death, as expected. Alternatively, we found that ADP induced mortality in mice was not able to reduce by heparin (1.5 U/g) treatment [32]. These data are consistent with the fact that platelet aggregation is a more crucial factor in inducing thromboembolism in rat animal model than fibrin formation. Furthermore, prolongation of hemostatic platelet plug formation (bleeding time) was observed in Ir-11-treated experimental mice. A cautious bleeding time analysis suggested that the elongation of bleeding time in humans does not predict the risk of hemorrhage or surgical bleeding, thereby questioning the rationale behind its use in the clinical evaluation of antiplatelet compounds [33].

4. Materials and Methods

4.1. Chemicals and Reagents

Thrombin, collagen, arachidonic acid (AA), luciferin–luciferase, U46619, phorbol 12, 13-dibutyrate (PDBu), nitroglycerin (NTG), heparin, prostaglandin E_1 (PGE$_1$), 5,5-dimethyl-1-pyrroline N-oxide (DMPO), SQ22536, ODQ, and bovine serum albumin (BSA) were purchased from Sigma (St. Louis, MO, USA). Fura-2AM was obtained from Molecular Probes (Eugene, OR, USA). An anti-phospho-p38 mitogen-activated protein kinase (MAPK) Ser^{182} monoclonal antibody (mAb) was purchased from Santa Cruz Biotechnology (Santa Cruz, CA, USA). Anti-p38 MAPK, anti-phospho-c-Jun N-terminal kinase (JNK) (Thr^{183}/Tyr^{185}), and anti-p44/42 extracellular signal-regulated kinase (ERK) mAbs, as well as anti-phospholipase Cγ2 (PLCγ2), anti-phospho (Tyr^{759}) PLCγ2, anti-phospho-(Ser) protein kinase C (PKC) substrate (pleckstrin; p-p47), anti-JNK, and anti-phospho-p44/p42 ERK (Thr^{202}/Tyr^{204}) polyclonal antibodies (pAbs) were purchased from Cell Signaling (Beverly, MA, USA). Anti-phospho-protein kinase B (Akt) (Ser^{473}) and anti-Akt mAbs were purchased from Biovision (Mountain View, CA, USA). An anti-pleckstrin (p47) pAb was purchased from GeneTex (Irvine, CA, USA). Hybond-P polyvinylidene fluoride (PVDF) membrane, enhanced chemiluminescence Western blotting detection reagent, horseradish peroxidase (HRP)-conjugated donkey anti-rabbit immunoglobulin G (IgG), and sheep anti-mouse IgG were purchased from Amersham (Buckinghamshire, UK). Fluorescein isothiocyanate (FITC) anti-human CD42P (P-selectin) mAb was obtained from BioLegend (San Diego, CA, USA).

4.2. Synthesis of 1-(2-Pyridyl)-3-(2-hydroxyphenyl)imidazo[1,5-a]pyridine (L)

A mixture of di-pyridin-2-yl-methanone (0.92 g, 5 mM), 2-hydroxybenzaldehyde (1.22 g, 10 mM), and ammonium acetate (1.93 g, 25 mM) in 30 mL of glacial acetic acid was refluxed for 24 h under a nitrogen atmosphere by using an oil bath. After completion of the reaction, the mixture was cooled to ambient temperature and poured into a beaker containing deionized water. The precipitate that formed was then filtered, washed in an excess of water, and dried. The solid obtained was further purified through column chromatography on silica gel using hexane/ethyl acetate (3:1) as an eluent. An off-white solid was finally obtained. Yield: 66%; m.p. 184–190 °C; ^{1}H NMR (400 MHz, CDCl$_3$) δ 11.78 (bs, 1H), 8.83–8.80 (d, 1H, J = 12 Hz), 8.66–8.64 (d, 1H, J = 8 Hz), 8.58–8.56 (d, 1H, J = 8 Hz), 8.15–8.13 (d, 1H, J = 8 Hz), 7.82–7.74 (m, 2H), 7.37–7.33 (t, 1H, J = 8 Hz), 7.21–7.19 (d, 1H, J = 8 Hz), 7.16–7.13 (t, 1H, J = 6 Hz), 7.06–7.0 (m, 2H), 6.81–6.77 (t, 1H, J = 8 Hz); UV–vis: λ$_{abs}$, nm: 227, 298, 387(sh); ESI-MS (m/z) 288.20 [M$^+$ + H] (Figure 1A).

4.3. Synthesis of [Ir(Cp*)(L)Cl]BF$_4$ (Ir-11)

A suspension of L (0.11 g, 0.4 mM) and [Ir(Cp*)(Cl)$_2$]$_2$ dimer (0.16 g, 0.2 mM) in 10 mL of methanol was stirred for 2 h. NH$_4$BF$_4$ was added, and the mixture was stirred overnight. The resulting orange solution was evaporated; the precipitate formed was redissolved in dichloromethane and filtered. Finally, the filtrate was evaporated and washed with diethyl ether, and it yielded an orange solid. Yield: 89%; ^{1}H NMR (400 MHz, dimethyl sulfoxide [DMSO]-d_6) δ 8.82–8.81 (d, 1H, J = 4 Hz), 8.54–8.48 (m, 2H), 8.16–8.14 (t, 1H, J = 4 Hz), 7.98–7.90 (m, 2H), 7.61–7.50 (m, 3H), 7.22–7.10 (m, 3H), 1.30 (s, 15H); UV–vis, λ$_{abs}$, nm (ε, M^{-1} cm^{-1}): 239 (2624), 282 (2856), 308 (2082), 358 (2102), 379 (2775), 395 (1933); ESI-MS (m/z) 650.05 [M$^+$-BF$_4$$^-$] (Figure 1B).

4.4. Platelet Aggregation

This study was approved by the Institutional Review Board of Taipei Medical University (TMU-JIRB-N201612050, 20 January 2017), and it conformed to the directives of the Declaration of Helsinki. All human volunteers involved in this study provided informed consent. Human platelet suspensions were prepared as described previously [34]. Blood samples were collected from adult human volunteers who had not taken any drugs or other substances for at least 14 days before collection; the collected blood samples were mixed with an acid–citrate–dextrose solution. After centrifugation, platelet-rich plasma (PRP) was mixed with 0.5 μM PGE$_1$ and 6.4 IU/mL heparin. Tyrode solution comprising 3.5 mg/mL BSA was used to prepare the final suspension of washed human platelets. The final Ca^{2+} concentration in the Tyrode solution was 1 mM. A platelet aggregation study was conducted using a lumiaggregometer (Payton Associates, Scarborough, ON, Canada), as described previously [33]. An isovolumetric solvent control (0.1% DMSO) or Ir-11 was preincubated with platelet suspensions (3.6 × 10^8 cells/mL) for 3 min before the addition of agonists (i.e., collagen). The extent of platelet aggregation was calculated as the percentage compared with individual control (without Ir-11) expressed in light transmission units, after the reaction proceeded for 6 min. For an ATP release assay,

20 µL of luciferin–luciferase was added 1 min before the addition of the collagen (1 µg/mL), and the amount of ATP released was compared with that released by the control (without Ir-11).

4.5. Measurement of Relative $[Ca^{2+}]i$ Mobilization by Using Fura-2AM Fluorescence

The relative $[Ca^{2+}]i$ concentration was determined using Fura-2AM as described previously [34]. Briefly, citrated whole blood was centrifuged at 120× g for 10 min, and the PRP was collected and incubated with Fura-2AM (5 µM) for 1 h. Human platelets were prepared as described in the preceding section. The Fura-2AM-loaded platelets were preincubated with various concentrations of Ir-11 (6 and 10 µM) in the presence of 1 mM $CaCl_2$ and then stimulated with collagen (1 µg/mL). The Fura-2 fluorescence was measured using a spectrofluorometer (Hitachi FL Spectrophotometer F-4500, Tokyo, Japan) at excitation wavelengths of 340 and 380 nm, and an emission wavelength of 510 nm.

4.6. Detection of Lactate Dehydrogenase

Washed platelets (3.6 × 10^8 cells/mL) were preincubated with the solvent control (0.1% DMSO) or Ir-11 (10–50 µM) for 20 min at 37 °C. An aliquot of the supernatant (10 µL) was deposited on a Fuji Dri-Chem slide LDH-PIII (Fuji, Tokyo, Japan), and the absorbance wavelength was read at 540 nm using a UV–vis spectrophotometer (UV–160; Shimadzu, Japan). A maximal value of lactate dehydrogenase (LDH) was recorded in the sonicated platelets (Max).

4.7. Flow Cytometric Analysis of Surface P-Selectin Expression

Washed platelets were prepared as described in the preceding section, and the aliquots of platelet suspensions (3.6 × 10^8 cells/mL) were preincubated with the solvent control (0.1% DMSO) or Ir-11 (6 and 10 µM) and FITC-P-selectin (2 µg/mL) for 3 min, and collagen (1 µg/mL) was added to trigger platelet activation. The suspensions were then assayed for fluorescein-labeled platelets by using a flow cytometer (FACScan System, Becton Dickinson, San Jose, CA, USA). Fifty thousand platelets/experimental group were used to collected data. To confirm reproducibility, all experiments repeated at least four times.

4.8. Immunoblotting of Protein Phosphorylation

Washed platelets (1.2 × 10^9 cells/mL) were preincubated with the solvent control (0.1% DMSO) or Ir-11 (6 and 10 µM) for 3 min. Subsequently, collagen (1 µg/mL) was added to stimulate platelet activation. After the reaction was stopped, the platelets were directly resuspended in 200 µL of lysis buffer. Samples comprising 80 µg of protein were separated through 12% sodium dodecyl sulfate gel electrophoresis, and the proteins were electrotransferred to PVDF membranes using a Bio-Rad semidry transfer unit (Bio-Rad, Hercules, CA, USA). The blots were then blocked by treating them with Tris-buffered saline in Tween 20 (TBST; 10 mM Tris-base, 100 mM NaCl, and 0.01% Tween 20) containing 5% BSA for 1 h, and were probed with various primary antibodies. The membranes were incubated for 1 h with HRP-conjugated anti-mouse IgG or anti-rabbit IgG (diluted 1:3000 in TBST). An enhanced chemiluminescence system was used to detect immunoreactive bands, and their optical density was quantified using Bio-profil Biolight (version V2000.01; Vilber Lourmat, Marne-la-Vallée, France).

4.9. Measurement of OH· Formation in Either Platelet Suspensions or the Fenton Reaction Solution through Electron Spin Resonance Spectrometry

Electron spin resonance (ESR) spectrometry was performed using a Bruker EMX ESR spectrometer (Bruker, Billerica, MA, USA) as described previously [35]. Suspensions of washed platelets (3.6 × 10^8 cells/mL) were preincubated with 0.1% DMSO or Ir-11 (6 and 10 µM) for 3 min. Subsequently, either collagen (1 µg/mL) or the Fenton reagent (50 µM $FeSO_4$ + 2 mM H_2O_2) was added, and incubation proceeded for 5 min. Before ESR spectrometry, 100 µM DMPO was added to both the solutions. The ESR spectra were recorded using a quartz flat cell designed for aqueous solutions. The spectrometer was operated under the following conditions: power, 20 mW; frequency, 9.78 GHz; scan range, 100 G; and receiver gain, 5×10^4. The modulation amplitude was 1G, the time constant was 164 ms, and scanning was performed for 42 s; each ESR spectrum obtained was the sum of four scans.

4.10. Measurement of Bleeding Time in Mouse Tail Vein

The bleeding time was measured through transection of the tails of male ICR mice. In brief, after 30 min of administering either 0.5 or 1.0 mg/kg Ir-11 intraperitoneally, the tails of mice were cut 3 mm from the tip. The tails were immediately placed into a tube filled with normal saline at 37 °C for measuring the bleeding time, which was recorded until the bleeding completely stopped. In the animal experiments, the method applied to the animal model conformed to the Guide for the Care and Use of Laboratory Animals (8th edition, 2011), and we received an affidavit of approval for the animal use protocol from Taipei Medical University (LAC-2016-0395).

4.11. ADP-Induced Acute Pulmonary Thromboembolism in Mice

A previously defined method was used to induce acute pulmonary [36]. Various doses of Ir-11 (0.5, 1.0 and 2.0 mg/kg) or 0.1% DMSO (all in 50 µL) were administered through intraperitoneal injection in mice. After 5 min, adenosine diphosphate (ADP, 0.7 mg/g) was injected into the tail vein. The mortality of mice in each group after injection was determined within 10 min.

4.12. Statistical Analysis

The results are stated as means ± standard error of the means, beside the number of observations (n). The values of n refer to the number of experiments; each experiment was performed using different blood donors. The unpaired Student's t test was used to determine the significance of differences between control and experimental mice. The differences between the groups in other experiments were assessed using analysis of variance (ANOVA). When the ANOVA results designated significant changes among group means, the groups were equated using the Student–Newman–Keuls method. A p value of <0.05 designated statistical significance. Statistical analyses were performed using SAS (version 9.2; SAS Inc., Cary, NC, USA).

5. Conclusions

The present, findings reveal that the novel Ir-11 compound powerfully inhibits platelet activation by inhibiting signaling pathways, such as the PLCγ2-PKC cascade, and subsequently suppressing Akt and MAPK activation. These alterations reduce granule secretion (i.e., ATP release, $[Ca^{2+}]i$ levels, and P-selectin expression) and ultimately inhibit platelet aggregation. However, additional studies are required to investigate the involvement of other unidentified mechanisms of the Ir-11-mediated inhibition of platelet activation. Ir-11 was intended to be used as a novel antitumor drug. However, it can be considered a new therapeutic agent that inhibits either arterial thrombosis or bidirectional cross talk between platelets and tumor cells.

Acknowledgments: This work was supported by grants from the Ministry of Science and Technology of Taiwan (MOST 104-2622-B-038-003, MOST 104-2320-B-038-045-MY2, MOST 106-2320-B-038-012), Cathay General Hospital-Taipei Medical University (103CGH-TMU-01-3), and the University Grants Commission, India (MRP-MAJOR-CHEM-2013-5144; 69/2014 F. No. 10-11/12UGC).

Author Contributions: Joen-Rong Sheu perceived the work and planned the experiments. Chih-Wei Hsia, Marappan Velusamya and Jeng-Ting Tsao carried out most of the experiments. Chih-Hsuan Hsia, Duen-Suey Chou, Thanasekaran Jayakumar, Lin-Wen Lee and Jiun-Yi Li. contributed interpretations and assistance on the manuscript. All authors were involved in editing the manuscript.

Conflicts of Interest: The authors declare no conflict of interest.

References

1. Jayakumar, T.; Yang, C.H.; Geraldine, P.; Yen, T.L.; Sheu, J.R. The pharmacodynamics of antiplatelet compounds in thrombosis treatment. *Expert Opin. Drug Metab. Toxicol.* **2016**, *12*, 615–632. [CrossRef] [PubMed]
2. Shah, B.H.; Lashari, I.; Rana, S.; Saeed, O.; Rasheed, H.; Arshad Saeed, S. Synergistic interaction of adrenaline and histamine in human platelet aggregation is mediated through activation of phospholipase, map kinase and cyclo-oxygenase pathways. *Pharmacol. Res.* **2000**, *42*, 479–483. [CrossRef] [PubMed]
3. Belloc, C.; Lu, H.; Fridman, C.R.; Legrand, Y.; Menashi, S. The effect of platelets on invasiveness and protease production of human mammary tumor cells. *Int. J. Cancer* **1995**, *60*, 413–417. [CrossRef] [PubMed]
4. Felding-Habermann, B.; Oooie, T.E.; Smith, J.W.; Fransvea, E.; Ruggeri, Z.M.; Ginsberg, M.H.; Hughes, P.E.; Pampori, N.; Shattil, S.J.; Saven, A.; et al. Integrin activation controls metastasis in human breast cancer. *Proc. Natl. Acad. Sci. USA* **2001**, *98*, 1853–1858. [CrossRef] [PubMed]
5. Boucharaba, A.; Serre, C.M.; Grès, S.; Saulnier-Blache, J.S.; Bordet, J.C.; Guglielmi, J.; Clézardin, P.; Peyruchaud, O. Platelet-derived lysophosphatidic acid supports the progression of osteolytic bone metastases in breast cancer. *J. Clin. Investig.* **2004**, *114*, 1714–1725. [CrossRef] [PubMed]
6. Iavicoli, I.; Cufino, V.; Corbi, M.; Goracci, M.; Caredda, E.; Cittadini, A.; Bergamaschi, A.; Sgambato, A. Rhodium and iridium salts inhibit proliferation and induce DNA damage in rat fibroblasts in vitro. *Toxicol. In Vitro* **2012**, *26*, 963–969. [CrossRef] [PubMed]
7. Iavicoli, I.; Fontana, L.; Marinaccio, A.; Alimonti, A.; Pino, A.; Bergamaschi, A.; Calabrese, E.J. The effects of iridium on the renal function of female Wistar rats. *Ecotoxicol. Environ. Saf.* **2011**, *74*, 1795–1799. [CrossRef] [PubMed]
8. Yellol, J.; Pérez, S.A.; Buceta, A.; Yellol, G.; Donaire, A.; Szumlas, P.; Bednarski, P.J.; Makhloufi, G.; Janiak, C.; Espinosa, A.; et al. Novel C,N-cyclometalated benzimidazole ruthenium(II) and iridium(III) complexes as antitumor and antiangiogenic agents: A structure–activity relationship study. *J. Med. Chem.* **2015**, *58*, 7310–7327. [CrossRef] [PubMed]
9. Schmitt, F.; Donnelly, K.; Muenzner, J.K.; Rehm, T.; Novohradsky, V.; Brabec, V.; Kasparkova, J.; Albrecht, M.; Schobert, R.; Mueller, T. Effects of histidin-2-ylidene vs. imidazol-2-ylidene ligands on the anticancer and antivascular activity of complexes of ruthenium, iridium, platinum, and gold. *J. Inorg. Biochem.* **2016**, *163*, 221–228. [CrossRef] [PubMed]
10. Harrison, P.; Cramer, E.M. Platelet α-granules. *Blood Rev.* **1993**, *7*, 52–62. [CrossRef]
11. Singer, W.D.; Brown, H.A.; Sternweis, P.C. Regulation of eukaryotic phosphatidylinositol-specific phospholipase C and phospholipase D. *Annu. Rev. Biochem.* **1997**, *6*, 475–509. [CrossRef] [PubMed]
12. Woulfe, D.S. Akt signaling in platelet and thrombosis. *Expert Rev. Hematol.* **2010**, *3*, 81–91. [CrossRef] [PubMed]
13. Bugaud, F.; Nadal-Wollbold, F.; Levy-Toledano, S.; Rosa, J.P.; Bryckaert, M. Regulation of c-jun-NH2 terminal kinase and extracellular-signal regulated kinase in human platelets. *Blood* **1999**, *94*, 3800–3805. [PubMed]
14. Tesfamariam, B. Involvement of platelets in tumor cell metastasis. *Pharmacol. Ther.* **2016**, *157*, 112–119. [CrossRef] [PubMed]
15. Lip, G.Y.; Chin, B.S.; Blann, A. Cancer and the prothrombotic state. *Lancet Oncol.* **2002**, *3*, 27–34. [CrossRef]
16. Ferroni, P.; Della-Morte, D.; Palmirotta, R.; McClendon, M.; Testa, G.; Abete, P.; Rengo, F.; Rundek, T.; Guadagni, F.; Roselli, M. Platinum-based compounds and risk for cardiovascular toxicity in the elderly: Role of the antioxidants in chemoprevention. *Rejuvenation Res.* **2011**, *14*, 293–308. [CrossRef] [PubMed]
17. Jafri, M.; Protheroe, A. Cisplatin-associated thrombosis. *Anticancer Drugs* **2008**, *19*, 927–929. [CrossRef] [PubMed]
18. Barni, S.; Labianca, R.; Agnelli, G.; Bonizzoni, E.; Verso, M.; Mandalà, M.; Brighenti, M.; Petrelli, F.; Bianchini, C.; Perrone, T.; et al. Chemotherapy-associated thromboembolic risk in cancer outpatients and effect of nadroparin thromboprophylaxis: Results of a retrospective analysis of the PROTECHT study. *J. Transl. Med.* **2011**, *9*, 179. [CrossRef] [PubMed]
19. Dasanu, C.A. Gemcitabine: Vascular toxicity and prothrombotic potential. *Expert Opin. Drug Saf.* **2008**, *7*, 703–716. [CrossRef] [PubMed]

20. Borsig, L.; Wong, R.; Feramisco, J.; Nadeau, D.R.; Varki, N.M.; Varki, A. Heparin and cancer revisited: Mechanistic connections involving platelets, P-selectin, carcinoma mucins, and tumor metastasis. *Proc. Natl. Acad. Sci. USA* **2001**, *98*, 3352–3357. [CrossRef] [PubMed]
21. Kaibuchi, K.; Sano, K.; Hoshijima, M.; Takai, Y.; Nishizuka, Y. Phosphatidylinositol turnover in platelet activation; calcium mobilization and protein phosphorylation. *Cell Calcium* **1982**, *3*, 323–335. [CrossRef]
22. Ragab, A.; Séverin, S.; Gratacap, M.P.; Aguado, E.; Malissen, M.; Jandrot-Perrus, M.; Malissen, B.; Ragab-Thomas, J.; Payrastre, B. Roles of the C-terminal tyrosine residues of LAT in GP VI-induced platelet activation: Insights into the mechanism of PLC gamma 2 activation. *Blood* **2007**, *110*, 2466–2474. [CrossRef] [PubMed]
23. Walter, U.; Eigenthaler, M.; Geiger, J.; Reinhard, M. Role of cyclic nucleotide-dependent protein kinases and their common substrate VASP in the regulation of human platelets. *Adv. Exp. Med. Biol.* **1993**, *344*, 237–249. [PubMed]
24. Chang, L.; Karin, M. Mammalian MAP kinase signaling cascades. *Nature* **2001**, *410*, 37–40. [CrossRef] [PubMed]
25. Adam, F.; Kauskot, A.; Rosa, J.P.; Bryckaert, M. Mitogen-activated protein kinases in hemostasis and thrombosis. *J. Thromb. Haemost.* **2008**, *6*, 2007–2016. [CrossRef] [PubMed]
26. Canobbio, I.; Reineri, S.; Sinigaglia, F.; Balduini, C.; Torti, M. A role for p38 MAP kinase in platelet activation by von Willebrand factor. *Thromb. Haemost.* **2004**, *91*, 102–110. [CrossRef] [PubMed]
27. Flevaris, P.; Li, Z.; Zhang, G.; Zheng, Y.; Liu, J.; Du, X. Two distinct roles of mitogen-activated protein kinases in platelets and a novel Rac1-MAPK-dependent integrin outside-in retractile signaling pathway. *Blood* **2009**, *113*, 893–901. [CrossRef] [PubMed]
28. Adam, F.; Kauskot, A.; Nurden, P.; Sulpice, E.; Hoylaerts, M.F.; Davis, R.J.; Rosa, J.P.; Bryckaert, M. Platelet JNK1 is involved in secretion and thrombus formation. *Blood* **2010**, *115*, 4083–4092. [CrossRef] [PubMed]
29. Chen, J.; De, S.; Damron, D.S.; Chen, W.S.; Hay, N.; Byzova, T.V. Impaired platelet responses to thrombin and collagen in AKT-1-deficient mice. *Blood* **2004**, *104*, 1703–1710. [CrossRef] [PubMed]
30. Jayakumar, T.; Chen, W.F.; Lu, W.J.; Chou, D.S.; Hsiao, G.; Hsu, C.Y.; Sheu, J.R.; Hsieh, C.Y. A novel antithrombotic effect of sulforaphane via activation of platelet adenylate cyclase: Ex vivo and in vivo studies. *J. Nutr. Biochem.* **2013**, *24*, 1086–1095. [CrossRef] [PubMed]
31. Wachowicz, B.; Olas, B.; Zbikowska, H.M.; Buczyński, A. Generation of reactive oxygen species in blood platelets. *Platelets* **2002**, *13*, 175–182. [CrossRef] [PubMed]
32. Sheu, J.R.; Chao, S.H.; Yen, M.H.; Huang, T.F. In vivo antithrombotic effect of triflavin, an Arg-Gly-Asp containing peptide on platelet plug formation in mesenteric microvessels of mice. *Thromb. Haemost.* **1994**, *72*, 617–621. [PubMed]
33. Lind, S.E. The bleeding time does not predict surgical bleeding. *Blood* **1991**, *77*, 2547–2552. [PubMed]
34. Sheu, J.R.; Lee, C.R.; Lin, C.H.; Hsiao, G.; Ko, W.C.; Chen, Y.C.; Yen, M.H. Mechanisms involved in the antiplatelet activity of Staphylococcus aureus lipoteichoic acid in human platelets. *Thromb. Haemost.* **2000**, *83*, 777–784. [PubMed]
35. Chou, D.S.; Hsiao, G.; Shen, M.Y.; Tsai, Y.J.; Chen, T.F.; Sheu, J.R. ESR spin trapping of a carbon-centered free radical from agonist-stimulated human platelets. *Free Radic. Biol. Med.* **2005**, *39*, 237–248. [CrossRef] [PubMed]
36. Sheu, J.R.; Hung, W.C.; Wu, C.H.; Lee, Y.M.; Yen, M.H. Antithrombotic effect of rutaecarpine, an alkaloid isolated from Evodia rutaecarpa, on platelet plug formation in in vivo experiments. *Br. J. Haematol.* **2000**, *110*, 110–115. [CrossRef] [PubMed]

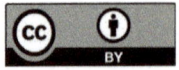 © 2017 by the authors. Licensee MDPI, Basel, Switzerland. This article is an open access article distributed under the terms and conditions of the Creative Commons Attribution (CC BY) license (http://creativecommons.org/licenses/by/4.0/).

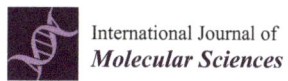

Article

Population-Specific Associations of Deleterious Rare Variants in Coding Region of *P2RY1–P2RY12* Purinergic Receptor Genes in Large-Vessel Ischemic Stroke Patients

Piotr K. Janicki [1], Ceren Eyileten [2], Victor Ruiz-Velasco [3], Khaled Anwar Sedeek [3], Justyna Pordzik [2], Anna Czlonkowska [2,4], Iwona Kurkowska-Jastrzebska [4], Shigekazu Sugino [1], Yuka Imamura-Kawasawa [5], Dagmara Mirowska-Guzel [2] and Marek Postula [1,2,*]

1. Perioperative Genomics Laboratory, Penn State College of Medicine, Hershey, PA 17033, USA; pjanicki@pennstatehealth.psu.edu (P.K.J.); ssugino@hmc.psu.edu (S.S.)
2. Department of Experimental and Clinical Pharmacology, Medical University of Warsaw, Center for Preclinical Research and Technology CEPT, 02-097 Warsaw, Poland; cereneyileten@gmail.com (C.E.); j.pordzik@yahoo.co.uk (J.P.); czlonkow@ipin.edu.pl (A.C.); dmirowska@wum.edu.pl (D.M.-G.)
3. Department of Anesthesiology and Perioperative Medicine, Penn State College of Medicine, Hershey, PA 17033, USA; vruizvelasco@psu.edu (V.R.-V.); ksedeek@pennstatehealth.psu.edu (K.A.S.)
4. 2nd Department of Neurology, Institute of Psychiatry and Neurology, 02-957 Warsaw, Poland; ikurkowska@ipin.edu.pl
5. Genome Sciences Facility, Penn State College of Medicine, Hershey, PA 17033, USA; imamura@hmc.psu.edu
* Correspondence: mpostula@wum.edu.pl; Tel.: +48-221-166-160

Received: 20 September 2017; Accepted: 7 December 2017; Published: 11 December 2017

Abstract: The contribution of low-frequency and damaging genetic variants associated with platelet function to ischemic stroke (IS) susceptibility remains unknown. We employed a deep re-sequencing approach in Polish patients in order to investigate the contribution of rare variants (minor allele frequency, MAF < 1%) to the IS genetic susceptibility in this population. The genes selected for re-sequencing consisted of 26 genes coding for proteins associated with the surface membrane of platelets. Targeted pooled re-sequencing (Illumina HiSeq 2500) was performed on genomic DNA of 500 cases (patients with history of clinically proven diagnosis of large-vessel IS) and 500 controls. After quality control and prioritization based on allele frequency and damaging probability, follow-up individual genotyping of deleterious rare variants was performed in patients from the original cohort. Gene-based analyses identified an association between IS and 6 rare functional and damaging variants in the purinergic genes (*P2RY1* and *P2RY12* locus). The predicted properties of the most damaging rare variants in *P2RY1* and *P2RY12* were confirmed by using mouse fibroblast cell cultures transfected with plasmid constructs containing cDNA of mutated variants (FLIPR on FlexStation3). This study identified a putative role for rare variants in *P2RY1* and *P2RY12* genes involved in platelet reactivity on large-vessel IS susceptibility in a Polish population.

Keywords: DNA sequencing; platelets; genetic polymorphism; cerebrovascular stroke; purinergic receptors; large-vessel ischemic stroke; Polish population

1. Introduction

The genetics of complex diseases, including ischemic stroke (IS), has been previously investigated in genome wide association studies (GWAS), which identified large numbers of common single nucleotide variants associated with disease susceptibility [1]. While relevant disease pathways have been identified by several GWAS, and one targeted re-sequencing study focused on common genetic variants, IS-associated common variants only explain <10% of variance in disease onset [2]. Therefore, research looking into the missing heritability in IS has been focused on the evaluation of the contribution of low frequency and rare variants [3]. Sequencing studies have revealed that low frequency (i.e., minor allele frequency or MAF between 1% and 5%), and in particular, rare (MAF < 1%) genetic variants, are more likely to have a deleterious effect on health compared to common variants [4,5]. Few re-sequencing studies investigating IS in European populations have been performed [6,7]. These studies showed that low frequency and rare protein coding variants in several genes are associated with stroke ($p < 1 \times 10^{-6}$) [7].

The pathogenesis of IS is strongly influenced by the activation of platelets and subsequent release of the bioactive materials they transport. Platelets can also exert a far-reaching influence, when activated, by releasing microparticles containing lipids, receptors, proteins, and genetic material into circulation. Apart from their well-established role in hemostasis, platelets have been identified as key players in inflammation, angiogenesis, and central nervous system repair [8]. For that reason, we have selected genes associated with platelet plasma membrane receptors as the target for this re-sequencing study. Only one previous re-sequencing study, in association with IS, was performed in the Polish population, and focused on platelets' common genetic variants [9].

Thus, we aimed to further investigate the contribution of rare, presumably large effect genetic variants within a selection of previously described 26 genes encoding platelet surface receptors, to IS susceptibility in the Polish population [10].

2. Results

The study design and flowchart is presented in Figure 1. Pooled targeted enrichment, with the custom Agilent SureSelect capturing kit, resulted in coverage of 99.6%. Sequencing of 10 pools (five each for control and stroke groups) was performed on the Illumina HiSeq2500 sequencer, and generated an average of 36.1 (22.7–45.9 range) million pair-end 101 bp reads, and 5.3 (3–7 range) Gbp per pooled sample consisting of 100 subjects. It corresponds to mean coverage per pool of 12000×, associated with a mean of 120× per individual sample (range 21–369).

The frequency of the investigated damaging allele was presented as combined MAF (cMAF) which encompassed all rare damaging variants in the sequenced gene or region. In total, 477 unique single nucleotide variants (SNVs) with sufficient quality coverage were detected after subsequent stringent quality control. Sixty nine percent (69%) of SNVs were known in the single nucleotide polymorphism (SNP) database (dbSNP) version dbSNP138 (see complete list of known variants in Tables S1 and S2). In all, 248 of the 477 variants (51.9%) were coding variants within target exons of sequenced genes, and the remainder was located in untranslated (introns) and intergenic regions. The final 38 rare and damaging variants were selected out of 129 non-synonymous coding variants based on MAF < 1%, and predicted deleteriousness of single variants, from significant gene-based tests using Combined Annotation Dependent Depletion (CADD), with a minimum scaled CADD score of 10 (corresponding to the top 10% deleterious variants in the genome, as indicated by authors) as a threshold for predicted deleteriousness or damaging properties [11]. The selected variants consisted of 28 known (by dbSNP149 November 2016) and 10 novel (previously not listed) variants.

The rare SNPs ($n = 38$, Table 1) with the most damaging properties were submitted for verification with individual genotyping, of which 31 passed the design of iPLEX Design suite. The individual genotyping was performed in all patients ($n = 1000$) from the original cohort of patients used for pooled targeted re-sequencing. The presence of all 31 variants was verified in at least one carrier from investigated cohorts. In addition, we repeated the calculations in the remaining 605 patients, after exclusion of subjects (from both groups) with a known medical history which could interfere with the burden analysis (including coronary artery disease—CAD, congestive heart failure—CHF, and diabetes mellitus—DM), because the prevalence of these conditions differ between control and stroke groups (Table S3).

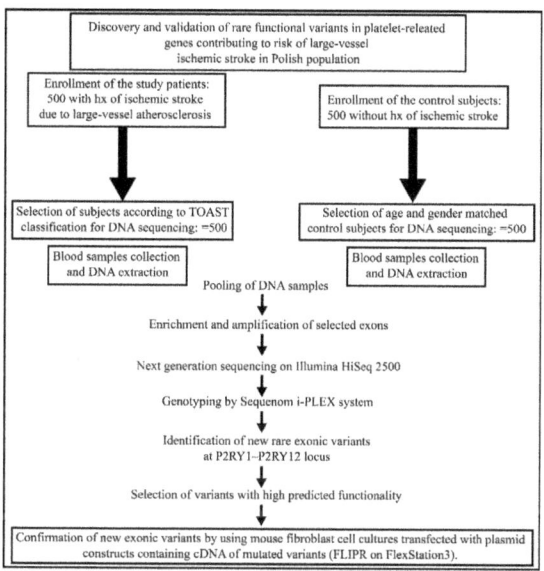

Figure 1. Study-flow diagram. TOAST; Trial of Org 10172 in Acute Stroke Treatment, hx; history.

Table 1. List of all rare (predicted MAF < 0.1%) non-synonymous and deleterious single nucleotide variants observed in the investigated Polish patients (n = 1000) after pooled resequencing of exons in 26 genes.

Chr	Gene	Position	Ref	Alt	dbSNP149	cDNA	Protein AA	CADD	MAF Ctrl	MAF Stroke
chr3	ITPR1	4714920	A	G	rs35789999	c.A2260G	p.M754V	15.92	0.0014	
chr3	ITPR1	4716885	C	T	rs201519806	c.C2687T	p.A896V	12.80		0.0011
chr3	ITPR1	4774887	G	T		c.G5147T	p.G1716V	15.77		0.0014
chr3	ITPR1	4821291	G	T	rs373973399	c.G6160T	p.A2054S	20.2		0.0013
chr3	ITPR1	4842276	G	A	rs201144431	c.G6910A	p.A2304T	16.91	0.0015	0.001
chr17	GP1BA	4837662	T	C	rs201408072	c.T1763C	p.V588A	15.12	0.0013	
chr3	RAF1	12641707	C	T	rs555034652	c.G934A	p.V312M	12.39		0.0017
chr1	PTAFR	28477192	T	C	rs138629813	c.A341G	p.N114S	20.8		0.0018
chr1	PTAFR	28477408	C	A		c.G125T	p.R42L	14.45	0.0015	
chr17	ITGA2B	42453084	C	T	rs74988902	c.G2602A	p.V868M	13.50		0.0014
chr17	ITGA2B	42455791	G	A	rs200481952	c.C2033T	p.A678V	20.4		0.0015
chr17	ITGA2B	42457474	G	A	rs548977341	c.C1648T	p.R550W	22.3	0.0018	
chr17	ITGA2B	42463054	G	C	rs76066357	c.C439G	p.L147V	11.09		0.0025
chr17	ITGB3	45363765	A	G	rs56173532	c.A754G	p.I252V	13.67	0.0012	
chr17	ITGB3	45376796	G	A	rs144884023	c.G1813A	p.G605S	35		0.0013
chr19	PTGIR	47126849	G	A	rs4987262	c.C634T	p.R212C	22.3		0.0034
chr5	ITGA2	52344487	A	G	rs55973669	c.A517G	p.I173V	12.10		0.0022
chr19	GP6	55543660	G	A	rs199588110	c.C172T	p.R58C	18.28	0.0025	0.0016
chr19	GP6	55543660	G	A	rs199588110	c.C172T	p.R58C	18.28	0.0023	
chr19	GP6	55543692	C	T	rs750889036	c.G140A	p.R47Q	10.75		0.0019
chr11	FERMT3	63974970	T	G	rs759179590	c.T134G	p.V45G	33	0.0035	0.0042
chr11	FERMT3	63974995	C	G	rs142815441	c.C159G	p.I53M	12.17	0.0013	
chr11	FERMT3	63978538	G	A	rs762181713	c.G409A	p.E137K	29.0		0.0014
chr11	P2RY2	72945434	T	C	rs148391446	c.T230C	p.V77A	14.97		0.0017
chr11	P2RY2	72945799	A	G	rs141776297	c.A595G	p.S199G	15.02		0.0021
chr11	P2RY2	72945799	A	G	rs141776297	c.A595G	p.S199G	15.02	0.0019	0.0026
chr11	P2RY2	72946279	T	C	rs74472890	c.T1075C	p.S359P	12.54	0.0024	
chr3	GP9	128781048	G	A	rs3796130	c.G466A	p.A156T	12.21	0.0015	
chr3	P2RY12 *	151055962	C	A		c.G672T	p.R224S	15		0.0021

Table 1. Cont.

Chr	Gene	Position	Ref	Alt	dbSNP149	cDNA	Protein AA	CADD	MAF Ctrl	MAF Stroke
chr3	P2RY12 *	151056084	G	T		c.C550A	p.L184I	15.13		0.0013
chr3	P2RY1 *	152554155	G	A		c.G584A	p.R195H	18.35	0.0012	0.0034
chr3	P2RY1 *	152554326	C	A		c.C755A	p.S252Y	22.4		0.0015
chr3	P2RY1 *	152554395	C	A		c.C824A	p.P275H	22.8		0.0013
chr3	P2RY1 *	152554482	C	T	rs868057570	c.C911T	p.A304V	12.84		0.0026
chr1	PEAR1	156878116	C	T		c.C1099T	p.R367W	18.01		0.0012
chr1	SELP	169576246	G	A		c.C1460T	p.A487V	12.76	0.0017	
chr1	SELP	169581608	G	A	rs139249907	c.C808T	p.R270X	13.86		0.0016
chr3	GP5	194117640	C	A		c.G1372T	p.A458S	10.81		0.0012

* Functional and damaging variants selected for FlexStation3 analyzes.

The initial statistical analysis was performed using Pearson's chi-squared test for the comparison of the total (cumulative) frequencies of all cMAF for rare deleterious variants in all sequenced genes between controls and IS cohort, as confirmed by individual genotyping. The obtained data are shown in Table 2. There was a highly statistically significant ($p = 0.0005$) increase in cMAF for all damaging variants in the IS group when compared with controls. Subsequent calculation of cMAF in the study patients remaining after removal of results of subjects with known CAD, CHF, and DM (in both groups) provided a similar difference in the cMAF for all deleterious variants between control and IS cohorts.

The pooled analysis of multiple variants within unique regions or genes, which was based on pooled association test (CMAT), demonstrated a statistically significant difference ($p = 0.0007$) between control and IS cohorts for the P2RY1–P2RY12 location on chromosome 3 (Table 2). It contained five novel and one known rare and deleterious (CADD score range 12.8–22.8) variant. The region-based, Bonferroni-corrected significance threshold was $p = 0.0021$ (0.05/24 analyzed regions). Similar results were obtained after repeating CMAT analysis for control and IS cohorts remaining after removal of patients with CAD and DM ($p = 0.03$).

Table 2. List of cumulative minor allele frequencies (cMAF) for damaging non-synonymous variants in the individually genotyped subjects from the control (ctrl) and study (stroke) groups in all patients used for pooled sequencing (left panel) and remaining patients after subtracting cardiac conditions (right panel).

Gene	All Individuals (n = 1000). Number of Variant Carriers for Each Locus and Cohort in Brackets			Subjects without Cardiac Disease (n = 605). Number of Variants Carriers for Each Locus and Cohort in Brackets		
Region	cMAF ctrl	cMAF stroke	CMAT P/Fisher	cMAF ctrl	cMAF stroke	CMAT P/Fisher
GP6	0.006 (3)	0.002 (1)	0.3700	0.000 (0)	0.000 (0)	NA
ITGA2	0.000 (0)	0.004 (2)	0.4900	0.0000 (0)	0.002 (2)	0.51
ITGA2B/ITGB3	0.004 (2)	0.014 (7)	0.1200	0.005 (2)	0.006 (5)	0.62
ITPR1	0.004 (2)	0.006 (3)	0.4900	0.0025 (1)	0.002 (2)	0.90
P2RY1/P2RY12	0.002 (1)	0.02 (10)	0.0007 **	0.0025 (1)	0.123 (10)	0.002 **
P2RY2	0.004 (2)	0.006 (3)	0.2100	0.0006 (1)	0.004 (3)	0.62
PEAR1	0.0000 (0)	0.002 (1)	1.0000	0.000 (0)	0.000 (0)	NA
PTAFR	0.0000 (0)	0.002 (1)	1.0000	0.0000 (0)	0.001 (1)	0.99
SELP	0.0000 (0)	0.004 (2)	0.1200	0.0000 (0)	0.002 (2)	0.14
PTGIR	0.0000 (0)	0.004 (2)	0.2500	0.0000 (0)	0.002 (2)	0.26
Total [#]	0.02 (10)	0.064 (32)	0.0005 *	0.0125 (5)	0.033 (27)	0.03 *
OR			3.4 (7.6–6.9)			2.8 (1.1–7.3)

** Statistical significance (p value) calculated using burden CMAT test (for data with cMAF for variants in present both control and stroke groups) or Fisher exact test (for variants with cMAF only in one studies group and not observed in another group). * Statistical analysis performed using Pearson's chi-squared test; [#]—combined cMAF for all observed damaging variants in one of the study group. OR—odds ratio.

To determine whether the SNPs exert a deleterious effect on *P2RY1* and *P2RY12* function, we chose the two presumably most damaging variants (with highest CADD) from each gene, and examined coupling between the heterologously expressed mutant receptors and G protein inwardly-rectifying K^+ (GIRK) channels in mouse fibroblast (L cells). Figure 2 shows the fluorescence signals of 3 individual wells with L cells expressing wild type *P2RY1* (black trace), *P2RY1* C755A (blue trace), and *P2RY1* C824A (red trace) before and following 2-methylthioadenosine diphosphate (MeSADP) (1 µM) exposure. Following MeSADP application, the fluorescence decreased rapidly, indicative of cell hyperpolarization. It can be seen that the decrease in fluorescence for the C824A variant is approximately half of that obtained with the wild type-expressing L cells. Similarly, the decreased magnitude in fluorescence of C755A *P2RY1*-expressing cells was not as high as that observed in control. The summary plot illustrates that MeSADP produced a dose-dependent increase in hyperpolarization for wild type *P2RY1*-expressing cells, while that obtained with C824A was significantly ($p < 0.05$) attenuated with application of 1 µM MeSADP. On the other hand, the MeSADP-mediated hyperpolarization in C755A-expressing mutants was lower when compared to wild type *P2RY1*, but did not reach significance ($p = 0.10$). The fluorescence tracings shown in Figure 2B depict the effect of MeSADP (1 µM) in L cells expressing wild type *P2RY12* (black trace), *P2RY12* C550A (blue trace), and *P2RY12* G672T (red trace) variants. The summary plot shows that MeSADP (1 µM) exposure produced a significantly ($p < 0.05$) lower change in *P2RY12* C550A-expressing cells than the wild type receptor. The *P2RY12* G672T-expressing cells also exhibited a diminished change ($p = 0.08$) following receptor activation.

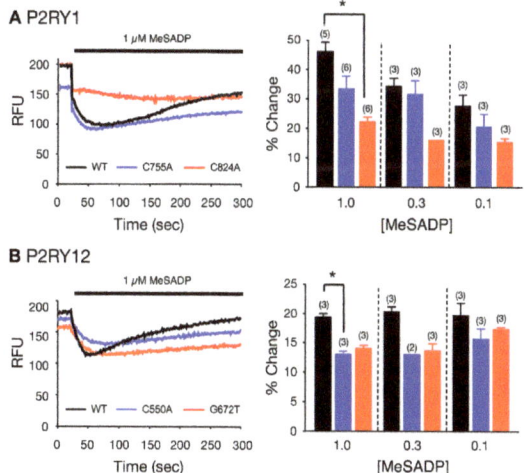

Figure 2. Effect of MeSADP-stimulated fluorescence changes in L cells heterologously expressing *P2RY1* (**A**) and *P2RY12* (**B**) wild type and variant receptors. The left panel (**A**) shows sample fluorescence signals (raw fluorescence units, RFU) from L cells transfected with wild type (black trace), C755A (blue), and C824A (red) *P2RY1* cDNA constructs, before and during MeSADP (1 µM solid line) application. Left panel (**B**) depicts the fluorescence signals (RFU) in cells expressing wild type (black trace), C550A (blue trace) and G672T *P2RY12* receptors. Panels on the right (**A**,**B**) are summary plots showing the mean (+SEM) changes of fluorescence signals following MeSADP application. * $p < 0.05$ employing ANOVA.

3. Discussion

In the present sequencing study of a relatively large cohort of 1000 Polish subjects, we investigated the contribution of rare non-synonymous variants in genes coding for platelet plasma membrane surface proteins, to the genetic susceptibility of large-vessel IS. The comparison of MAF for all rare and damaging non-synonymous variants across all sequenced genes and regions demonstrated that there was a statistically significant increase in the cumulative frequency of these variants in the IS group when compared with controls. These results allowed us to examine the contribution of rare coding variants to population variation in IS. By prioritizing rare variants using gene- and region-based tests, we identified novel associations, not previously detected by GWAS. We found association of 6 rare non-synonymous variants in *P2RY1–P2RY12* coding region with large-vessel IS. Grouping rare variants by gene units allowed us to observe associations we were underpowered to detect when only examining single variants, as shown in previous studies of other traits [9]. By doing so, we had not only been gaining insight into the biology underlying platelet membrane proteins, but show that grouping variants by functional annotations could be an effective future strategy. It is important to note that, with exception of one variant, all of the other five investigated rare non-synonymous variants in the *P2RY1–P2RY12* were novel, and never reported before (based on review of >300 rare non-synonymous variants in dbSNP149, and 1000 Genome database listings in March 2017). This might raise the possibility that the observed variants might be specific for the Polish cohort. It is important to mention that Polish patients have been poorly, or not at all, represented in 1000 Genomes and dbSNP. In addition, the recent work of Visschedijk et al. indicates that, at least in case of rare damaging variants associated with ulcerative colitis, the associated variants in the Dutch population could not be replicated in a German replication cohort [12]. Moreover, the first trans-ancestry association study in inflammatory bowel disease performed in several thousands of European individuals and individuals from East Asia, India, or Iran show that the majority of the loci based on MAF > 5% were shared between different ancestry groups [13]. However, this study also found genetic heterogeneity between different ancestry groups for less frequent alleles. Rare variants are even more likely to be specific to a particular population, as was demonstrated by a recent sequencing study in Korean population [14]. It was also demonstrated that the rare variants differ strongly among populations, even between closely related UK populations [15]. As far as the results of our study are concerned, it is interesting that we were able to confirm the presence only one (out of several hundreds) of previously listed rare non-synonymous variants in the *P2RY1–P2RY12* region, which either indicated population-specific distribution of these variants, or might also indicate the limited power of this study. Further studies in both Polish and other populations are obviously needed to confirm that the rare deleterious variants in the purinergic receptor genes region on chromosome 3 are associated with large-vessel stroke, but also with other types of IS (small-vessel and embolic).

Different coding and non-coding SNPs (mostly common type) in *P2RY1* and *P2RY12* were previously evaluated in various IS population, however, the reported results have been conflicting so far [16–19]. It is worth mentioning that the possible associations of *P2RY12* genetic variants, in a "gain-of-function" haplotype H2 of *P2Y12*, with thromboembolic events (myocardial infarction (MI), IS, or deep venous thromboembolism/pulmonary embolism (DVT/PE)), were not confirmed in a prospective analysis of 14,916 initially healthy American men [17]. The reported conflicting findings could be partly attributable to allelic heterogeneity, case-control selection criteria, phenotype/trait definition, and different population backgrounds.

The hyperpolarization response observed in the cell culture model served as a measure of adenine diphosphate (ADP)-induced purinergic activation, and was significantly attenuated by the investigated variants. Therefore, it can be assumed that the mutations, when expressed in platelets, could cause subsequent alterations in aggregation and clot formation. The reverse situation (more loss-of-function mutations in the IS group), as observed in this study, indicates that other mechanisms could be responsible for pro-stroke activity associated with P2RY1/P2RY12 receptors. It was previously demonstrated that the ADP-initiated activation of purinergic receptors causes release of endothelium-derived relaxing factor and nitric oxide, with subsequent activation of GIRK channel, hyperpolarization, and vasodilatation of small arteries [20,21]. It can be therefore hypothesized that the attenuation of this mechanism (presence of loss-of-function mutations in P2RY1/P2RY12 receptors) could produce a greater tendency to vasospasm and hypoperfusion associated with IS. It is interesting to note, in this regard, that a protective role for SNVs within coding regions of *P2RY1* in MI was postulated by Ignatovica et al. in the Latvian population [22].

No previous studies addressed the impact or association of rare damaging polymorphisms in *P2RY* genes and IS. On the other hand, different SNPs (mostly common type) in *P2RY1* and *P2RY12* were previously evaluated in various IS cohorts, however, the reported results have been conflicting so far [16–20]. Out of all P2RY receptors, the greatest focus has been put on *P2RY12*, which is expressed in megakaryocyte/platelet lineage, and contributes to progression of thrombosis and hemostasis to cerebrovascular events [23]. To date, most of the studies focused on association between common SNPs within *P2RY12* gene and antiplatelet drug response, mainly clopidogrel [24]. However, only few studies aimed to evaluate the relation between genetic polymorphism within *P2RY* receptor genes' family, and risk of stroke and data are conflicting. Ziegler et al. found increased risk of ischemic cerebrovascular events in patients with peripheral artery disease treated with clopidogrel, that was associated with of rs6785930 (which is not part of the "H2" haplotype), but not rs6809699 (which is part of the "H2" haplotype) [16]. In the latest study performed in order to investigate the relationship between genetic polymorphisms and poor clinical outcomes in IS patients who underwent stenting for extracranial or intracranial arterial stenosis, four common SNPs within *P2RY12* gene were included (i.e., rs6787801, rs6798347, rs2046934, and rs6801273). Only A-allele carriers of rs2046934 of *P2RY12* had a significant association with an increased risk of clinical outcome events (transient ischemic attack (TIA), IS, MI, and death). In another study, the C allele in *P2RY12* (rs2046934) was predicted to be a protective factor for clopidogrel resistance in IS patients [25]. The latest study aimed to evaluate the association of 2 common SNPs in *P2RY12* (i.e., rs16863323, and rs9859538), 3 common SNPs in *P2RY1* (i.e., rs701265, rs1439010, and rs1371097), and 2 SNPs in *GPIIIa* gene, as well as their interactions with antiplatelet drug responsiveness, and adverse clinical events after minor IS. The high-risk interactive genotypes (i.e., rs16863323TT in *P2RY12*) were independently associated with poor antiplatelet drug responsiveness and increased risk of primary outcomes, defined as composite adverse events of recurrent IS, MI, and death within 90 days after treatment [26]. However, in a prospective analysis of 14,916 American men, there was no evidence for an association of any of the variants or the haplotype H2 (composed of dbSNP rs10935838, rs2046934, rs5853517, and rs6809699) tested with risk of MI, or IS [17].

It has been previously reported that genetic variability of P2RY2 receptor had substantial influence on occurrence of IS. In 237 Japanese patients with a history of IS, five single SNPs within *P2RY2* gene (rs4944831, rs1783596, rs4944832, rs4382936, rs10898909) were genotyped, and using a dominant model for rs4944832 phenotype, it was found that the GG genotype of this SNP is a genetic marker for IS, particularly in women. Moreover, the overall distribution of the haplotype defined by rs1783596–rs4382936–rs10898909 was significantly different between IS and the control groups [27]. The reported conflicting findings could be partly attributable to allelic heterogeneity, case-control selection criteria, phenotype/trait definition, and different population backgrounds.

Our confirmatory in vitro results also indicate that the MeSADP-mediated hyperpolarization of L cells expressing *P2RY1* and *P2RY12* variants was attenuated when compared to cells expressing the wild type receptors. These findings suggest that the signaling is likely altered in platelets expressing the mutant P2RY receptors.

4. Materials and Methods

4.1. Patients

The local ethics committee of the Institute of Psychiatry and Neurology, Warsaw, Poland, approved both the study protocol (including DNA sample collection and genotyping) and the informed consent form (identification code KB IPiN 06/2011). The study was conducted in accordance with the current version of the Declaration of Helsinki at the time when the study was designed, and informed written consent was obtained from all enrolled patients. The study population consisted of 500 patients with the diagnosis of the acute IS based on clinical features according to the World Health Organization definition and always supported by brain imaging (CT or MRI) that was selected for the existing dataset, as previously described [9,28–30]. Briefly, it included information about patients' demographics, comorbidities, laboratory findings, and the course of stroke. Based on the Trial of Org 10172 in Acute Stroke Treatment (TOAST) classification, we included (i) all patients classified as having IS due to large-vessel atherosclerosis, and (ii) a subset of patients classified as having IS of unknown etiology, provided they had at least 50% stenosis of the carotid artery ipsilateral to the infarct side, and no evidence or no history of atrial fibrillation. The controls consisted of 500 age- and gender-matched patients, free of stroke, with multiple risk factors for cardiovascular disease or present CAD. Blood sampling and DNA extraction was performed as described before [9].

4.2. Genotyping

The target for genotyping consisted of 26 genes (Table 3) coding for platelet plasma membrane functions and containing total of 241 exons, as well as 10 flanking bases beyond each exon on both sides, which were selected using the human (*Homo sapiens*, hg19, GRCh37, February 2009) database. Pooled targeted enrichment of DNA, from 500 Polish large-vessel IS patients (100 individuals per pool × 5 pools) and 500 age-, gender-matched control patients (without any type of stroke history) (100 individuals per pool × 5 pools), was performed using a custom-made kit (SureSelect from Agilent Santa Clara, CA, USA) in accordance with the manufacturer's instructions. The customized library was created by the SureDesign platform from Agilent Technologies, with average coverage of 99.6% of the selected exons. A detailed description of sequencing and data analysis is given in the Materials and Methods Supplementary Materials.

Table 3. List of sequenced genes involved with the platelet membrane functions.

Gene	Protein Product	Chr Location
P2RY2	purinergic receptor P2Y, G-protein coupled, 2	11q13.5-q14.1
P2RY12	purinergic receptor P2Y, G-protein coupled, 12	3q25.1
P2RY1	Purinergic receptor P2Y, G-protein coupled, 1	3q25.2
ITGB3	integrin, beta 3 (platelet glycoprotein IIIa, antigen CD61)	17q21.32
ITGA2B	integrin, alpha 2b (platelet glycoprotein IIb of IIb/IIIa complex, antigen CD41)	17q21.32
GP5	glycoprotein V	3q29
GP9	glycoprotein IX	3q21.3
GP6	glycoprotein VI	19q13.42
GP1Bα	glycoprotein 1bα	17p13.2
GP1BB	glycoprotein Ib (platelet), beta polypeptide, antigen CD42c	22q11.21
ITGA2 (GPIa)	integrin, alpha 2 (alpha 2 subunit of VLA-2 receptor, antigen CD49B)	5q11.2
ADRA2A	adrenoceptor alpha 2A	10q25.2
TBXA2R	thromboxane A2 receptor	19p13.3
HTR2A	5-hydroxytryptamine (serotonin) receptor 2A, G protein-coupled	13q14-q21
F2R (PAR-1)	proteinase-activated receptor 1 (PAR1), coagulation factor II (thrombin) receptor	5q13
F2RL3 (PAR-4)	protease activated receptor 4 (PAR-4), coagulation factor II (thrombin) receptor-like 3	19p12
PEAR1	platelet endothelial aggregation receptor-1	1q23.1
GNB3	guanine nucleotide binding protein (G protein), beta polypeptide 3	12p13
CD148	receptor-type protein tyrosine phosphatase	11p11.1
ITPR1	inositol 1,4,5-trisphosphate receptor, type 1	3p26.1
CD36	thrombospondin receptor, antigen CD36	7q11.2
CD40	TNF receptor superfamily member 5, antigen CD40	20q12-q13.2
EPR1	effector cell peptidase receptor 1	17q25
PECAM-1	platelet/endothelial cell adhesion molecule 1	17q23.3
FERMT3	ferritin family member 3	11q13.1
PTAFR	platelet-activating factor receptor	1p35-p34.3
PTGIR	prostaglandin I2 (prostacyclin) receptor (IP)	19q13.

4.2.1. Statistical Tests and Calculations

The initial analysis was performed by Pearson's chi-squared test to ascertain statistical significance for the difference in the total number of alleles in re-sequenced genes containing damaging, rare, non-synonymous variants between controls and patients with large-vessel ischemia. The frequency of the investigated damaging allele was presented as cMAF, which encompassed all rare damaging variants in the sequenced gene or region. Since all observed genes were selected for MAF < 0.05, gene- or region-based burden analysis with the cumulative minor-allele test (CMAT) test (10,000× permutations) was performed in all targeted regions separately, to estimate the statistical significance of the observed differences in the accumulation of non-synonymous SNVs in large-vessel stroke in the investigated cohort when compared to controls. Statistical significance threshold was adjusted to number of target regions re-sequenced in the study (Bonferroni correction).

4.2.2. Sample Size and Power Considerations

In power calculations, instead of using individual rare variants, we decided to use predicted cMAF for all deleterious rare variants in single genes or regions. In this study, we have followed a self-sufficient, closed-form, maximum-likelihood estimator for allele frequencies that account for errors associated with sequencing, and a likelihood-ratio test statistic that provides a simple means for evaluating the null hypothesis of monomorphism [31,32]. Unbiased estimates of allele frequencies $10/n$ (where n is the number of individuals sampled) appear to be achievable, and near-certain identification of a SNP requires a cMAF (which is 10 variants for all pooled samples in the given cohort cMAF ~0.01). In addition, because the power to detect significant allele-frequency differences between two populations is limited, we set both the number of sampled individuals (500 in the cohort) and depth of sequencing coverage in excess of 100. The level of significance ($p = 0.001$) was assumed for a Fisher's exact test for frequency differences in cMAF between populations.

4.3. Fluorescence-Based Functional Assay for P2RY1 and P2RY12 Receptor Activation in L Cells

Mouse fibroblast (L cells) cultures were transiently transfected by electroporation with cDNA constructs of the identified purinergic receptor genes within the pcDNA3.1 plasmid vector. GIRK channels, effectors for purinergic receptors, are not natively expressed in L cells. Thus, L cells were co-transfected with the *GIRK4* S143T cDNA construct. The heterologously expressed purinergic receptors were stimulated with the *P2Y1* and *P2Y12* selective agonist, MeSADP. Purinergic receptor stimulation in this system cause specific G proteins to activate GIRK channels, resulting in membrane hyperpolarization (details provided in the Materials and Methods Supplementary Materials).

5. Limitations

The main limitation of the study is the lack of verification of observed variants and its association with IS in the independent verification cohort. It should be, however, noted that several previous studies demonstrated that the rare variant associations, because of their private character, are often limited to very limited populations, and are very hard to reproduce, unless the verification groups are very large (in this case, several tens of thousands patients). The other limitation of the study is that only a fraction of all known relevant genes related to platelet reactivity were sequenced in this study. Since the aim of our study was to analyze the impact of rare variants within genes related to platelet reactivity on IS risk, we did not measure platelet reactivity and its association with genetic polymorphism. Also, important limitation of the study was that we matched controls based on gender and age; however, comorbid clinical factors such as DM, CAD, or heart failure were observed more often in the control group. Based on the results of the multivariate logistic regression, after correcting for these clinical factors, one can conclude that the impact of observed polymorphism is unrelated to well-known risk factors for atherothrombotic disease, which further increases the strength of the results. Finally, the iPLEX-Sequenom method used with individual genotyping has a very high level of specificity (~100%), and its sensitivity depends very much on the primer design and stringency, which is usually optimized for detection of frequent SNPs, but not so much for singletons (e.g., only one mutated allele among hundreds of wild type alleles). We did our own spot check to confirm the heterozygous calls, and they were made with high confidence. However, because neither original Sequenom's calling algorithm nor our post-processing scripts have been optimized for detection of very rare variants, we may have missed other samples with heterozygous or alternate allele homozygous genotypes.

6. Conclusions

In summary, the results of our study indicate that the distributions of investigated rare deleterious variants in the coding regions of selected platelet membrane genes (and in particular, located in the region of purinergic receptor P2RY1–P2RY12), in the cohort of Polish patients, could be associated with the large-vessel IS. The mechanisms by which these variants interact with the purinergic transmission and IS remains unclear, and will require further investigations. It is also not certain if our findings could be translated directly to other populations, as the variants driving the observed associations are rare, and appear to be limited to the Polish population. Further studies in larger, and also different populations, would be needed to clarify this question.

Supplementary Materials: Supplementary materials can be found at www.mdpi.com/1422-0067/18/12/2678/s1.

Acknowledgments: Research subject was implemented with CEPT infrastructure financed by the European Union—the European Regional Development Fund within the Operational Program "Innovative economy" for 2007–2013. The study was supported financially as part of the research grant from the Ministry of Science and Higher Education "Iuventus Plus" research grant (grant number IP2014 038473). The authors would like to thank Michal Karlinski, Agnieszka Cudna, Lukasz Milanowski, Marta Solarska, and Pawel Wylezol for preparing samples and database for further analysis.

Author Contributions: Piotr K. Janicki substantial contribution to concept and design, analysis and interpretation of data, critical writing or revising the intellectual content, and final approval of the version to be published. Ceren Eyileten analysis and interpretation of data, critical writing or revising the intellectual content, final approval of the version to be published. Victor Ruiz-Velasco substantial contribution to concept and design, analysis and interpretation of data, critical writing or revising the intellectual content, and final approval of the version to be published. Khaled Anwar Sedeek analysis and interpretation of data, final approval of the version to be published. Justyna Pordzik analysis and interpretation of data, final approval of the version to be published. Anna Czlonkowska substantial contribution to concept and design, final approval of the version to be published. Iwona Kurkowska-Jastrzebska substantial contribution to concept and design, final approval of the version to be published. Shigekazu Sugino analysis and interpretation of data, final approval of the version to be published. Yuka Imamura-Kawasawa substantial contribution to concept and design, analysis of data, final approval of the version to be published. Dagmara Mirowska-Guzel substantial contribution to concept and design, final approval of the version to be published. Marek Postula substantial contribution to concept and design, analysis and interpretation of data, critical writing or revising the intellectual content, and final approval of the version to be published.

Conflicts of Interest: The authors declare no conflict of interest.

Abbreviations

IS	Ischemic stroke
GWAS	Genome wide association studies
MAF	Minor allele frequency
SNVs	Single nucleotide variants
SNPs	Single nucleotide polymorphism
CADD	Combined Annotation Dependent Depletion
TOAST	Trial of Org 10172 in Acute Stroke Treatment
CAD	Coronary artery disease
CHF	Congestive heart failure
DM	Diabetes mellitus
cMAF	Combined MAF
CMAT	Cumulative minor-allele test
SNP	Single nucleotide polymorphism
GIRK	G protein inwardly-rectifying K$^+$
MeSAD	2-Methylthioadenosine diphosphate
TIA	Transient ischemic attack

References

1. Welter, D.; MacArthur, J.; Morales, J.; Burdett, T.; Hall, P.; Junkins, H.; Klemm, A.; Flicek, P.; Manolio, T.; Hindorff, L.; et al. The NHGRI GWAS Catalog, a curated resource of SNP-trait associations. *Nucleic Acids Res.* **2014**, *42*, D1001–D1006. [CrossRef] [PubMed]
2. Holliday, E.G.; Maguire, J.M.; Evans, T.J.; Koblar, S.A.; Jannes, J.; Sturm, J.W.; Hankey, G.J.; Baker, R.; Golledge, J.; Parsons, M.W.; et al. Common variants at 6p21.1 are associated with large artery atherosclerotic stroke. *Nat. Genet.* **2012**, *44*, 1147–1151. [CrossRef] [PubMed]
3. Bevan, S.; Traylor, M.; Adib-Samii, P.; Malik, R.; Paul, N.L.; Jackson, C.; Farrall, M.; Rothwell, P.M.; Sudlow, C.; Dichgans, M.; et al. Genetic heritability of ischemic stroke and the contribution of previously reported candidate gene and genomewide associations. *Stroke* **2012**, *43*, 3161–3167. [CrossRef] [PubMed]
4. Gibson, G. Rare and common variants: Twenty arguments. *Nat. Rev. Genet.* **2011**, *13*, 135–145. [CrossRef] [PubMed]
5. Francioli, L.C.; Menelaou, A.; Pulit, S.L.; van Dijk, F.; Palamara, P.F.; Elbers, C.C.; Neerincx, P.B.; Ye, K.; Guryev, V.; Kloosterman, W.P.; et al. Whole-genome sequence variation, population structure and demographic history of the Dutch population. *Nat. Genet.* **2014**, *46*, 818–825. [CrossRef] [PubMed]
6. Cheng, Y.C.; Cole, J.W.; Kittner, S.J.; Mitchell, B.D. Genetics of ischemic stroke in young adults. *Circ. Cardiovasc. Genet.* **2014**, *7*, 383–392. [CrossRef] [PubMed]
7. Auer, P.L.; Nalls, M.; Meschia, J.F.; Worrall, B.B.; Longstreth, W.T., Jr.; Seshadri, S.; Kooperberg, C.; Burger, K.M.; Carlson, C.S.; Carty, C.L.; et al. Rare and Coding Region Genetic Variants Associated With Risk of Ischemic Stroke: The NHLBI Exome Sequence Project. *JAMA Neurol.* **2015**, *72*, 781–788. [CrossRef] [PubMed]
8. Anyanwu, C.; Hahn, M.; Nath, M.; Li, J.; Barone, F.C.; Rosenbaum, D.M.; Zhou, J. Platelets Pleiotropic Roles in Ischemic Stroke. *Austin J. Cerebrovasc. Dis. Stroke* **2016**, *3*, 1048.
9. Postula, M.; Janicki, P.K.; Milanowski, L.; Pordzik, J.; Eyileten, C.; Karlinski, M.; Wylezol, P.; Solarska, M.; Czlonkowka, A.; Kurkowska-Jastrzebka, I.; et al. Association of frequent genetic variants in platelet activation pathway genes with large-vessel ischemic stroke in Polish population. *Platelets* **2017**, *28*, 66–73. [CrossRef] [PubMed]
10. Milanowski, L.; Pordzik, J.; Janicki, P.K.; Postula, M. Common genetic variants in platelet surface receptors and its association with ischemic stroke. *Pharmacogenomics* **2016**, *17*, 953–971. [CrossRef] [PubMed]
11. Kircher, M.; Witten, D.M.; Jain, P.; O'Roak, B.J.; Cooper, G.M.; Shendure, J. A general framework for estimating the relative pathogenicity of human genetic variants. *Nat. Genet.* **2014**, *46*, 310–315. [CrossRef] [PubMed]
12. Visschedijk, M.C.; Alberts, R.; Mucha, S.; Deelen, P.; de Jong, D.J.; Pierik, M.; Spekhorst, L.M.; Imhann, F.; van der Meulen-de, A.E.; van der Woude, C.J.; et al. Pooled Resequencing of 122 Ulcerative Colitis Genes in a Large Dutch Cohort Suggests Population-Specific Associations of Rare Variants in *MUC2*. *PLoS ONE* **2016**, *11*, e0159609. [CrossRef] [PubMed]
13. Liu, J.Z.; van Sommeren, S.; Huang, H.; Ng, S.C.; Alberts, R.; Takahashi, A.; Ripke, S.; Lee, J.C.; Jostins, L.; Shah, T.; et al. Association analyses identify 38 susceptibility loci for inflammatory bowel disease and highlight shared genetic risk across populations. *Nat. Genet.* **2015**, *47*, 979–986. [CrossRef] [PubMed]
14. Hong, K.W.; Shin, M.S.; Ahn, Y.B.; Lee, H.J.; Kim, H.D. Genomewide association study on chronic periodontitis in Korean population: Results from the Yangpyeong health cohort. *J. Clin. Periodontol.* **2015**, *42*, 703–710. [CrossRef] [PubMed]
15. Prescott, N.J.; Lehne, B.; Stone, K.; Lee, J.C.; Taylor, K.; Knight, J.; Papouli, E.; Mirza, M.M.; Simpson, M.A.; Spain, S.L.; et al. Pooled Sequencing of 531 Genes in Inflammatory Bowel Disease Identifies an Associated Rare Variant in *BTNL2* and Implicates Other Immune Related Genes. *PLoS Genet.* **2015**, *11*, e1004955. [CrossRef] [PubMed]
16. Ziegler, S.; Schillinger, M.; Funk, M.; Felber, K.; Exner, M.; Mlekusch, W.; Sabeti, S.; Amighi, J.; Minar, E.; Brunner, M.; et al. Association of a functional polymorphism in the clopidogrel target receptor gene, *P2Y12*, and the risk for ischemic cerebrovascular events in patients with peripheral artery disease. *Stroke* **2005**, *36*, 1394–1399. [CrossRef] [PubMed]

17. Zee, R.Y.; Michaud, S.E.; Diehl, K.A.; Chasman, D.I.; Emmerich, J.; Gaussem, P.; Aiach, M.; Ridker, P.M. Purinergic receptor P2Y, G-protein coupled, 12 gene variants and risk of incident ischemic stroke, myocardial infarction, and venous thromboembolism. *Atherosclerosis* **2008**, *197*, 694–699. [CrossRef] [PubMed]
18. Wang, Z.; Nakayama, T.; Sato, N.; Yamaguchi, M.; Izumi, Y.; Kasamaki, Y.; Ohta, M.; Soma, M.; Aoi, N.; Ozawa, Y.; et al. Purinergic receptor P2Y, G-protein coupled, 2 (*P2RY2*) gene is associated with cerebral infarction in Japanese subjects. *Hypertens. Res.* **2009**, *32*, 989–996. [CrossRef] [PubMed]
19. Yi, X.; Zhou, Q.; Wang, C.; Lin, J.; Liu, P.; Fu, C. Platelet receptor Gene (*P2Y12, P2Y1*) and platelet glycoprotein Gene (*GPIIIa*) polymorphisms are associated with antiplatelet drug responsiveness and clinical outcomes after acute minor ischemic stroke. *Eur. J. Clin. Pharmacol.* **2017**, *73*, 437–443. [CrossRef] [PubMed]
20. You, J.; Johnson, T.D.; Marrelli, S.P.; Mombouli, J.V.; Bryan, R.M., Jr. P2u receptor-mediated release of endothelium-derived relaxing factor/nitric oxide and endothelium-derived hyperpolarizing factor from cerebrovascular endothelium in rats. *Stroke* **1999**, *30*, 1125–1133. [CrossRef] [PubMed]
21. Marrelli, S.P. Altered endothelial Ca^{2+} regulation after ischemia/reperfusion produces potentiated endothelium-derived hyperpolarizing factor-mediated dilations. *Stroke* **2002**, *33*, 2285–2291. [CrossRef] [PubMed]
22. Ignatovica, V.; Latkovskis, G.; Peculis, R.; Megnis, K.; Schioth, H.B.; Vaivade, I.; Fridmanis, D.; Pirags, V.; Erglis, A.; Klovins, J. Single nucleotide polymorphisms of the purinergic 1 receptor are not associated with myocardial infarction in a Latvian population. *Mol. Biol. Rep.* **2012**, *39*, 1917–1925. [CrossRef] [PubMed]
23. Abbracchio, M.P.; Burnstock, G.; Boeynaems, J.-M.; Barnard, E.A.; Boyer, J.L.; Kennedy, C.; Knight, G.E.; Fumagalli, M.; Gachet, C.; Jacobson, K.A.; et al. International Union of Pharmacology LVIII: Update on the P2Y G Protein-Coupled Nucleotide Receptors: From Molecular Mechanisms and Pathophysiology to Therapy. *Pharmacol. Rev.* **2006**, *58*, 281–341. [CrossRef] [PubMed]
24. Cui, G.; Zhang, S.; Zou, J.; Chen, Y.; Chen, H. *P2Y12* receptor gene polymorphism and the risk of resistance to clopidogrel: A meta-analysis and review of the literature. *Adv. Clin. Exp. Med.* **2017**, *26*, 343–349. [PubMed]
25. Liu, R.; Zhou, Z.; Chen, Y.; Li, J.L.; Jin, J.; Huang, M.; Zhao, M.; Yu, W.B.; Chen, X.M.; Cai, Y.F.; et al. Associations of *CYP3A4*, *NR1I2*, *CYP2C19* and *P2RY12* polymorphisms with clopidogrel resistance in Chinese patients with ischemic stroke. *Acta Pharmacol. Sin.* **2016**, *37*, 882–888. [CrossRef] [PubMed]
26. Yi, X.; Lin, J.; Wang, Y.; Zhou, J.; Zhou, Q. Interaction among *CYP2C8*, *GPIIIa* and *P2Y12* variants increase susceptibility to ischemic stroke in Chinese population. *Oncotarget* **2017**, *8*, 70811–70820. [CrossRef] [PubMed]
27. Wang, Z.; Nakayama, T.; Sato, N.; Izumi, Y.; Kasamaki, Y.; Ohta, M.; Soma, M.; Aoi, N.; Ozawa, Y.; Ma, Y. The purinergic receptor P2Y, G-protein coupled, 2 (*P2RY2*) gene associated with essential hypertension in Japanese men. *J. Hum. Hypertens.* **2010**, *24*, 327–335. [CrossRef] [PubMed]
28. WHO Task Force on Stroke and Other Cerebrovascular Diseases. Recommendations on stroke prevention, diagnosis, and therapy. Report of the WHO task force on stroke and other cerebrovascular disorders. *Stroke* **1989**, *20*, 1407–1431.
29. Foulkes, M.; Wolf, P.; Price, T.; Mohr, J.; Hier, D. The Stroke Data Bank: Design, methods, and baseline characteristics. *Stroke* **1988**, *19*, 547–554. [CrossRef] [PubMed]
30. Grabska, K.; Gromadzka, G.; Członkowska, A. Infections and ischemic stroke outcome. *Neurol. Res. Int.* **2011**, *2011*, 691348. [CrossRef] [PubMed]
31. Lee, S.; Abecasis, G.R.; Boehnke, M.; Lin, X. Rare-variant association analysis: Study designs and statistical tests. *Am. J. Hum. Genet.* **2014**, *95*, 5–23. [CrossRef] [PubMed]
32. Lynch, M.; Bost, D.; Wilson, S.; Maruki, T.; Harrison, S. Population-genetic inference from pooled-sequencing data. *Genome Biol. Evol.* **2014**, *6*, 1210–1218. [CrossRef] [PubMed]

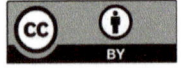

© 2017 by the authors. Licensee MDPI, Basel, Switzerland. This article is an open access article distributed under the terms and conditions of the Creative Commons Attribution (CC BY) license (http://creativecommons.org/licenses/by/4.0/).

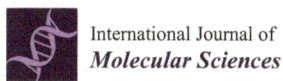

Article

Neuroprotective Effects of Platonin, a Therapeutic Immunomodulating Medicine, on Traumatic Brain Injury in Mice after Controlled Cortical Impact

Ting-Lin Yen [1,2], Chao-Chien Chang [2,3], Chi-Li Chung [4,5], Wen-Chin Ko [3], Chih-Hao Yang [2] and Cheng-Ying Hsieh [2,*]

1. Department of Medical Research, Cathay General Hospital, Taipei 22174, Taiwan; d119096015@tmu.edu.tw
2. Department of Pharmacology, College of Medicine, Taipei Medical University, Taipei 11031, Taiwan; change@seed.net.tw (C.-C.C.); chyang@tmu.edu.tw (C.-H.Y.)
3. Department of Cardiology, Cathay General Hospital, Taipei 10630, Taiwan; wckcgh@ms17.hinet.net
4. Division of Pulmonary Medicine, Department of Internal Medicine, Taipei Medical University Hospital, Taipei 11031, Taiwan.; clchung@tmu.edu.tw
5. School of Respiratory Therapy, Division of Thoracic medicine, Department of Internal Medicine, School of Medicine, College of Medicine, Taipei Medical University, Taipei 11031, Taiwan
* Correspondence: hsiehcy@tmu.edu.tw; Tel.: +886-2-2736-1661 (ext. 3194)

Received: 31 January 2018; Accepted: 3 April 2018; Published: 6 April 2018

Abstract: Traumatic brain injury (TBI) is one of the leading causes of mortality worldwide and leads to persistent cognitive, sensory, motor dysfunction, and emotional disorders. TBI-caused primary injury results in structural damage to brain tissues. Following the primary injury, secondary injuries which are accompanied by neuroinflammation, microglial activation, and additional cell death subsequently occur. Platonin, a cyanine photosensitizing dye, has been used to treat trauma, ulcers, and some types of acute inflammation. In the present study, the neuroprotective effects of platonin against TBI were explored in a controlled cortical impact (CCI) injury model in mice. Treatment with platonin (200 µg/kg) significantly reduced the neurological severity score, general locomotor activity, and anxiety-related behavior, and improved the rotarod performance of CCI-injured mice. In addition, platonin reduced lesion volumes, the expression of cleaved caspase-3, and microglial activation in TBI-insulted brains. Platonin also suppressed messenger (m)RNA levels of caspase-3, caspase-1, cyclooxygenase-2, tumor necrosis factor-α, interleukin-6, and interleukin-1β. On the other hand, free radical production after TBI was obviously attenuated in platonin-treated mice. Treatment with platonin exhibited prominent neuroprotective properties against TBI in a CCI mouse model through its anti-inflammatory, anti-apoptotic, and anti-free radical capabilities. This evidence collectively indicates that platonin may be a potential therapeutic medicine for use with TBIs.

Keywords: traumatic brain injury; platonin; neuroinflammation; microglial activation; free radical

1. Introduction

Traumatic brain injury (TBI) is defined as damage to the brain resulting from an external mechanical force, such as that caused by rapid acceleration or deceleration, blast waves, crushing, impacts, or penetration by a projectile [1]. Over the past decade, TBI has been one of the main causes of mortality and one of the most serious public health problems worldwide. TBI not only causes a burden to medical resources but also contributes to approximately one-third of all injury-related deaths [2,3]. Persistent dysfunctions after TBI include cognitive, sensory, motor dysfunction, and emotional function disorders. Patients who suffer from TBI may confront excruciating pain for a few days to their entire lifetime. Consequently, these issues affect individuals and have lasting effects on their families and communities [2,4]. Brain damage caused by TBI is usually subdivided into primary and secondary injuries. The primary injury results in structural damage to the brain that occurs after exposure to an external force and includes contusions, subsequent damage to blood vessels (hemorrhaging, edema, and hypoxia), and diffuse axonal injury. Following the primary injury, secondary brain injuries occur through a complex cascade of biochemical and cellular changes that are accompanied by neuroinflammation, reactive oxygen species (ROS) generation, and additional cell death for a few minutes to many months [5,6].

Microglia are resident immune cells of the central nervous system and play a critical role in neuroinflammation. After TBI, microglia become highly activated and deliver cytokines and chemokines, which leads to apoptosis, neuroinflammation, and neurodegeneration due to neuron trauma [7,8]. Apoptosis of neurons and glia results in the pathology of TBI in both humans and animals [9]. The participation of caspase-3 in the neuronal apoptotic process after TBI has been previously examined [10,11]. Caspase-3 activation leads to cleavage of cytoskeletal proteins and proteolysis of DNA repair proteins, ultimately causing apoptosis and cell loss. Therefore, the abrogation of caspase-3 activation in brain tissues after TBI may help diminish the death of brain cells and maintain better neurological outcomes [12]. Previous studies have revealed that, in the postmortem human brain, messenger (m)RNA levels of proinflammatory cytokines, such as interleukin (IL)-6, IL-8, tumor necrosis (TNF)-α, and IL-1β, significantly increase in the brain following TBI insult [13]. Reductions in IL-1β, IL-6, monocyte chemoattractant protein (MCP)-1, and macrophage inflammatory protein (MIP)-2 in the injured brain revealed the neuroprotective effect in a controlled cortical impact (CCI) animal study [14]. In addition, experimental and clinical studies have provided additional evidence that neuroinflammation in TBIs involves the upregulation of ROS, cyclooxygenase (COX) enzyme, prostaglandin E2 (PGE_2), and caspase-1, which contribute to cellular damage and subsequent apoptosis [15–17]. ROS scavengers and COX-2 inhibitors were suggested for use in treating neurological disorders such as stroke and TBIs [15,18], which indicated that ROS and COX-2 might be important targets of TBI therapy.

Platonin, a photosensitive trithiazolepentamethine cyanine dye, has been reported to have antioxidant, antimicrobial, and immunomodulatory activities [19–21] and is used for treating immune diseases [21]. Previous studies have indicated that platonin can moderate circulatory failure and downregulate mortality in septic rats [22] and attenuate sepsis-caused loss of an intact blood–brain barrier (BBB) [23]. Notably, the neuroprotective effect of platonin was demonstrated in a mouse model of ischemic stroke. Furthermore, the neuroprotective ability of platonin in ischemic brain injury may be attributed to its anti-inflammatory, antithrombotic, and free radical-scavenging effects [24].

On the basis of the anti-inflammatory and neuroprotective properties of platonin, which are intimately related to brain injuries, we hypothesized that platonin might be a potential therapeutic agent against TBIs. Moreover, in consideration of the critical role of the formation of excessive free radicals in the pathology of TBI, the in vivo scavenging activity of platonin against ROS was determined in the present study.

2. Results

2.1. Platonin Improves Neurobehavioral Functions in Mice Subjected to TBI

TBI has been known to lead to several long-term harmful symptoms including cognitive, sensory, motor dysfunction, and emotional disorders [2,4]. In order to determine the neuroprotective potential of platonin against TBI, a CCI animal model, a widely used animal model in TBI studies [25], was utilized to mimic pathological phenomena of TBI in this study.

Neurological deficits were examined and scored on an 18-point scale before and 1, 2, 7, 14, 21, 28, and 120 days after the TBI. The varieties of neurological severity scoring of different groups are illustrated in Figure 1B. After the TBI, neurological severity scoring obviously increased compared to those before the TBI; nevertheless, treatment with platonin (200 µg/kg) significantly ameliorated these increased scores (### $p < 0.001$; $n = 6$, compared to the sham group; ** $p < 0.01$ and *** $p < 0.001$; $n = 6$, compared to the phosphate-buffered saline (PBS) group). Rotarod tests and grip strength tests are widely used to evaluate sensorimotor functions in experimental models of TBI [26,27]. Figure 1C shows that the TBI resulted in a significant impairment in the rotarod test, and the decrease in the rotarod duration was reversed in the platonin-treated (200 μg/kg) group. ($^{###}$ $p < 0.001$; $n = 6$, compared to the sham group; * $p < 0.05$, ** $p < 0.01$ and *** $p < 0.001$; $n = 6$, compared to the PBS group). In addition, mice that had received the CCI exhibited decreased grip strength compared to control mice (Figure 1D). Although it did not reach statistical significance, there was a trend showing that treatment with platonin (200 μg/kg) may ameliorate the impairment of grip force.

On the other hand, an open field test [28] was used to measure the general locomotor activity (LMA) and anxiety-like behavior in the present study. TBI significantly induced LMA in the vehicle-treated group at 24 h ($^{#}$ $p < 0.05$; $n = 10$, compared to the pre-operated group); treatment with 200 μg/kg platonin extensively reversed the hyperactivity of LMA that occurred at 24 h after the TBI (* $p < 0.05$; $n = 10$, compared to the PBS group; Figure 1E,F). In addition, the time spent in the central zone of the open field decreased in mice with TBI. However, platonin-treated animals showed more extended times in the central zone than did vehicle-treated animals at 48 h after the TBI ($^{###}$ $p < 0.001$; $n = 10$, compared to the 0 h group; ** $p < 0.01$; $n = 10$, compared to the PBS group; Figure 1G).

The body weight and mortality of mice used in this study were recorded during the 0–120 day period. Neither the vehicle (PBS) nor the platonin-treated (200 μg/kg, one-dose treatment on the first day) groups revealed a significant difference in body weight (Figure 1H) or mortality during the experimental period.

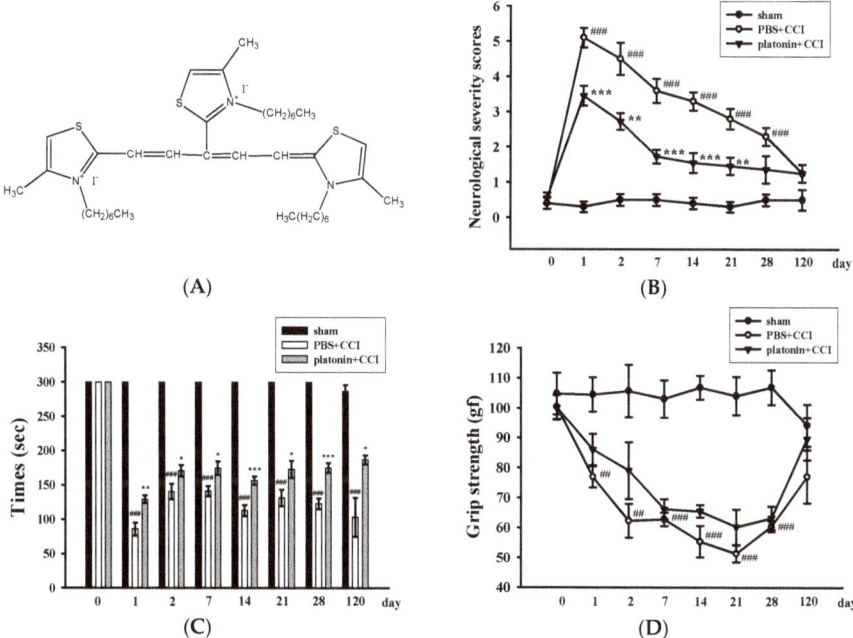

Figure 1. Cont.

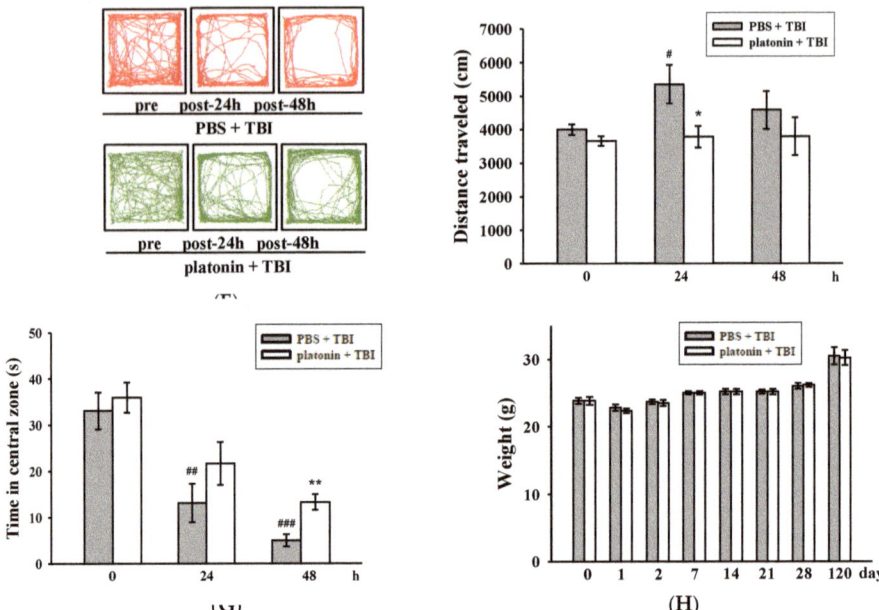

Figure 1. Alleviation of neurobehavioral deficits after platonin treatment in a mouse traumatic brain injury (TBI) model. Mice were treated with an isovolumetric solvent control (phosphate-buffered saline (PBS), intraperitoneally (ip)) or platonin (200 µg/kg, ip) for 30 min and then subjected to TBI. (**A**) The chemical structure of platonin. Assays of neurobehavioral functions including neurological severity scoring (**B**), a rotarod test (**C**), and a grip strength test (**D**) were performed before and 1, 2, 7, 14, 21, 28, and 120 days after TBI. All data are presented as the mean ± SEM ($n = 6$). ## $p < 0.01$, ### $p < 0.001$, compared to the sham group; * $p < 0.05$, ** $p < 0.01$ and *** $p < 0.001$, compared to the PBS group. Locomotor activity (**E**,**F**) and anxiety-like behavior (**G**) were evaluated before and 24 and 48 h after TBI. All data are presented as the mean ± SEM ($n = 10$). # $p < 0.05$, ## $p < 0.01$ and ### $p < 0.001$, compared to the presurgery group; * $p < 0.05$ and ** $p < 0.01$, compared to the PBS group. (**H**) Body weight of mice only treated with the isovolumetric solvent control (PBS, ip) or platonin (200 µg/kg, ip) after TBI, recorded for 0–120 days.

2.2. Platonin Attenuates Lesion Volumes and Caspase-3 Activation in Mice Subjected to TBI

The histological assessment of lesion volume of brain tissues was conducted 28 days after the TBI. No groups exhibited pathological changes in the contralateral brain site, whereas apparent potholes were revealed in the ipsilateral site (Figure 2A). As shown in Figure 2B, serial brain sections after the TBI showed severe contusion injuries, with substantial tissue loss in the cortex and damage to the hippocampal region. Treatment with platonin (200 µg/kg) resulted in a significant reduction (Figure 2A–C) in the cortical lesion volume; platonin-treated mice (17.88 ± 0.57 mm^3) revealed an approximate 14% reduction in brain damage compared to vehicle-treated mice (21.21 ± 0.85 mm^3). In the microscopic analysis (Figure 2D,E), cleaved caspase-3 expression had obviously increased at 24 h in mice exposed to the TBI, and treatment with platonin (200 µg/kg) potently attenuated the expression of cleaved caspase-3. Furthermore, the induction of caspase-3 mRNA expressions in TBI mice was significantly attenuated by treatment with platonin (Figure 2F) (### $p < 0.001$; $n = 6$, compared to the sham group; * $p < 0.05$; $n = 6$, compared to the PBS group).

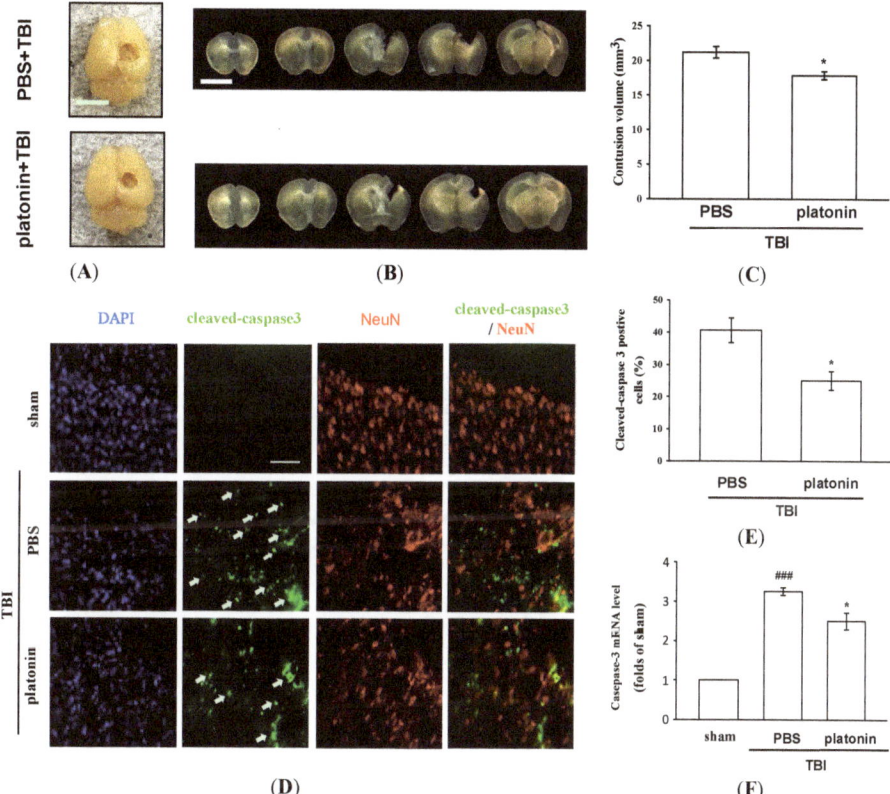

Figure 2. Mitigation of TBI-induced brain contusion volume and caspase-3 activation by platonin treatment in mice. (**A**) The photos represent the TBI impact location and exterior of brains of vehicle-(phosphate-buffered saline (PBS), ip) and platonin-treated (200 µg/kg, ip) mice on the 28th day after the TBI. The white bar indicates 5 mm. (**B**) Coronal brain sections (1 mm thick) showing the lesion volume, and quantitative analytical results are illustrated (**C**). The white bar indicates 5 mm. Data are presented as the mean ± SEM ($n = 4$). * $p < 0.05$, compared to the PBS group. (**D**,**E**) Mice were treated with the isovolumetric solvent control (PBS, ip) or platonin (200 µg/kg, ip) for 30 min and then subjected to TBI. The expression of cleaved-caspase-3 and NeuN was determined at 24 h after the impact by fluorescence microscopy as described in "Materials and Methods." Fluorescence images are typical of those obtained in three separate experiments demonstrating caspase-3 activation (arrows) near the lesion portion in mice subjected to the TBI. Blue depicts the nucleus, green depicts cleaved caspase-3, and red depicts NeuN. The white bar indicates 75 µm. (**F**) The mRNA from contralateral brain homogenates at 24 h after TBI subjected to an RT-qPCR assay. Data are presented as the mean ± SEM ($n = 6$). ### $p < 0.001$, compared to the sham group; * $p < 0.05$, compared to the PBS group.

2.3. The Anti-Neuroinflammatory Effects of Platonin in Mice Subjected to TBI

Neuroinflammation is an important component of secondary injury after TBI and has been linked to various sequelae such as neurodegenerative diseases [29]. The hallmark of TBI-induced cerebral inflammatory responses includes microglial activation, blood–brain barrier (BBB) dysfunction, release of inflammatory cytokines, and recruitment of peripheral leukocytes into brain parenchyma [30,31]. To evaluate microglial activation in a mice model of TBI, we identified expression of the ionized calcium-binding adaptor molecule 1 (Iba1), a specific marker of microglia/macrophages, to distinguish morphological changes in microglia following the TBI. As shown in Figure 3A, resting (ramified) microglia were present in the sham-operated brain, while activated and amoeboid-form microglia had arisen in mouse brains at 24 h after being subjected to TBI. Treatment with platonin (200 µg/kg) significantly attenuated the expression of activated microglia (Figure 3B) (### $p < 0.05$; $n = 3$, compared to the sham group; * $p < 0.05$; $n = 3$, compared to the PBS group).

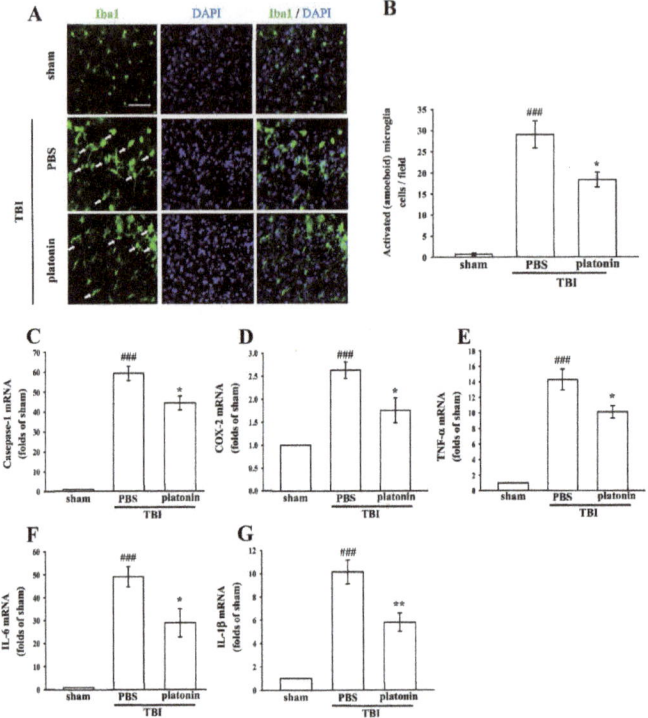

Figure 3. Treatment with platonin suppressed microglial activation and mRNA expressions of cyclooxygenase (COX)-2, caspase-1, and inflammatory cytokines in mice after a TBI. Mice were treated with the isovolumetric solvent control (phosphate-buffered saline (PBS), ip) or platonin (200 µg/kg, ip) for 30 min and then subjected to TBI. Brain slices were harvested at 24 h after surgery. (**A**) The expression of the ionized calcium-binding adaptor molecule (Iba1) was determined by a fluorescence microscopic analysis as described in "Materials and Methods." Fluorescence images are typical of those obtained in three separate experiments demonstrating expression of the Iba1 near the lesion portion of mice subjected to TBI. Blue depicts the nucleus, and green depicts the Iba1. The white bar indicates 75 µm. (**B**) The number of activated microglia (arrows) was quantified, and data are illustrated. Data are presented as the mean ± SEM ($n = 3$). ### $p < 0.001$, compared to the sham group; * $p < 0.05$, compared to the PBS group. mRNA from the contralateral brain was purified and subjected to an RT-qPCR assay to evaluate mRNA expressions of (**C**) caspase-1, (**D**) cyclooxygenase (COX)-2, (**E**) tumor necrosis factor (TNF)-α, (**F**) interleukin (IL)-6, and (**G**) IL-1β at 24 h post-TBI. Data are presented as the mean ± SEM ($n = 5$). ### $p < 0.001$, compared to the sham group; * $p < 0.05$ and ** $p < 0.01$ compared to the PBS group.

We next evaluated expressions of several critical inflammatory factors, including COX-2, caspase-1, IL-1β, IL-6, and TNF-α in the present study. As shown in Figure 3C–G, mRNA levels of COX-2, caspase-1, IL-1β, IL-6, and TNF-α were significantly upregulated in brain tissues of mice subjected to TBI (*** $p < 0.001$; $n = 5$, compared to the sham control group). Increases in TBI-stimulated inflammatory factors were substantially inhibited by treatment with platonin (200 μg/kg) ($^{\#}\,p < 0.05$, $^{\#\#}\,p < 0.01$; n = 5, compared to the PBS group) (Figure 3C–G).

2.4. Platonin Suppresses TBI-Induced Free Radical Formation in Mice through Upregulating Heme Oxygenase (HO)-1

Previous studies reported that TBI induced excessive free radical production, possibly exacerbating neuron injury by oxidizing lipids, proteins, and DNA, which contributes to further cellular damage and apoptosis [32]. In this study, the IVIS Imaging System was utilized to investigate the anti-free radical property of platonin in mice after TBI. Figure 4A reveals higher free radical production in brains of TBI-insulted mice than in those of the sham control group. The administration of platonin (200 μg/kg) markedly reduced TBI-induced free radical formation (Figure 4A). The statistical results are illustrated in Figure 4B ($^{\#\#}\,p < 0.01$; n = 6, compared to the sham group; $^{*}\,p < 0.05$, compared to the PBS group).

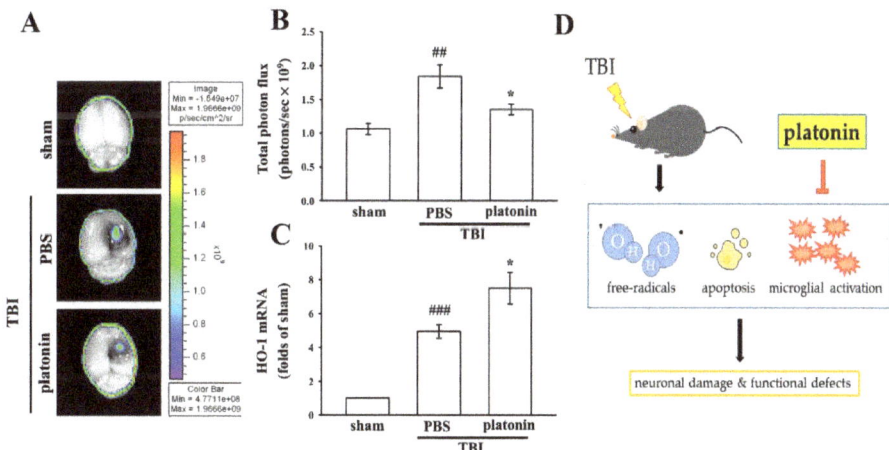

Figure 4. Reduction of free radicals and enhancement of heme oxygenase (HO)-1 expression after a TBI in mice treated with platonin. Mice were treated with the isovolumetric solvent control (phosphate-buffered saline (PBS), ip) or platonin (200 μg/kg, ip) for 30 min and then subjected to TBI. (**A,B**) The superoxide marker, dihydroethidium (DHE), was used to determine free radical production at 24 h post-TBI with the IVIS Imaging System. The color bar indicates the intensity of DHE fluorescence (total photon flux, photons/s). (**C**) mRNA from the contralateral brain was purified and subjected to an RT-qPCR assay to evaluate mRNA expression of HO-1 at 6 h post-TBI. Data are presented as the mean ± SEM (n = 5). $^{\#\#}\,p < 0.01$ and $^{\#\#\#}\,p < 0.001$, compared to the sham group; $^{*}\,p < 0.05$ compared to the PBS group. (**D**) Diagram of the neuroprotective mechanism of platonin against TBI in mice.

Heme oxygenase 1 (HO-1) is a phase II detoxifying/antioxidant enzyme and has been reported to have neuroprotective effects in brain injury. HO-1 provides protection in part through degrading its pro-oxidant substrate, heme, and releasing biliverdin and bilirubin as antioxidants [33]. Figure 4C demonstrates that HO-1 mRNA was upregulated in the vehicle-treated group at 6 h post-TBI ($^{\#}\,p < 0.05$, compared to the sham group). Treatment with platonin (200 μg/kg) further enhanced HO-1 mRNA expression compared to that of the vehicle-treated group ($^{*}\,p < 0.05$; n = 6, compared to the PBS group).

3. Discussion

Traumatic brain injury is a frequent and clinically highly heterogeneous neurological disorder with enormous economic consequences and burdens to both individuals and society.

Neuroinflammation, apoptosis, and oxidative stress are considered major causes that link brain damage and neurodegeneration after TBI. Although advances in technology and treatment over the last few decades have improved the quality of life and longevity of patients with TBI, no effective drugs or preventative treatments currently exist. The present study used mouse CCI [34], a well-established experimental TBI model, to identify the neuroprotective effect of platonin. The results demonstrated that pretreatment of platonin exerts neuroprotective effects against TBI. Although posttreatment is the proper experimental design for clinical application in TBI or other acute brain injury such as ischemic stroke, this study still indicates the neuroprotective potential of platonin. In the future, we must change the timing of drug administration and perform the experiments in different animal species and animal models. In addition, even though the clinical application of platonin pretreatment is limited in acute TBI and ischemic stroke. The pretreatment of platonin may be advantageous in the prevention of chronic TBI or secondary ischemic stroke.

Psychiatric disturbances, including anxiety disorders and depressive disorders, are reported to occur significantly more frequently among individuals with TBI compared to healthy controls, regardless of the injury severity [35,36]. It was found that anxiety disorders were the most prevalent psychiatric outcome in patients at both 3 and 12 months post-injury [37]. In addition, TBI has been reported to induce hyperactive symptoms in both humans and mice [38,39]. Children with TBI may result in attentional deficits, response inhibition, and hyperactivity [40]. Due to the high incidence of TBIs and the common diagnosis of anxiety and hyperactivity following TBI, physical and pharmaceutical interventions should be identified to improve the psychosocial functioning and life quality of patients. We demonstrated that platonin significantly ameliorated general locomotor activity and anxiety-like behavior using an open field test. Figure 2E,F showed that the manifestation of hyperactivated locomotion after TBI had significantly decreased in platonin-treated mice. Anxiety-like behavior (Figure 2G) also improved in platonin-treated animals. These results suggest that platonin may have the effect of reducing anxiety disorders after TBI. However, based on the complexity of emotional diseases, more animal models should be used to confirm the impacts of platonin on anxiety. In this study, platonin was also found to inhibit expressions of proinflammatory cytokines after the TBI (Figure 3C–G). According to a previous study, neuroinflammation may be involved in the development and maintenance of anxiety-like behaviors after TBI [41]. The anti-neuroinflammatory effect may be an underlying mechanism in platonin's improvement of TBI symptoms.

TBI-induced cell death is a major cause of neurological deficits and mortality. According to previous studies, cell apoptosis, microglial activation, and neuroinflammation are mediators of neuronal cell death and tissue loss after TBI [7,11,15,17]. After an acute TBI, apoptosis occurs in areas that are not severely affected by the injury; a biochemical cascade activates caspase-3 to destroy molecules that are required for cell survival and others that mediate a program of cell suicide [42]. Cell fragments and enzymatically cleaved chromosomes recruit activated microglia to the injured area for clearance of dying cells by phagocytosis [43]. Moreover, activated microglia secrete multiple neurotoxic factors including cytokines, chemokines, and ROS to drive progressive neuron damage [44]. In the present study, platonin showed an antiapoptotic property by reducing caspase-3 activation and caspase-3 mRNA expression after the TBI (Figure 2D–F). Microglial activation was also alleviated by treatment with platonin (Figure 3A). Moreover, mRNA expressions of IL-1β, IL-6, TNF-α, caspase-1, and COX-2 (Figure 3B–F) were also attenuated by platonin in mice subjected to TBI. As a result, treatment with platonin decreased the brain lesion volume (Figure 2A–C), and these results suggest that platonin may achieve neuroprotective effects by inhibiting neuron cell mortality and neuroinflammation after TBI.

In the past decade, major advances found that ROS are generated and harm the brain after TBI insult [16]. Platonin was shown to significantly attenuate increased ROS levels in collagen-induced platelets and the Fenton reaction system [24]. A previous study also indicated that endotoxemia was ameliorated by platonin through decreasing NO and free radical formation in a rat model [45]. In the present study, we further investigated the role of platonin in the endogenous antioxidant system. HO-1 is one of the phase II enzymes and was reported to have the most antioxidant response elements on its promoter, making it a highly effective therapeutic target for protecting against neurodegenerative diseases [46]. Figure 4A,B show that platonin downregulated free radical production at the injury lesion. In addition, a boost in HO-1 mRNA expression was observed in the platonin-treated group (Figure 4C). These findings are consistent with our previous study in which HO-1 played a vital role in neuroprotection against brain injury by inhibiting ROS production [33]. The neuroprotective effects of platonin after TBI might not only occur by scavenging ROS but also be due to moderation of the endogenous antioxidant system.

In conclusion, this study showed for the first time that platonin has therapeutic potential against brain injury after TBI. We evaluated the neuroprotective effects of platonin through a CCI animal model, and demonstrated that platonin treatment significantly improved neurobehavioral function and reduced the lesion volume after TBI. The antiapoptotic, anti-inflammatory, and free radical-inhibitory effects of platonin may contribute to its neuroprotective potential in TBI-insulted brains (Figure 4D). These results indicate that platonin may be a promising therapeutic drug for treating TBI.

4. Materials and Methods

4.1. Materials

Platonin was synthesized by and obtained from Gwo Chyang Pharmaceuticals (Tainan, Taiwan; Figure 1A). Primary antibody against cleaved-caspase-3 was purchased from Abcam (Cambridge, UK). The anti-Iba1 antibody was purchased from Wako Chemicals USA (Richmond, VA, USA). The anti-NeuN antibody was from Merck Millipore (Darmstadt, Germany). For immunostaining, CF488A donkey anti-mouse IgG and CF488A donkey anti-rabbit IgG were purchased from Biotium (Fremont, CA, USA). Dihydroethidium (DHE) was purchased from Cayman Chemical (Ann Arbor, MI, USA). Platonin was dissolved in phosphate-buffered saline (PBS) and stored at 4 °C.

4.2. Animals

Ten-week-old male C57BL/6 mice were purchased from BioLASCO (Taipei, Taiwan). All animal experiments and care procedures were approved by the Institutional Animal Care and Use Committee of Taipei Medical University. Before undergoing the experimental procedures, all animals were clinically normal and free from apparent infection, inflammation, or neurological deficits.

4.3. Controlled Cortical Impact (CCI) Injury

TBI was induced using a CCI device, and the injury procedure was performed as described previously [25]. Briefly, a mouse was anesthetized with isoflurane (induced at 4% and maintained at 3%) evaporated in a mixture containing 75% air and 25% oxygen, and then positioned in a stereotaxic frame with a heating pad to maintain its body temperature. After the mouse head was mounted, the scalp and fascia were retracted and a 3.5 mm circular craniotomy was performed on the right cerebral hemisphere (2.0 mm posterior to the bregma and 2.0 mm lateral to the sagittal suture) to expose the intact dura. For moderate-TBI induction, a 3-mm-flat impactor tip was used to impact the exposed dura (impact parameters: a velocity of 5.25 m/s, a depth of 2 mm, and a dwell time of 100 ms). After the CCI injury was performed, the scalp incision was sutured, and the mouse was placed on a heating pad until it had recovered from anesthesia. Mice were divided into three groups: (1) a sham-operated group; (2) a group treated with an isovolumetric solvent (PBS; intraperitoneally (ip)), followed by CCI; and (3) a group treated with platonin (200 µg/kg ip), followed by CCI. All treatments were administered 30 min before the CCI in all the groups except the sham-operated group, which received no injury.

4.4. Neurological Severity Examination

A neurological examination was performed on each mouse immediately before and at 1, 2, 7, 14, 21, and 28 days after the TBI. Neurological severity scores (NSSs) were derived using an 18-point sliding scale (normal score, 0; maximal deficit score, 18) [24]. The NSS examination includes motor tests (flexion of forelimb and hindlimb, head movements, and walking ability), reflex tests (pinna, corneal, and startle reflexes, and epileptic seizures), sensory tests (placing and proprioceptive tests), and balance tests (beam balance tests). In an NSS test, 1 point represents an inability to perform the test or the lack of a tested reflex (Table 1). Therefore, a higher score indicates a more severe injury.

Table 1. Neurological severity scores (NSSs).

Tests	Points
Motor tests	6
Raising mice by the tail (normal = 0; maximum = 3)	3
Flexion of forelimb	1
Flexion of hindlimb	1
Head moved >10° to vertical axis within 30 s	1
Placing mice on the floor (normal = 0; maximum = 3)	3
Normal walk	0
Inability to walk straight	1
Circling toward the paretic side	2
Fall down to the paretic side	3
Sensory tests	2
Placing test (visual and tactile test)	1
Proprioceptive test (deep sensation, pushing the paw against the table edge to stimulate limb muscles)	2
Beam balance tests (normal = 0; maximum = 6)	6
Balances with steady posture	0
Grasps side of beam	1
Hugs the beam and one limb falls down from the beam	2
Hugs the beam and two limbs fall down from the beam, or spins on beam (>60 s)	3
Attempts to balance on the beam but falls off (>40 s)	4
Attempts to balance on the beam but falls off (>20 s)	5
Falls off: No attempt to balance or hang on to the beam (<20 s)	6
Reflexes absent and abnormal movements	4
Pinna reflex (head shake when touching the auditory meatus)	1
Corneal reflex (blink when lightly touching the cornea with cotton)	1
Startle reflex (motor response to a brief noise from snapping a clipboard paper	1
Seizures, myoclonus, myodystony	1
Maximum points	18

4.5. Spontaneous Locomotor Activity and Rotarod Assessments

Before neurobehavioral testing, the mice were trained daily for 3 days. They were then trained to stay on an accelerating rotarod (4~40 rpm over 5 min, with increasing increments of 4 rpm at 30 s intervals) for three trials daily before being subjected to TBI surgery. Before and 24 and 48 h after the TBI, each mouse was placed in the center of the open field apparatus (50 × 50 × 40 cm). Locomotor activity (LMA) was automatically recorded with an activity monitor (Noldus Information Technology, Wageningen, the Netherlands) in the test period to count the total distance traveled, time spent in the center (25 × 25 cm), and the number of beam-break counts. After the LMA assessment, the rotarod performance was assessed to test the balance and coordination (UGO Basile, Varese, Italy). The rotarod was rotated from 4 to 40 rpm within 3 min. The time (in seconds) at which each mouse fell from the drum was determined for up to 300 s with a stopwatch and recorded.

4.6. Grip Strength Assessment

Neuromuscular strength was tested with grip strength tests. A grip strength meter (UGO Basile, Varese, Italy) was used to assess the forelimb grip strength. A mouse was lifted and held by its tail so that its forepaws could grasp a wire grid. The mouse was then gently pulled backward by its tail with its body parallel to the surface of the table until it released the grid. The peak force applied by the forelimbs of the mouse was recorded in gram-force (gf). Each mouse was tested three times, and the mean of the measured value was used for the statistical analysis.

4.7. Measurement of Brain Lesion Volume

At 28 days after TBI, the mice were anesthetized and perfused with 4% paraformaldehyde in phosphate buffer (PB), and the brains were then transferred into 4% paraformaldehyde overnight and immersed by 30% sucrose for 24 h. Each brain was sliced into five 1-mm-thick slices and analyzed by utilizing the ImageJ 1.50i software (National Institutes of Health, Bethesda, MD, USA). The volume measurement was calculated by summation of the lesion areas: [(area of the intact contralateral left hemisphere) − (area of the intact ipsilateral right hemisphere)] × slice thickness (1 mm).

4.8. Immunofluorescent Staining of Brain Tissues

Animals of each group were euthanized and perfused with 4% paraformaldehyde in PB. Brains were post-fixed with 4% paraformaldehyde in PB overnight. Before sectioning, the brains were immersed in 30% sucrose in PB for cryoprotection. The brains were sliced in the coronal plane at 50 μm and permeabilized with PB containing 0.2% Triton X-100 and 6% donkey serum for 60 min. These slices were incubated overnight at 4 °C with primary antibodies including anti-caspase-3, anti-NeuN, and anti-Iba-1 antibodies. Subsequently, samples were washed three times with 0.2% Tween 20 in PB and then exposed to secondary antibodies overnight. The prepared slices were then counterstained with DAPI (30 mM) and mounted with mounting buffer (Vector Laboratories, Burlingame, CA, USA) on a glass coverslip. Samples were detected under an Evos FL Auto 2 imaging system using the LED fluorescence light cubes (Thermo Fisher Scientific, Waltham, MA, USA).

4.9. Real-Time Reverse-Transcription Quantitative Polymerase Chain Reaction (RT-qPCR)

Approximately 10 mg of fresh brain tissue was immediately collected from the ipsilateral (injured) hemisphere of a euthanized mouse and processed for a real-time RT-qPCR. Total RNA was isolated using the NucleoSpin RNA isolation kit (Macherey-Nagel, Düren, Germany). The purity and quality of RNA were confirmed by defining the ratio of absorbance levels at wavelengths of 260 and 280 nm (NanoDrop ND-1000, Thermo Fisher Scientific). A sample of 1 μg of total RNA was treated with the high-capacity cDNA reverse transcription kit (Thermo Fisher Scientific) and reverse-transcribed into complementary (c)DNA. For mRNA measurements, diluted cDNA was amplified using a QuantiNova SYBR Green PCR Kit (Qiagen, Hilden, Germany) in a Rotor-Gene Q 2plex HRM Platform (Qiagen). Reaction conditions were carried out for 35~40 cycles (5 min at 95 °C, 5 s at 95 °C, and 10 s at 60 °C). Quantified values of RNA were normalized with those of glyceraldehyde 3- phosphate dehydrogenase (GAPDH). The primers used for the RT-qPCR assay were as follows: caspase-3: 5′-GGGCCTGTTGAACTGAAAAA-3′ (forward) and 5′-CCGTCCTTTG AATTTCTCCA-3′ (reverse); caspase-1: 5′-AGGAATTCTGGAGCTTCAATCAG-3′ (forward) and 5′-TGGAAATGTGCCATCTTCTTT-3′ (reverse); COX-2: 5′-CCACTTCAAGGGAGTCTGGA-3′ (forward) and 5′-AGTCATCTGCTACGGGAGGA-3′ (reverse); TNF-α: 5′-TCTTCTGTCTACTGAA CTTCGG-3′ (forward) and 5′-AAGATGATCTGAGTGTGAGGG-3′ (reverse); IL-6: 5′-CCTCTCTGC AAGAGACTTCCATCCA-3′ (forward) and 5′-GGCCGTGGTTGTCACCAGCA-3′ (reverse); IL-1β: 5′-AACCTGCTGGTGTGTGACGTTC-3′ (forward) and 5′-CAGCACGAGGCTTTTTTGTTGT-3′ (reverse); HO-1: 5′-GCACTATGTAAAGCGTCTCC-3′ (forward) and 5′-GACTCTGGTCTTTGTGTT CC-3′ (reverse); GAPDH: 5′-AGACAGCCGCATCTTCTTGT-3′ (forward) and 5′-CTTGCCGTGGGT AGAGTCAT-3′ (reverse).

4.10. Evaluation of Free Radical Production in Brain Tissues

Dihydroethidium (DHE) was used to detect brain damage-induced free radical production [33]. Sham-operated and TBI-insulted (including the PBS and platonin-treated groups) mice were administered DHE (0.5 mg in 100 µL of DMSO) through a tail vein injection 23.5 h after TBI treatment. The mice were euthanized 24 h after the TBI and perfused with cold saline from the left ventricle for 10 min. Subsequently, whole-brain tissues were immediately viewed under the IVIS Imaging System 200 Series (Xenogen Corporation, Alameda, CA, USA) to monitor ROS production. They were from separate groups of animals, and data are expressed as the total photon flux in a region of interest and expressed as photons per second.

4.11. Statistical Analysis

Data are expressed as the mean ± standard error of the mean (SEM) of the results and are accompanied by the number of observations. The normality of the data was first tested using the Kolmogorov–Smirnov test. Continuous variables were compared using an analysis of variance (ANOVA). When the analysis indicated significant differences among group means, each group was compared using the Newman–Keuls method. $p < 0.05$ was considered statistically significant.

Acknowledgments: This work was supported by grants provided by the Ministry of Science and Technology of Taiwan (MOST-105-2320-B-038-015, MOST-106-2320-B-038-060-MY2), the Taipei Medical University (TMU)-TMU Hospital (105 TMU-TMUH-02-02), and Cathay General Hospital (CGH-MR-A106020).

Author Contributions: Chao-Chien Chang, Chi-Li Chung, and Cheng-Ying Hsieh conceived and designed the experiments. Ting-Lin Yen, Chih-Hao Yang, and Wen-Chin Ko performed the experiments and analyzed the data. Ting-Lin Yen and Cheng-Ying Hsieh wrote the manuscript. All authors discussed, edited, and approved the final version.

Conflicts of Interest: The authors declare no conflict of interest.

References

1. Xiong, Y.; Mahmood, A.; Chopp, M. Animal models of traumatic brain injury. *Nat. Rev. Neurosci.* **2013**, *14*, 128–142. [CrossRef] [PubMed]
2. Rubiano, A.M.; Carney, N.; Chesnut, R.; Puyana, J.C. Global neurotrauma research challenges and opportunities. *Nature* **2015**, *527*, S193–S197. [CrossRef] [PubMed]
3. CDC. *Traumatic Brain Injury in the United States: Fact Sheet*; US Department of Health and Human Services: Atlanta, GA, USA, 2016. Available online: http://www.cdc.gov/traumaticbraininjury/get_the_facts.html (accessed on 30 December 2017).
4. Adelson, P.D.; Dixon, C.E.; Robichaud, P.; Kochanek, P.M. Motor and cognitive functional deficits following diffuse traumatic brain injury in the immature rat. *J. Neurotrauma* **1997**, *14*, 99–108. [CrossRef] [PubMed]
5. Andriessen, T.M.; Jacobs, B.; Vos, P.E. Clinical characteristics and pathophysiological mechanisms of focal and diffuse traumatic brain injury. *J. Cell Mol. Med.* **2010**, *14*, 2381–2392. [CrossRef] [PubMed]
6. Corps, K.N.; Roth, T.L.; McGavern, D.B. Inflammation and neuroprotection in traumatic brain injury. *JAMA Neurol.* **2015**, *72*, 355–362. [CrossRef] [PubMed]
7. Guadagno, J.; Xu, X.; Karajgikar, M.; Brown, A.; Cregan, S.P. Microglia-derived TNF-α induces apoptosis in neural precursor cells via transcriptional activation of the Bcl-2 family member Puma. *Cell Death Dis.* **2013**, *4*, e538. [CrossRef] [PubMed]
8. Guadagno, J.; Swan, P.; Shaikh, R.; Cregan, S.P. Microglia-derived IL-1β triggers p53-mediated cell cycle arrest and apoptosis in neural precursor cells. *Cell Death Dis.* **2015**, *6*, e1779. [CrossRef] [PubMed]
9. Raghupathi, R.; Graham, D.I.; McIntosh, T.K. Apoptosis after traumatic brain injury. *J. Neurotrauma* **2000**, *17*, 927–938. [CrossRef] [PubMed]
10. Clark, R.S.; Kochanek, P.M.; Watkins, S.C.; Chen, M.; Dixon, C.E.; Seidberg, N.A.; Melick, J.; Loeffert, J.E.; Nathaniel, P.D.; Jin, K.L.; et al. Caspase-3 mediated neuronal death after traumatic brain injury in rats. *J. Neurochem.* **2000**, *74*, 740–753. [CrossRef] [PubMed]
11. Lau, A.; Arundine, M.; Sun, H.S.; Jones, M.; Tymianski, M. Inhibition of caspase-mediated apoptosis by peroxynitrite in traumatic brain injury. *J. Neurosci.* **2006**, *26*, 11540–11553. [CrossRef] [PubMed]

12. Knoblach, S.M.; Nikolaeva, M.; Huang, X.; Fan, L.; Krajewski, S.; Reed, J.C.; Faden, A.I. Multiple caspases are activated after traumatic brain injury: Evidence for involvement in functional outcome. *J. Neurotrauma* **2002**, *19*, 1155–1170. [CrossRef] [PubMed]
13. Frugier, T.; Morganti-Kossmann, M.C.; O'Reilly, D.; McLean, C.A. In situ detection of inflammatory mediators in post mortem human brain tissue after traumatic injury. *J. Neurotrauma* **2010**, *27*, 497–507. [CrossRef] [PubMed]
14. Chen, C.C.; Hung, T.H.; Lee, C.Y.; Wang, L.F.; Wu, C.H.; Ke, C.H.; Chen, S.F. Berberine protects against neuronal damage via suppression of glia-mediated inflammation in traumatic brain injury. *PLoS ONE* **2014**, *9*, e115694. [CrossRef] [PubMed]
15. Roth, T.L.; Nayak, D.; Atanasijevic, T.; Koretsky, A.P.; Latour, L.L.; McGavern, D.B. Transcranial amelioration of inflammation and cell death after brain injury. *Nature* **2014**, *505*, 223–228. [CrossRef] [PubMed]
16. Wong, C.H.; Crack, P.J. Modulation of neuro-inflammation and vascular response by oxidative stress following cerebral ischemia reperfusion injury. *Curr. Med. Chem.* **2008**, *15*, 1–14. [PubMed]
17. Abdul-Muneer, P.M.; Long, M.; Conte, A.A.; Santhakumar, V.; Pfister, B.J. High Ca^{2+} influx during traumatic brain injury leads to caspase-1-dependent neuroinflammation and cell death. *Mol. Neurobiol.* **2017**, *54*, 3964–3975. [CrossRef] [PubMed]
18. Glushakov, A.V.; Fazal, J.A.; Narumiya, S.; Doré, S. Role of the prostaglandin E2 EP1 receptor in traumatic brain injury. *PLoS ONE* **2014**, *9*, e113689. [CrossRef] [PubMed]
19. Ishihara, M.; Kadoma, Y.; Fujisawa, S. Kinetic radical-scavenging activity of platonin, a cyanine photosensitizing dye. *In Vivo* **2006**, *20*, 845–848. [PubMed]
20. Komori, T.; Yamaoka, S. Kanko-so and its antimicrobial action. *Koushyokaishi* **1984**, *8*, 43–59.
21. Motoyoshi, F.; Kondo, N.; Ono, H.; Orii, T. The effect of photosensitive dye platonin on juvenile rheumatoid arthritis. *Biotherapy* **1991**, *3*, 241–244. [CrossRef] [PubMed]
22. Hsiao, G.; Lee, J.J.; Chou, D.S.; Fong, T.H.; Shen, M.Y.; Lin, C.H.; Sheu, J.R. Platonin, a photosensitizing dye, improves circulatory failure and mortality in rat models of endotoxemia. *Biol. Pharm. Bull.* **2002**, *25*, 995–999. [CrossRef] [PubMed]
23. Yeh, C.T.; Kao, M.C.; Chen, C.H.; Huang, C.J. Platonin preserves blood-brain barrier integrity in septic rats. *Acta Anaesthesiol. Taiwan* **2015**, *53*, 12–15. [CrossRef] [PubMed]
24. Sheu, J.R.; Chen, Z.C.; Jayakumar, T.; Chou, D.S.; Yen, T.L.; Lee, H.N.; Pan, S.H.; Hsia, C.H.; Yang, C.H.; Hsieh, C.Y. A novel indication of platonin, a therapeutic immunomodulating medicine, on neuroprotection against ischemic stroke in mice. *Sci. Rep.* **2017**, *7*, 42277. [CrossRef] [PubMed]
25. Washington, P.M.; Forcelli, P.A.; Wilkins, T.; Zapple, D.N.; Parsadanian, M.; Burns, M.P. The effect of injury severity on behavior: A phenotypic study of cognitive and emotional deficits after mild, moderate, and severe controlled cortical impact injury in mice. *J. Neurotrauma* **2012**, *29*, 2283–2296. [CrossRef] [PubMed]
26. Fujimoto, S.T.; Longhi, L.; Saatman, K.E.; Conte, V.; Stocchetti, N.; McIntosh, T.K. Motor and cognitive function evaluation following experimental traumatic brain injury. *Neurosci. Biobehav. Rev.* **2004**, *28*, 365–378. [CrossRef] [PubMed]
27. Larcher, T.; Lafoux, A.; Tesson, L.; Remy, S.; Thepenier, V.; François, V.; Le Guiner, C.; Goubin, H.; Dutilleul, M.; Guigand, L.; et al. Characterization of Dystrophin Deficient Rats: A New Model for Duchenne Muscular Dystrophy. *PLoS ONE* **2014**, *9*, e110371. [CrossRef] [PubMed]
28. Prut, L.; Belzung, C. The open field as a paradigm to measure the effects of drugs on anxiety-like behaviors: A review. *Eur. J. Pharmacol.* **2003**, *463*, 3–33. [CrossRef]
29. Chen, W.W.; Zhang, X.; Huang, W.J. Role of neuroinflammation in neurodegenerative diseases (Review). *Mol. Med. Rep.* **2016**, *13*, 3391–3396. [CrossRef] [PubMed]
30. Morganti-Kossmann, M.C.; Rancan, M.; Stahel, P.F.; Kossmann, T. Inflammatory response in acute traumatic brain injury: A double-edged sword. *Curr. Opin. Crit. Care* **2002**, *8*, 101–105. [CrossRef] [PubMed]
31. Lee, J.; Costantini, T.W.; D'Mello, R.; Eliceiri, B.P.; Coimbra, R.; Bansal, V. Altering leukocyte recruitment following traumatic brain injury with ghrelin therapy. *J. Trauma Acute Care Surg.* **2014**, *77*, 709–715. [CrossRef] [PubMed]
32. Chen, H.; Yoshioka, H.; Kim, G.S.; Jung, J.E.; Okami, N.; Sakata, H.; Maier, C.M.; Narasimhan, P.; Goeders, C.E.; Chan, P.H. Oxidative stress in ischemic brain damage: Mechanisms of cell death and potential molecular targets for neuroprotection. *Antioxid. Redox. Signal* **2011**, *14*, 1505–1517. [CrossRef] [PubMed]

33. Yen, T.L.; Chen, R.J.; Jayakumar, T.; Lu, W.J.; Hsieh, C.Y.; Hsu, M.J.; Yang, C.H.; Chang, C.C.; Lin, Y.K.; Lin, K.H.; et al. Andrographolide stimulates p38 mitogen-activated protein kinase-nuclear factor erythroid-2-related factor 2-heme oxygenase 1 signaling in primary cerebral endothelial cells for definite protection against ischemic stroke in rats. *Transl. Res.* **2016**, *170*, 57–72. [CrossRef] [PubMed]
34. Romine, J.; Gao, X.; Chen, J. Controlled cortical impact model for traumatic brain injury. *J. Vis. Exp.* **2014**, *90*, e51781. [CrossRef] [PubMed]
35. McAllister, T.W.; Green, R.L. Traumatic Brain Injury: A Model of Acquired Psychiatric Illness? *Semin. Clin. Neuropsychiatry* **1998**, *3*, 158–159. [PubMed]
36. Fann, J.R.; Burington, B.; Leonetti, A.; Jaffe, K.; Katon, W.J.; Thompson, R.S. Psychiatric illness following traumatic brain injury in an adult health maintenance organization population. *Arch. Gen. Psychiatry* **2004**, *61*, 53–61. [CrossRef] [PubMed]
37. Bryant, R.A.; O'Donnell, M.L.; Creamer, M.; McFarlane, A.C.; Clark, C.R.; Silove, D. The psychiatric sequelae of traumatic injury. *Am. J. Psychiatry* **2010**, *167*, 312–320. [CrossRef] [PubMed]
38. Sinopoli, K.J.; Dennis, M. Inhibitory control after traumatic brain injury in children. *Int. J. Dev. Neurosci.* **2012**, *30*, 207–215. [CrossRef] [PubMed]
39. Kane, M.J.; Angoa-Perez, M.; Briggs, D.I.; Viano, D.C.; Kreipke, C.W.; Kuhn, D.M. A mouse model of human repetitive mild traumatic brain injury. *J. Neurosci. Methods* **2012**, *203*, 41–49. [CrossRef] [PubMed]
40. Konrad, K.; Gauggel, S.; Manz, A.; Schöll, M. Inhibitory control in children with traumatic brain injury (TBI) and children with attention deficit/hyperactivity disorder (ADHD). *Brain Inj.* **2000**, *14*, 859–875. [PubMed]
41. Rodgers, K.M.; Deming, Y.K.; Bercum, F.M.; Chumachenko, S.Y.; Wieseler, J.L.; Johnson, K.W.; Watkins, L.R.; Barth, D.S. Reversal of established traumatic brain injury-induced, anxiety-like behavior in rats after delayed, post-injury neuroimmune suppression. *J. Neurotrauma* **2014**, *31*, 487–497. [CrossRef] [PubMed]
42. Friedlander, R.M. Apoptosis and caspases in neurodegenerative diseases. *N. Engl. J. Med.* **2003**, *348*, 1365–1375. [CrossRef] [PubMed]
43. Elliott, M.R.; Ravichandran, K.S. The dynamics of apoptotic cell clearance. *Dev. Cell* **2016**, *38*, 147–160. [CrossRef] [PubMed]
44. Lull, M.E.; Block, M.L. Microglial activation and chronic neurodegeneration. *Neurotherapeutics* **2010**, *7*, 354–365. [CrossRef] [PubMed]
45. Lee, J.J.; Huang, W.T.; Shao, D.Z.; Liao, J.F.; Lin, M.T. Platonin, a cyanine photosensitizing dye, inhibits pyrogen release and results in antipyresis. *J. Pharmacol. Sci.* **2003**, *93*, 376–380. [CrossRef] [PubMed]
46. Shah, Z.A.; Li, R.C.; Ahmad, A.S.; Kensler, T.W.; Yamamoto, M.; Biswal, S.; Doré, S. The flavanol (−)-epicatechin prevents stroke damage through the Nrf2/HO1 pathway. *J. Cereb. Blood Flow Metab.* **2010**, *30*, 1951–1961. [CrossRef] [PubMed]

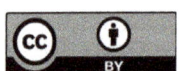 © 2018 by the authors. Licensee MDPI, Basel, Switzerland. This article is an open access article distributed under the terms and conditions of the Creative Commons Attribution (CC BY) license (http://creativecommons.org/licenses/by/4.0/).

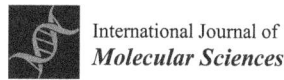

Article

Effects of Protocatechuic Acid (PCA) on Global Cerebral Ischemia-Induced Hippocampal Neuronal Death

A Ra Kho [1], Bo Young Choi [1], Song Hee Lee [1], Dae Ki Hong [1], Sang Hwon Lee [1], Jeong Hyun Jeong [2], Kyoung-Ha Park [3,†], Hong Ki Song [4,†], Hui Chul Choi [4,†] and Sang Won Suh [1,*]

1. Department of Physiology, College of Medicine, Hallym University, Chuncheon 24252, Korea; rnlduadkfk136@hallym.ac.kr (A.R.K.); bychoi@hallym.ac.kr (B.Y.C.); sshlee@hallym.ac.kr (S.H.L.); zxnm01220@gmail.com (D.K.H.); bluesea3616@naver.com (S.H.L.)
2. Department of Medical Science, College of Medicine, Hallym University, Chuncheon 24252, Korea; jd1422@hanmail.net
3. Division of Cardiovascular Disease, Hallym University Medical Center, Anyang 14068, Korea; pkhmd@naver.com
4. College of Medicine, Neurology, Hallym University, Chuncheon 24252, Korea; hksong0@hanmail.net (H.K.S.); dohchi@naver.com (H.C.C.)
* Correspondence: swsuh@hallym.ac.kr; Tel.: +82-10-8573-6364; Fax: +82-33-248-2580
† These authors contributed equally to this work.

Received: 11 April 2018; Accepted: 8 May 2018; Published: 9 May 2018

Abstract: Global cerebral ischemia (GCI) is one of the main causes of hippocampal neuronal death. Ischemic damage can be rescued by early blood reperfusion. However, under some circumstances reperfusion itself can trigger a cell death process that is initiated by the reintroduction of blood, followed by the production of superoxide, a blood–brain barrier (BBB) disruption and microglial activation. Protocatechuic acid (PCA) is a major metabolite of the antioxidant polyphenols, which have been discovered in green tea. PCA has been shown to have antioxidant effects on healthy cells and anti-proliferative effects on tumor cells. To test whether PCA can prevent ischemia-induced hippocampal neuronal death, rats were injected with PCA (30 mg/kg/day) per oral (p.o) for one week after global ischemia. To evaluate degenerating neurons, oxidative stress, microglial activation and BBB disruption, we performed Fluoro-Jade B (FJB), 4-hydroxynonenal (4HNE), CD11b, GFAP and IgG staining. In the present study, we found that PCA significantly decreased degenerating neuronal cell death, oxidative stress, microglial activation, astrocyte activation and BBB disruption compared with the vehicle-treated group after ischemia. In addition, an ischemia-induced reduction in glutathione (GSH) concentration in hippocampal neurons was recovered by PCA administration. Therefore, the administration of PCA may be further investigated as a promising tool for decreasing hippocampal neuronal death after global cerebral ischemia.

Keywords: global ischemia; neuron death; protocatechuic acid; oxidative stress; blood–brain barrier; microglial activation

1. Introduction

Cerebrovascular disorders encompass a diverse range of neurological diseases, such as stroke, myocardial infarction, vascular dementia, and chronic cerebral hypoperfusion [1]. Particularly, ischemic stroke causes one of the most severe cerebropathologic conditions, accounts for 88% of all stroke patients, and represents various clinical signs of focal or global cerebral dysfunction [2]. While focal ischemia can cause local damage and identify infarct volume, the advantage of global cerebral ischemia is that we can confirm the selective and delayed neuronal cell death of, especially, the cornu ammonis 1 (CA1) region in the hippocampus [3]. Global cerebral ischemia (GCI) accompanies the degeneration of the neural tissues, leading to hippocampal neuron death and cognitive deficits. Ischemia-induced brain damage can be recovered via early reperfusion, but this reperfusion can, itself, become an initiation mechanism of a cell death pathway that is caused by blood reperfusion, blood–brain barrier (BBB) disruption, microglia activation and zinc release. Furthermore, ischemia-reperfusion injury is due to free radical production at the onset of blood reintroduction after global cerebral ischemia [4]. Superoxide and other reactive oxygen species produced by the ischemic insult and zinc release can lead to the production of oxidative stress. Reactive oxygen species (ROS) reverses the protein-mediated sequestration of zinc and thus increases the intracellular free zinc levels, which increases activation of ROS formation. If it becomes elevated for sustained periods, it can cause neuronal death. The brain is especially susceptible to oxidative stress because neurons have high levels of polyunsaturated fatty acids and, on the other hand, the concentration of endogenous antioxidant enzymes found in neuronal tissues are too low to buffer against this increased ROS activity. Therefore, oxidative stress may lead to hippocampal neuronal cell death owing to ischemia and subsequent blood reperfusion.

Protocatechuic acid (PCA), a type of the major benzoic acid or phenols, a derivative from vegetables, fruits, and many Chinese herbal medicines, is a primary metabolite of antioxidant substance. Some studies with animal models have stated that PCA shows antitumor promotion effects and strong anti-oxidant behavior [5–7]. It has been suggested that PCA may be regarded as a therapeutic candidate for the administration of neurodegenerative diseases, such as Parkinson's disease [8]. The mechanism is mainly related with antioxidant activity, including prevention of free radical production, as well as removing free radicals and up-regulation of enzymes that are involved in their neutralization. A recent in vivo study demonstrated that PCA protected hepatic cells from hepatic injury caused by tertbutyl hydroperoxide [9,10]. Therefore, this experimental evidence has confirmed that phenolic compounds may offer several biological effects, such as anti-inflammatory, antibacterial, antioxidant, anti-diabetic, and neuroprotective properties [11,12].

Although information about PCA's protective property in tissue and organs has been widely reported [13], the effect of PCA on global cerebral ischemia-induced hippocampal neuronal death has not been studied. Thus, the present study investigates the possible neuroprotective effects of PCA on GCI-induced hippocampal neuron death.

2. Results

2.1. PCA Reduces Neuronal Death after Global Ischemia

Severe neuronal death is produced at seven days after ischemia. To investigate whether PCA has neuroprotective effects after ischemia, the rats were sacrificed at 1 week after ischemia with or without PCA treatment. After insult, we conducted NeuN staining in order to detect surviving neurons, and also FJB (Fluoro-Jade B) staining in order to detect degenerating neurons in the hippocampal subiculum (Sub), the cornu ammonis 1 (CA1), the cornu ammonis 3 (CA3) and dentate gyrus (DG) area. Firstly, FJB staining showed broad neuronal death in the subiculum (sub), CA1, CA3, and dentate gyrus (DG) of the hippocampus (Figure 1) ($p < 0.05$). This staining provides a selective marker of degenerating neurons. No degenerating neurons were present in the sham-operated brain sections. The number of degenerating neurons between the sham and ischemia-induced groups was highly contrasting. Compared to the vehicle-treated group, rats given PCA (30 mg/kg, p.o) after ischemia displayed a remarkable low number of degenerating neurons in the hippocampus (Figure 1A). As depicted in Figure 1B, PCA-treated group had 51%, 75%, and 76% fewer degenerating neurons in the CA1, CA3, and DG, and 58% in the subiculum than in the vehicle-treated group, respectively (Figure 1B). Moreover, NeuN staining confirmed that PCA treatment showed an increased number of live neurons compared to the vehicle-treated group, 43%, 50%, 40%, and 51% more live neurons in subiculum, CA1,

CA3, and dentate gyrus than the vehicle-treated group (Figure 2A,B) ($p < 0.05$). These results indicate that PCA treatment shows neuroprotective effects after transient cerebral ischemia.

2.2. PCA Reduces Ischemia-Induced Oxidative Injury

To determine the degree of oxidative damage after ischemia, we evaluated oxidative stress via 4-hydroxynonenal (4HNE) staining. Brain samples were immunohistochemically stained with a 4HNE antibody at one week after global cerebral ischemia induction to find whether oxidative stress had occurred in hippocampal neurons. In case of the sham-operated group, saline or PCA-injected sections had no difference in the intensity of 4HNE staining in the hippocampus. 4HNE intensity was increased in the hippocampus of ischemia-induced rats due to insult. However, 4HNE intensity was reduced in the PCA-treated rats after ischemia (Figure 3A) ($p < 0.05$). As demonstrated in Figure 3B, the group treated with PCA had around 47% and 49% reductions in the intensity of 4HNE staining in CA1 and CA3, 50% in the DG, and 43% in the subiculum than the vehicle-treated group (Figure 3B).

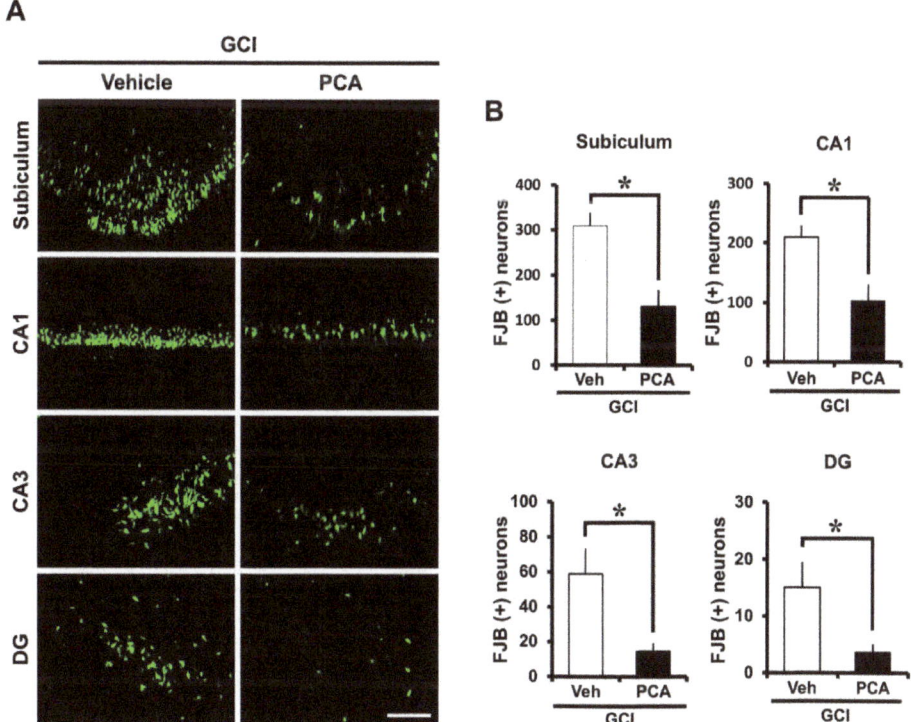

Figure 1. PCA treatment reduces ischemia-induced hippocampal neuronal death. Global ischemia induced neuronal death in the hippocampal areas: subiculum (Sub), CA1, CA3, and dentate gyrus (DG) one week after ischemic insult. Figure (**A**) shows FJB (+) neurons in the CA1, CA3, subiculum and DG. Oral post-treatment of PCA (30 mg/kg) for one week observed neuroprotective effect in the CA1, CA3, subiculum, and DG after ischemia ($n = 9$). Scale bar = 100 μm. (**B**) Bar graph indicating the quantification of degenerating neurons in the hippocampus. The number of FJB (+) neurons is reduced in PCA (30 mg/kg)-treated group in the subiculum, CA1, CA3, and DG compared to the vehicle-injected group. Data are mean ± S.E.M., $n = 5$ from each sham group. $n = 9$ from each ischemia group. * Significantly different from the vehicle-treated group, $p < 0.05$.

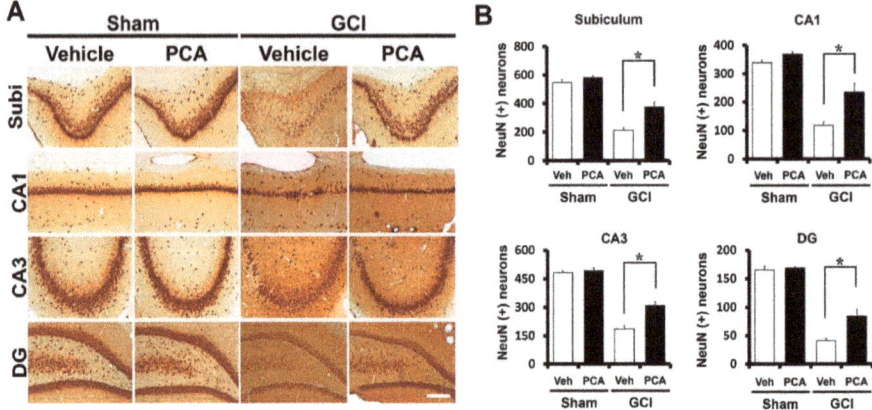

Figure 2. PCA treatment promotes neuronal survival following ischemia. Ischemia-induced neuronal loss was measured by NeuN staining at one week after global ischemia or sham operation. Figure (**A**) representative photomicrographs show significant neuronal loss in the CA1, CA3, subiculum, and DG after ischemia (n = 9). However, ischemia-induced NeuN (+) neurons were preserved by PCA treatment in the hippocampal regions compared to vehicle treatment. Scale bar = 100 μm. (**B**) This graph represents the quantitated live neurons (NeuN (+) neuron) in the hippocampus. Data reflect the mean ± S.E.M., n = 5 from each sham group. n = 9 from each ischemia group. * Significantly different from the vehicle-treated group, $p < 0.05$.

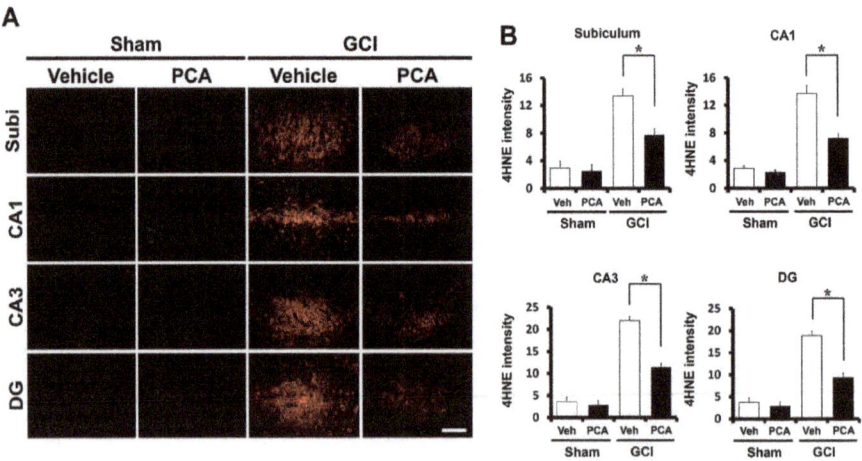

Figure 3. PCA treatment reduces oxidative damage after ischemia. Neuronal oxidative damage was detected by 4HNE (red color) staining in the hippocampal CA1, CA3, DG (dentate gyrus) and subiculum area at seven days following ischemia. As shown in Figure 2, PCA treatment alleviated damage by oxidative stress in the CA1, CA3, DG, and subiculum after insult. (**A**) Sham-operated groups display minimal 4HNE staining in the hippocampus. Oral injection of PCA for 1 week reduced the intensity of the 4HNE fluorescence compared to the saline-treated group after ischemia. Scale bar indicates 100 μm. (**B**) The bar graph shows the 4HNE fluorescence intensity in the CA1, CA3, DG, and subiculum. The fluorescence intensity reflects a significant distinction between saline- and PCA-treated groups. Data reflect the mean ± S.E.M., n = 5 from each sham group. n = 9 from each global ischemia group. * Significantly different from the vehicle-treated group, $p < 0.05$.

2.3. PCA Prevents Ischemia-Induced Blood–Brain Barrier (BBB) Disruption

To evaluate the degree of blood–brain barrier disruption, we stained brain sections to detect extravasation of serum IgG by using immunohistochemistry as described previously [14,15]. In sham-operated brain sections, leakage of IgG was shown to be minimal. However, in ischemia-induced rats, we observed significant extravascular IgG leakage in the hippocampus. Leaked IgG made coronas with a concentration gradient around vessels in the hippocampus region, infiltration of IgG in the hippocampus was seen across broad areas in whole brain sections. Ischemia-induced rats had around 90% more extravasation of serum IgG compared to sham-operated rats in the hippocampus. However, PCA-treated brain sections showed 58% lower immunoglobulin leakage compared to vehicle-treated group in the hippocampus after ischemic injury. Based on the results of the above IgG leakage from the hippocampus, it showed great dissimilarity between the two groups, ischemia-induced rat with saline, and with PCA (Figure 4) ($p < 0.05$).

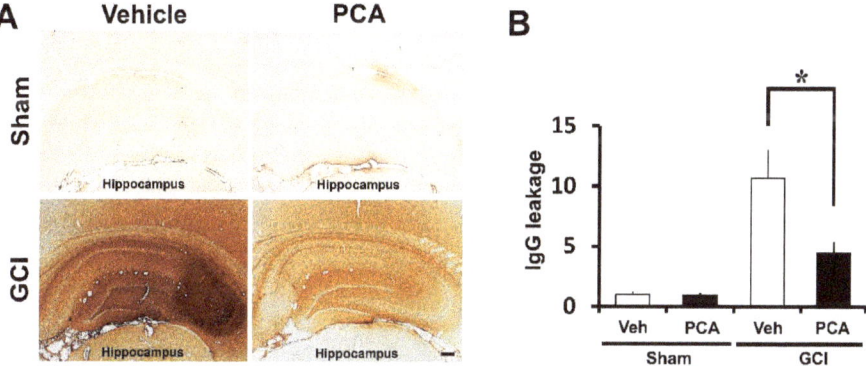

Figure 4. PCA administration reduces BBB disruption after ischemia. Images display a leakage of immunoglobulin through the blood–brain barrier (BBB) disruption in the hippocampus after global ischemia. Figure (**A**) shows low magnification (4×) photomicrographs of IgG staining in the hippocampus. At one week after ischemia, the entire hippocampus showed a high degree of immunoglobulin leakage, suggesting that serious BBB breakdown has occurred in ischemia-induced rats ($n = 9$). PCA (30 mg/kg)-injected rats ($n = 9$) for 1 weeks after ischemia decreases the IgG leakage in the whole hippocampus compared to the ischemia vehicle group ($n = 9$). Scale bar = 200 μm. (**B**) The bar graph shows the degree of IgG leakage in the whole hippocampus. The degree of IgG extravasation was reduced in the PCA (30 mg/kg)-treated group. Data reflect the mean ± S.E.M., $p < 0.05$.

2.4. PCA Decreases Ischemia-Induced Inflammatory Responses Mediated by Microglia and Astrocytes

Global ischemia is usually followed by inflammation induced by microglia and astrocytes. It is mentioned that inflammation contributes to ischemia injury [16,17]. The effect of the PCA treatment on activation of microglia and astrocyte after ischemia were detected by using the surface marker CD11b and GFAP at seven days after insult. We conducted assessment of microglial morphology, number, and intensity and intensity of astrocytes in the four groups (Sham (Vehicle, PCA) and ischemia (Vehicle, PCA)). Sham-operated groups had resting microglia and small astrocyte. Global cerebral ischemia triggered microglial activation, which reflecting macrophage activity. Also, activated astrocytes in ischemia are potentially harmful because they can express NOS and produce the neurotoxic NO [18]. In the present study, we discovered that microglial and astrocytes activation in CA1 region were rose around 64% and 43% respectively in the ischemia group in comparison to the sham-operated group. Microglial activation and reactive astrocytes were reduced around 35% and 23% in the PCA-treated group compared to the saline-treated group following ischemia. Therefore, this result demonstrates that

PCA reduces microglial activation and reactive astrocytes after global cerebral ischemia (Figure 5A–D) ($p < 0.05$).

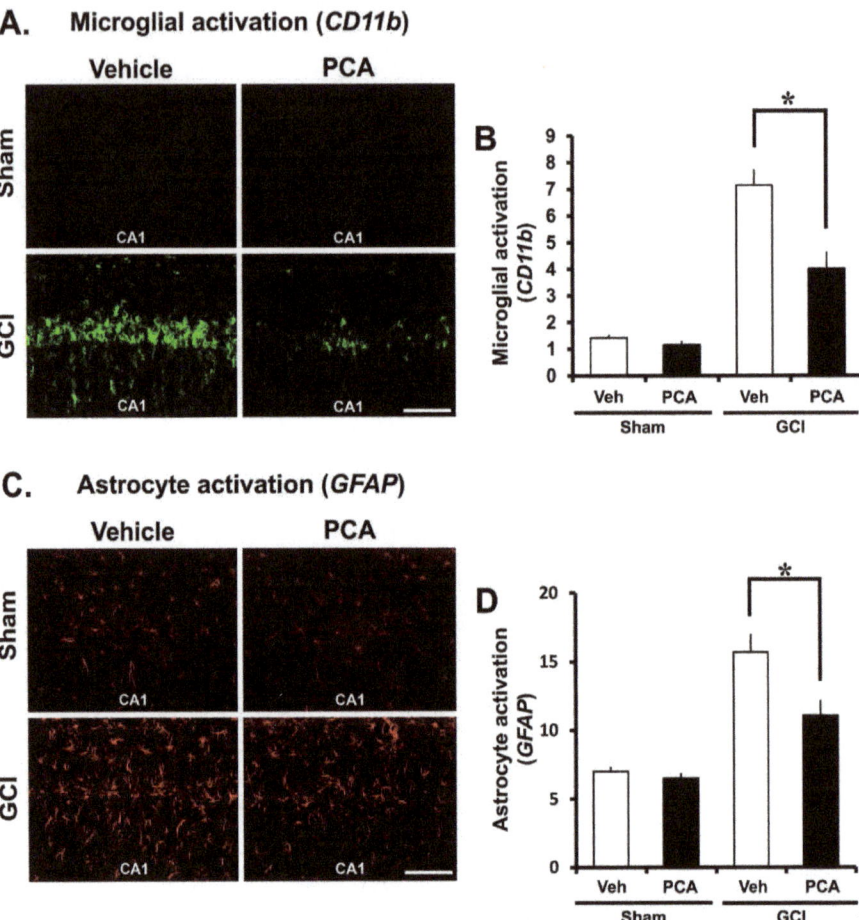

Figure 5. PCA treatment reduces microglia and astrocyte activation. Global ischemia induces an inflammatory response by promoting microglia activation and activated astrocytes, in the damaged region. In this figure, PCA treatment for one week prevents microglia and astrocyte activation in CA1 following global ischemia. (**A**) shows microglia activation and (**C**) shows astrocyte activation in the CA1 of hippocampus from sham-operated or ischemia-induced rats. It was increased in the ischemia-induced group in comparison to the sham-operated group. However, PCA administration prevented microglia and astrocyte activation in the PCA-treated groups after ischemia. Scale bar = 100 μm. (**B,D**) The bar graph represents the grade of microglia activation and the intensity of activated astrocytes in the CA1 region. Data reflect the mean ± S.E.M., $n = 5$ from each sham group. $n = 9$ from each ischemia group. $p < 0.05$.

2.5. PCA Reverses Ischemia-Induced Glutathione (GSH) Deprivation

Glutathione, an endogenous antioxidant, is important in controlling the redox response under the physiological environment of the human body. Brain damage owing to ischemia, seizure, and hypoglycemia reduce glutathione levels and then disrupt the overall redox system [19]. Thus, to investigate the effects of PCA on GSH reduction in a global ischemia setting, we performed GE-NEM staining with brain samples (30 µM) (Figure 6A) ($p < 0.05$). Then, we detected the GSH levels in the hippocampal CA1 region (Figure 6B). As a result, GSH levels were decreased in the CA1 at seven days following ischemia. However, GSH levels in the same region was increased around 37% thanks to PCA treatment compared to the saline-treated group in global cerebral ischemia.

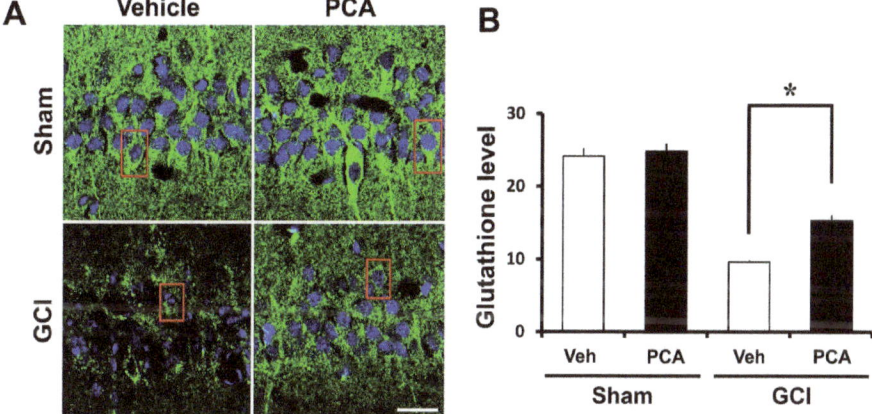

Figure 6. PCA administration rescues glutathione depletion after ischemia. This image displays gaps in glutathione (GSH) levels. (**A**) The sham-operated group include a mostly plentiful glutathione grade in the hippocampus. This image indicates GS-NEM (+) neurons of four groups; sham-vehicle ($n = 3$), sham-PCA ($n = 3$), ischemia-vehicle ($n = 3$), and ischemia-PCA ($n = 3$). Oral injection of PCA for one week after global ischemia improved GS-NEM fluorescent intensity in the CA1 region more than the saline-treated group. Scale bar = 20 µm. (**B**) The bar graph shows that the evaluation of GS-NEM fluorescence intensity in the CA1 region of four groups. The fluorescence intensity is significantly different between the vehicle and PCA-treated group. Data reflect the mean ± S.E.M., $n = 3$ from each sham group and the ischemia group. * Significantly different from the vehicle-treated group, $p < 0.05$.

2.6. PCA Reduces Intracellular Free Zinc Level

Global cerebral ischemia induces zinc release in CA1. This zinc release is known to promote both neuronal NADPH oxidase activity, which is the primary source of ROS responsible for the neuronal cell death seen in this setting. Therefore, intracellular zinc levels need to be tightly controlled. Under physiological conditions, cellular zinc levels are regulated by zinc transporters, zinc binding proteins and zinc sensors [20]. However, under conditions such as ischemia/reperfusion injury, traumatic brain injury or seizure, zinc homeostasis is destroyed and thus neuronal death occurs. Therefore, we performed TSQ fluorescence staining to reveal whether PCA can decrease intracellular zinc level in hippocampal CA1. As quantified in Figure 7, the intensity of TSQ staining within the intracellular CA1 region was decreased in the PCA-treated group compared to the saline-treated group after ischemia (Figure 7A,B) ($p < 0.05$).

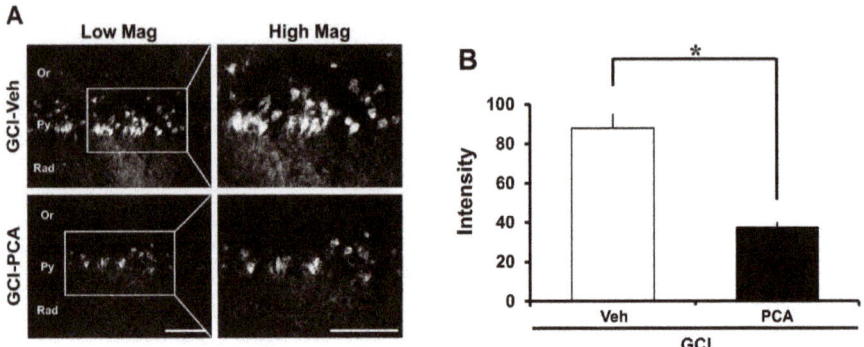

Figure 7. PCA administration decreases the intracellular free zinc level in the CA1 region. Ischemic neuronal death is promoted by zinc release and accumulation. However, oral treatment with PCA for 3 days reduces the intracellular free zinc level. (**A**) displays photomicrographs of TSQ fluorescence staining in CA1. After insult, the intracellular free zinc levels were increased. However, we confirmed that zinc levels were significantly decreased in the group that was administered PCA after ischemia. Scale bar = 100 μm (**B**) the bar graph indicates the TSQ fluorescence intensity from CA1. Data are mean ± S.E.M., n = 4 from each global cerebral ischemia group and ischemia group with PCA. * Significantly different from the vehicle-treated group, $p < 0.05$.

2.7. PCA Improves Cognitive Function after Ischemia

To test whether oral treatment of PCA showed improvement of cognitive function after ischemia, we analyzed behavior using a standard adhesive removal test protocol. The adhesive removal test (also referred to as the tape removal test) has commonly been used as a measure of motor co-ordination and sensory neglect after ischemia in experimental research using rats and mice [21–26]. We conducted this test for six days, starting the next day after surgery. As a result, the ischemia-induced group failed to get rid of the tape for maximum 120 s. However, the PCA treated group showed improved performance and removed the tape faster than in the vehicle-treated group after ischemia (Figure 8).

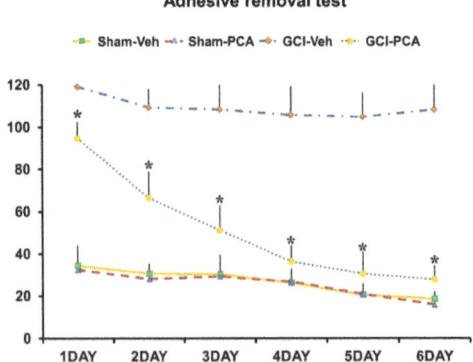

Figure 8. PCA administration improves cognitive function after ischemia. Rats administered PCA for 7 days after ischemia were evaluated for changes in cognitive and sensory function by the adhesive removal test. The graphs show the measured cognitive ability from each group. As a result, injection of PCA lead to increased improvement of ischemia-induced cognitive impairment, compared to the vehicle-treated group. Data reflect the mean ± S.E.M., n = 5 from each sham group and n = 8 form each ischemia group. * Significantly different from the vehicle-treated group, $p < 0.05$.

3. Discussion

The present study investigated the potential therapeutic effects of protocatechuic acid (PCA), one of the major phenol derivatives, on global cerebral ischemia-induced neuronal death. So far, we found that PCA significantly reduced oxidative stress, blood–brain barrier breakdown, activation of microglia and astrocytes, and neuronal death. These results suggest that reduction of oxidative stress by PCA may be used as a new therapeutic tool for preventing ischemic neuronal death.

The molecular mechanisms of global cerebral ischemia-induced neuronal death are highly complex. Although several laboratories have extensively investigated these mechanisms over the decades the precise mechanisms of ischemic neuronal death are still not clear. Previous studies have demonstrated that neuronal death was initiated during blood reperfusion period after certain period of ischemic state [27,28]. This ischemic-reperfusion can cause blood–brain barrier (BBB) breakdown and subsequently promote leukocyte infiltration and brain inflammatory process activation. Our previous study demonstrated that superoxide production by NADPH oxidase activation occurred during the blood reperfusion period after ischemia, which led to a series of neuronal death processes [27].

The present study was performed to prove the question of whether administration of PCA, known as an antioxidant, can prevent ischemia-induced hippocampal neuronal death. Muley et al. showed that a high concentration of PCA (200 mg/kg) reduced infarct volume, brain edema, and reactive oxygen species production [29]. However, they did not show individual hippocampal neuronal death, microglia activation, BBB disruption, and lipid peroxidation, as shown in our present study. In the present study we used a low dose of PCA (30 mg/kg) to see if this chemical has any neuroprotective effects after global cerebral ischemia. Kakkar et al. showed that a high dose of PCA induced GSH depletion and liver toxicity. They suggested that 100 mg/kg of PCA showed no toxicity [5]. Since PCA shows poor absorption by intestine, less than 100 mg/kg of PCA is nontoxic and a relatively safe. Therefore, we selected a dose of 30 mg/kg of PCA for use in this study to investigate whether oral administration has any neuroprotective effect on global ischemia-induced hippocampal neuronal death. Our previous studies have also demonstrated that a low dose of PCA (30 mg/kg) has neuroprotective effects after seizure or after traumatic brain injury [30,31]. We hypothesized that PCA may prevent BBB disruption, microglial activation, and neuronal death through reduction of ROS production by regeneration of glutathione contents. PCA is unusually effective in inhibiting neuronal cell death through oxidative stress in cultured PC12 cells [32]. Thus, PCA decreased neuronal death and prevented cognitive impairment by decreased oxidative stress [33]. PCA also showed protective effects on blood-brain barrier disruption, leading to neuroprotection [34]. With these previous studies, we hypothesized that administration of PCA can prevent ischemia-induced hippocampal neuronal death by scavenging or decreasing the production of ROS.

In the present study, we detected that PCA significantly lessened ischemia-induced neuronal death. The consequence of FJB staining demonstrated a marked decline of number of degenerating neurons in the hippocampal subiculum, CA1, CA3, and dentate granule cells in the PCA-administrated group compared to the vehicle-administered group after ischemia. This trend correlated with the NeuN staining results, which represented an increased number of live neurons in the PCA group. The consequences of FJB and NeuN staining reflected neuroprotective effects of PCA after global cerebral ischemia.

Ischemia/reperfusion produces a burst of free radical production, which eventually drives oxidative stress and subsequent brain injury. This formation of ROS occurs because of (i) iron-associated free radical formation; (ii) depletion of antioxidant enzymes; (iii) increase of lipids and fatty acids; and (iv) production of brain edema [35]. PCA, extracted from green tea, shows protective effects on H_2O_2-induced apoptosis and oxidative stress through increased glutathione (GSH) levels in cultured PC12 cells [36]. One study concluded that the neuroprotective mechanism of PCA was via functioning as endogenous antioxidants, where PCA promoted cell growth by quenching H_2O_2 [37]. They concluded that PCA can exert protective effects against tissue damage caused from superoxide formation and ROS-dependent stress [38]. Another study stated that the reduction of GSH levels in metal-treated animals suggests that a metal potentially binds to the ROS-related enzyme active site or interacts with the active amino acids of this enzyme and, thus, promotes the accumulation of free radicals [39]. Thus, they observed improvement in antioxidant enzymatic activity owing to PCA treatment and concluded that PCA can prevent production of reactive oxygen species and inhibit expansion of tissue injury [6]. Given this, PCA may act as a therapeutic tool for brain recovery and, thus, may be responsible for neurodegenerative disease repair [40]. The blood-brain barrier (BBB) balances nutrients and ions at necessary levels for proper neuronal function, and takes the neurotoxic substrates away from the brain. After global ischemia insult, the BBB can be disrupted, leading to plasma components, such as leukocytes and erythrocytes, crossing the BBB. This BBB disruption gradually increases intracerebral hemorrhage, neurodegenerative processes, inflammation, trauma, and vascular disruption. This process generates neurotoxic substrates that damage synaptic and neural transmission and brain function [41,42]. Furthermore, brain ischemia further breaks the BBB permeability and severely worsens brain edema, which leads to the development of brain penumbra and neurological disorder [43]. Therefore, BBB protection is a principal aim in alleviating brain edema and inhibiting cerebral ischemia. Additionally, brain injury induced by ischemia, hypoglycemia, and seizure leads to more severe neuroinflammation [44,45]. The inflammatory markers, such as microglia, ROS, IL-1β, and TNF-α, were detected in patents who experienced brain injuries. These inflammatory factors may penetrate the BBB and then enter intracerebral circulation. These factors may promote activation of peripheral immune responses [46], causing disruption of the blood-brain barrier and then serum IgG release from the cerebral blood vessels. Therefore, to evaluate the effects of PCA on BBB disruption, we performed IgG staining on brain sections. In the present study, we found that IgG-stained intensity as a function of area was reduced in the PCA-administered group compared to the vehicle-treated group after ischemia. This result suggests that neuroprotection by PCA administration might be associated with recovery or protection from BBB disruption, which is one of the central mechanisms associated with ischemic neuronal injury [47]. PCA displayed protective effects against early ischemic BBB disruption via regulation of tight junctions (TJs) and the protein kinase C-alpha (PKCα) signal pathway. Furthermore, PCA has the ability to prevent BBB damage in ischemia-reperfusion injury by controlling MMP-9, which is a key contributing factor of BBB disruption and TJ proteins. PCA decreased oxidative stress-induced BBB damage through reduction of oxidative stress [48,49].

Astrocytes and microglia play an important role in hypoxemia, inflammation, and neurodegenerative diseases, such as ischemia, in the central nervous system (CNS). Under ischemic conditions, astrocytes and microglia can be rapidly activated by neurotoxic compounds or pro-inflammatory factors, such as TNF-α and IL-1β, which cause neuroinflammation [50]. A previous study demonstrated that regulation of astrocyte activation can reduce cytokine formation and thus protect neurons from ischemic injury [51]. Therefore, brain inflammation has been regarded as a potential target to treat stroke for several years, and a wide variety of approaches have been conducted to suppress ischemia-induced brain inflammation. The CA1 region of the hippocampus is vulnerable to microglial activation and reactive astrocytes in our global ischemia model. Thus, the present study evaluated microglial activation by CD11b and astrocyte activation by GFAP immunofluorescent staining. In the present study, we found that PCA treatment reduced microglial activation and reactive astrocytes after ischemia. This result suggests that PCA can prevent inflammatory processes after stroke.

Glutathione (GSH), composed of glutamate, glycine and cysteine, is a cysteine-containing tripeptide and is regarded as the most significant cellular redox molecule and acts by scavenging ROS molecules [52]. Specifically, lipid peroxides and hydrogen peroxides produced by ischemic injury are eliminated by glutathione and it functions as a significant antioxidant element in this setting. There is significant evidence that brain damage, such as traumatic brain injury, seizure, ischemia, or hypoglycemia lead to a reduction of glutathione levels [53,54]. Therefore, we investigated whether administration of PCA can restore glutathione levels in hippocampal neurons after global cerebral ischemia. In the present study, we discovered that PCA prevents ischemia-induced glutathione (GSH) decrease in the CA1 region. Therefore, restoration of glutathione levels via PCA administration may exhibit neuroprotective effects. However, it is uncertain how PCA inhibits glutathione reduction after ischemic injury. This question will be investigated in future studies.

Zinc is well known as an important trace element because of its structural and catalytic functions. Thus, under physiological conditions intracellular zinc levels are very tightly controlled by zinc transporters, zinc binding molecules, and zinc sensors. However, under pathologic conditions such as ischemia, traumatic brain injury or seizure, zinc homeostasis is destroyed. Impairment of zinc homeostasis leads to cognitive impairment and neuronal cell death. In neurons, if there is brain damage, synaptically-released zinc can migrate to neighboring cells [55]. Zinc can directly regulate various intracellular signaling pathways by interacting with protein kinase, receptors, and transcription factors [56]. Moreover, previous studies have suggested that zinc may act as an intracellular signaling molecule or a second messenger in these cells [57,58]. Released zinc stimulates protein kinase C (PKC), p47, NADPH oxidases, ROS production [59]. Zinc-induced ROS formation destroys the sequestration of zinc by zinc-binding proteins, and thus free zinc levels are significantly increased in the intracellular space. Therefore, we evaluated the intracellular free zinc levels with TSQ staining and found that PCA reduced free zinc by scavenging ROS (Figure 9).

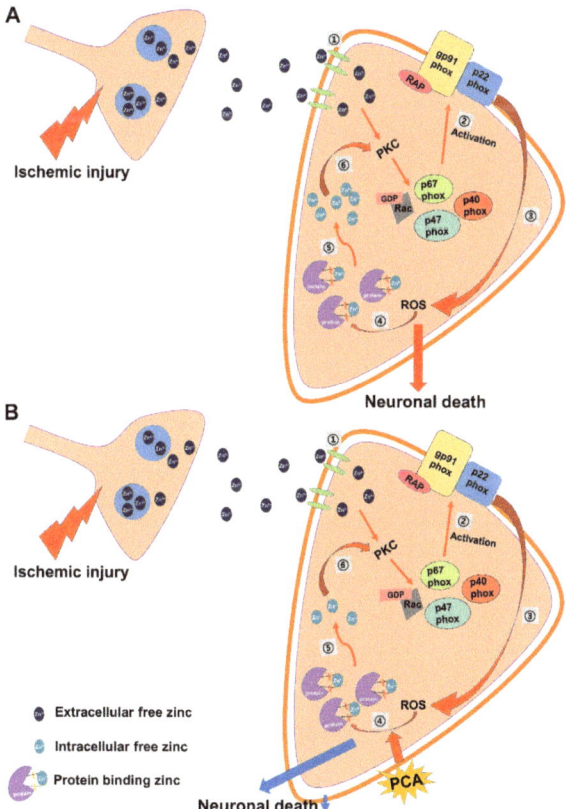

Figure 9. Possible association of zinc, PCA and neuronal death under ischemic conditions. This schematic illustration demonstrates neuronal death by ischemic-induced zinc release. (**A**) (1) Zinc is released into the intracellular space through zinc receptors. (2) PKC and p47 activation and NADPH oxidase activation. (3) Increased ROS formation. (4) ROS inhibits protein zinc binding. (5) Increase of intracellular free zinc. (6) Exacerbated neuronal death by increased intracellular free zinc. When these conditions dominate neuronal death is more likely to occur. (**B**) However, administration of PCA can reduce the intracellular free zinc level by scavenging ROS and thus decrease ischemia-induced neuronal death.

Finally, we conducted the adhesive removal test (tape removal test) in order to confirm whether administration of PCA can improve cognitive and sensory function. In our study, we observed that PCA improved ischemia-induced cognitive impairment. Therefore, the present study suggests that PCA administration may be a promising therapeutic tool for reducing hippocampal neuronal death after stroke.

4. Materials and Methods

4.1. Ethics Statement

The present study is conducted in accordance with the manuals in the Guide for the Use and Care of Laboratory Animals, approved by the National Institutes of Health. Animal studies were in accordance with the stipulation offered by the Committee on Animal Use for Study and Education at Hallym University (Protocol number Hallym-2016-66). We sacrificed animals under isoflurane anesthesia and all procedures were executed to minimize suffering.

4.2. Experimental Animals

This study used eight-week old adult male Sprague-Dawley rats (280–330 g, DBL Co., Chungcheongbuk-do, Eumseong-gun, Korea). Animals were maintained one per cage under conditions of constant room temperature (20 ± 2 °C) and humidity (55 ± 5%). Room lights were controlled automatically, turned on and off in a 12 h cycle (on at 06:00 and off at 18:00).

4.3. Global Cerebral Ischemia Surgery

Transient global cerebral ischemia was produced under the method introduced by Smith et al. [60]. Rats weighing 280–330 g were anesthetized with 2–3% isoflurane. The body temperature was kept at 37 ± 1.0 °C using a heating pad and heating machine is regulated by a rectal thermistor. A catheter was inserted into the femoral artery to monitor blood pressure and to collect blood samples. We revealed and clamped both common carotid arteries, and the systemic average arterial pressure (MAP) was diminished to 40 ± 5 mmHg by extracting blood (7–10 mL) from the femoral artery into a heparinized syringe for 7 min while maintaining temperature at 37 °C. Successful induction of global brain ischemia was checked by the monitoring of iso-electricity on an electroencephalograph (EEG) (BIOPAC system Inc., Santa Barbara, CA, USA) [27,61]. To monitor EEG patterns, we made bilateral holes in the temporal areas of the skull and then inserted the EEG probes beneath the dura and a reference needle was placed in the neck muscle. The onset of iso-electricity was defined as the point of the last three cortical bursts within a 60 s interval. We conducted reperfusion of blood that was recovered by unclamping both common carotid arteries and reinfusing the extracted blood through the femoral artery after seven minutes of the isoelectric EEG. After reperfusion, and confirmation by the restoration of the baseline EEG signal, rats were given an oral injection of PCA (30 mg/kg, p.o) at recovery of ischemia state. Controls were given 1 mL of 0.9% saline only and the sham operation groups (Vehicle, PCA) (n = 5) also received 1 mL of 0.9% saline and PCA (30 mg/kg, p.o). After recuperation from global ischemia, the rats moved their body to the temperature-controlled recovery room and ate a Purina diet (Purina, Gyeonggi, Korea) normally. With severe brain injury, there is the uncommon possibility of neuronal death or seizure in the post-ischemic condition; any animals showing seizure were ruled out from these data analyses. Twelve animals per ischemia group were used in this study. In the entire experiment, the mortality rate was 16.6% and the excluding rate due to seizure was 8.3% (less than 10% after ischemia).

4.4. PCA (Protocatechuic Acid) Administration

To confirm the effect of PCA (protocatechuic acid) on neuronal death after global ischemia, the experimental group was divided into four groups (Sham (Vehicle, PCA) and global ischemia (Vehicle, PCA)). The control group was given 0.9% normal saline instead of PCA. After ischemia, animals were injected with PCA (30 mg/kg, p.o.) once a day for one week. All groups were sacrificed at one week after ischemia.

4.5. Brain Sample Procedure

Animals were sacrificed at one week after global ischemia, using urethane (1.5 g/kg, i.p.) in order to deeply anesthetize animals. Brains were perfused transcardially with 0.9% saline, and then by 4% paraformaldehyde. Brains were separated after perfusion and then post-fixed in the identical fixative for one hour. The brain samples were cryoprotected by 30% sucrose solution for overnight. When the brain completely sank to the bottom of sucrose solution, we froze and cut whole brains with cryostats at 30 µm thicknesses and kept them in the storage solution until histological evaluation.

4.6. Analysis of Hippocampal Neuronal Death

To investigate degenerating neurons after ischemia, brain sections (30 µM) were laid on gelatin-coated slides to stain (Fisher Scientific, Pittsburgh, PA, USA). Fluoro-Jade B staining was performed as depicted by Hopkins and Schmued [62]. Firstly, the slides were put into a 100% alcohol solution for three minutes, 70% alcohol solution for one minute, distilled water, and then into 0.06% potassium permanganate for 15 min. Secondly, the slides were put into 0.001% Fluoro-Jade B (Histo-Chem Inc., Jefferson, AR, USA) solution for 30 min and then washed three times for 10 min in distilled water. We dried brain sample, covered with a cover slide and checked under a fluorescence microscope via blue (450–490 nm) excitation light. To quantify neuronal death, we choose five coronal brain parts from 4.0 mm posterior to the bragma; five brain sections from each animal were then used for analysis. These samples were concealed with encoding of their groups and then offered to a second, blinded tester. A blind tester counted the number of degenerating neurons in constant area (magnification = 10×) of the hippocampal subiculum (900 × 1200 µm), CA1 (900 × 400 µm), CA3 (900 × 1200 µm) and dentate gyrus (900 × 1200 µm) from both hemispheres. The total average number of degenerating neurons from each region was used for statistical evaluation.

4.7. Analysis of Live Neurons

To confirm live neurons, we conducted NeuN staining with monoclonal anti-NeuN, clone A60 antibody (diluted 1:500, EMD Millipore, Billerica, MA, USA). It was used as the primary antibody in PBS with 0.3% Triton X-100 overnight at 4 °C. The brain sections were washed three times for 10 min with PBS, and then incubated in biotinylated anti-mouse IgG secondary antibody (diluted 1:250) for two hours at room temperature (Vector Laboratories, Burlingame, CA, USA) and then were washed again Next, the sections were put into the ABC solution (Burlingame, Vector, CA, USA) for two hours at RT on the shaker. Afterwards, the tissues were washed repeatedly three times for 10 min. The immune responses occurred with 3,3′-diaminobenzidine (0.06% DAB agar, Sigma-Aldrich Co., St. Louis, MO, USA) in 0.01 M PBS buffer (100 mL) and 30% H_2O_2 (50 µL) for 1 min. We put the brain samples on the gelatin-coated slides. We analyzed the immunoreactions by using an Axioscope microscope [63]. A blind tester counted the number of live neurons in a constant area (magnification = 10×) of the hippocampal subiculum (900 × 1200 µm), CA1 (900 × 400 µm), CA3 (900 × 1200 µm), and dentate gyrus (900 × 1200 µm) from both hemispheres.

4.8. Analysis of Oxidative Stress

To evaluate level of oxidative stress in the hippocampus, we conducted immunofluorescence staining with paraformaldehyde-fixed brain tissue. Oxidative stress was detected by measuring the presence of the lipid peroxidation product, 4HNE (4-hydroxy-2-nonenal). Immunohistochemistry with 4HNE (Alpha Diagnostic Intl. Inc., San Antonio, TX, USA) antibodies was conducted according as previously described manual [64]. Brain sections were immersed in a polyclonal rabbit anti-4HNE serum (diluted 1:500, Alpha Diagnostic Intl. Inc., San Antonio, TX, USA) with the PBS containing 0.3% TritonX-100 for overnight in a 4 °C incubator. After we washed the sections three times for

10 min with PBS, these sections were also immersed in a solution of Alexa Fluor 594-conjugated goat anti-rabbit IgG secondary antibody (diluted 1:250, Invitrogen, Grand Island, NY, USA) for two hours at RT. The sections were laid on gelatin-coated slides in order to observe under a microscope. To measure the oxidative injury, we used Image J (v. 1.47c.) program and measured the mean gray value [63].

4.9. Analysis of Blood–Brain Barrier Disruption

We measured the degree of leakage of endogenous serum IgG after ischemia in order to investigate the effects of PCA [65,66]. As previously explained, we perfused whole brains. By using fixed brain samples (30 μm thicknesses), we conducted IgG staining with anti-rat IgG (diluted 1:250, Burlingame, Vector, CA, USA), which represents a level of IgG leakage caused by BBB breakdown. The sections were washed as previously described and put into ABC solution (Burlingame, Vector, CA, USA) for two hours at RT on the shaker. The immune responses occurred by 3,3′-diaminobenzidine (DAB in 0.1 M PBS buffer and 0.015% H_2O_2). The immune responses were observed through an Axioscope microscope and the whole brain was quantified for the degree of endogenous serum IgG infiltration by using Image J software. The sequence of use is as follows: First, the image is loaded into Image J and the following sequence is applied: Click Image → Adjust → color threshold. Check the threshold color is black and remove the check in the blank of dark background. Then, adjust the brightness and saturation with the same value (the researcher can set this to a value useful to their dataset, but the same value should be used in all images being analyzed from an experiment). Click the menu option Image → Type → 8 bits and then, edit → invert. To measure the area, the menu option Analyze → Measure was selected. We use mean gray value (magnification = 4×).

4.10. Analysis of Microglia and Astrocytes Activation

To investigate microglial activation and activated astrocytes, we conducted CD11b and GFAP staining. After washing in PBS, staining was conducted with a mixture of mouse antibody to rat CD11b (diluted 1:500, Serotec) and of goat antibody to rat GFAP (diluted 1:1000, Abcam). Following incubation in PBS containing 0.3% TritonX-100, we left it overnight in a 4 °C incubator. After rinsing, the sections were submerged into secondary antibody (Alexa Fluor 488-conjugated donkey anti-mouse IgG secondary antibody, Alexa Fluor 594-conjugated donkey anti-goat IgG secondary antibody respectively, both diluted 1:250, Molecular Probes, Invitrogen) for two hours at RT. A randomly blinded researcher then measured the intensity of astrocytes in the CA1 region. In the case of microglia, five sections from each brain were scored with same area (magnification = 20×) of the hippocampal CA1 region. Functional standards of microglial activation were their morphology, the number, and intensity of microglial cells. Morphology score of 0: no activated morphology (amoeboid morphology with enlarged soma and thickened processes); 1: 1–45% of microglia; 2: 45–90% of microglia; and 3: >90% of microglia with the activated morphology. CD11b-immunoreactive cell score of 0: no cells are present; 1: 1–9 cells; 2: 10–20 cells; and 3: >20 cells with continuous processes per 100 μm^2. Intensity score of 0: no expression; 1: weak expression; 2: average expression; and 3: intense expression. Therefore, the total score sums up the three scores (microglial morphology, cell number, and intensity) depending on the categories, ranging from zero to nine (magnification = 20×) [67,68].

4.11. Analysis of GSH Levels

To measure glutathione levels, we conducted GS-NEM staining and incubated brain samples with a solution including 10 mM N-ethylmaleimide (NEM, Sigma-Aldrich, St. Louis, MO, USA) for 4 h in a 4 °C incubator. After rinsing in PBS, we stained samples in order to measure glutathione production levels with the primary GS-NEM antibody (diluted 1:100, GS-NEM, Millipore). After this, it was put into a secondary antibody (Alexa Fluor 488-conjugated goat anti-mouse IgG, diluted 1:400, Molecular Probes, Invitrogen) for two hours at RT in darkness. Then we measured GSH levels of selected sections of hippocampus using Image-J software. To measure the concentration of glutathione, we loaded the image into Image J (v. 1.47c) and the following steps were executed: select 5 cells in one brain tissue and then click the menu option Analyze → Measurement. This produced the mean value (generally, in sham group, glutathione was at maximal cellular levels. However, in the ischemia-induced group, glutathione was reduced in degenerating or degenerated neuronal cells) (magnification = 80×) (NCBI, Bethesda, MD, USA).

4.12. Analysis of Intracellular Free Zinc Level

Intracellular free zinc was detected using *N*-(6-methoxy-8-quinolyl)-*para*-toluene sulfonamide (TSQ) staining [69]. Rats were euthanized at 3 days after PCA (30 mg/kg, p.o) administration and then the fresh frozen (but not fixed) brains were coronally sectioned at 10 µm thickness in a −15 °C cryostat, then put on gelatin-coated slides and dried. Five evenly spaced sections were selected in the hippocampal region from each brain and dipped in a solution of 4.5 mmol/L TSQ (Enzo Life Science, Enzo Biochem, Inc, Farmingdale, New York, USA, ENZ-52153) for 1 min, then washed for 1 min in 0.9% saline. We observed and photographed each sample with a microscope under 360 nm UV light and 500 nm long-pass filter. To measure zinc intensity, we used the Image J (v. 1.47c.) program and measured the mean gray value.

4.13. Behavioral Test

Adhesive removal test. To test whether oral treatment of PCA showed improvement of cognitive function after ischemia, we conducted an adhesive removal test for six days from day after the surgery. After an initial adjustment time in a transparent test box (45 × 35 × 20 cm), the rat was lightly restrained to allow adherence of 1 cm square stickers to the palm of each forepaw. And then, we moved the rat quickly into the test box and measured the time to remove the tape. Five trials were undertaken in each test session, with a break time for at least 1 min between trials. A maximum time of 120 s was assigned for each trial. If the stickers could not be removed within this period, a maximum time was recorded.

4.14. Data Analysis

Comparisons among experimental groups were executed using analysis of variance (ANOVA) in accordance with the Bonferroni post hoc test. Data were displayed as the mean ± S.D., and differences were regarded significant at $p < 0.05$.

5. Conclusions

In the present study, we studied whether PCA known as antioxidant has neuroprotective effects on global ischemia neuronal death. To sum up, we found the following: (1) Administration of PCA decreased degenerating neuron in the hippocampus after ischemic injury; (2) Administration of PCA reduced ischemia-induced oxidative stress; (3) Administration of PCA prevented ischemia-induced blood-brain barrier disruption; (4) Administration of PCA lessened ischemia-induced microglial activation and activated astrocytes in the hippocampus; (5) Administration of PCA prevented ischemia-induced reduction of GSH concentration in the hippocampal neurons; (6) Administration of PCA reduced the intracellular free zinc level in the CA1 region; (7) Administration of PCA improved cognitive and sensory function after ischemia.

Taken together, our present study proposes that PCA has the strongly antioxidant and neuroprotective effects and thus we suggest that PCA can be therapeutic treatment for global ischemia-induced neuronal death.

Author Contributions: A.R.K. researched data and reviewed and edited the manuscript. K.-H.P., H.K.S., and H.C.C. reviewed and edited the manuscript. B.Y.C., S.H.L., D.K.H., S.H.L., and J.H.J. researched the data. S.W.S. contributed to the discussion and wrote/reviewed and edited the overall manuscript. S.W.S., MD, PhD is the person who takes full responsibility for the manuscript and its originality. All authors read and approved the final manuscript.

Acknowledgments: This work was support by Brain Research Program through the National Research Foundation of Korea (NRF) funded by the Ministry of Science, ICT and Future Planning (NRF-2017R1D1A3B03028830) to K.H.P. and (NRF-2017M3C7A1028937) to S.W.S. This study was also supported by Hallym University Research Fund (HRF-201801-014).

Conflicts of Interest: The authors declare no conflict of interest.

References

1. Ste-Marie, L.; Vachon, P.; Vachon, L.; Bemeur, C.; Guertin, M.C.; Montgomery, J. Hydroxyl radical production in the cortex and striatum in a rat model of focal cerebral ischemia. *Can. J. Neurol. Sci.* **2000**, *27*, 152–159. [PubMed]
2. Wan, L.; Cheng, Y.; Luo, Z.; Guo, H.; Zhao, W.; Gu, Q.; Yang, X.; Xu, J.; Bei, W.; Guo, J. Neuroprotection, learning and memory improvement of a standardized extract from Renshen Shouwu against neuronal injury and vascular dementia in rats with brain ischemia. *J. Ethnopharmacol.* **2015**, *165*, 118–126. [CrossRef] [PubMed]
3. Nagel, S.; Papadakis, M.; Hoyte, L.; Buchan, A.M. Therapeutic hypothermia in experimental models of focal and global cerebral ischemia and intracerebral hemorrhage. *Expert Rev. Neurother.* **2008**, *8*, 1255–1268. [CrossRef] [PubMed]
4. Dirnagl, U.; Lindauer, U.; Them, A.; Schreiber, S.; Pfister, H.W.; Koedel, U.; Reszka, R.; Freyer, D.; Villringer, A. Global cerebral ischemia in the rat: Online monitoring of oxygen free radical production using chemiluminescence in vivo. *J. Cereb. Blood Flow Metab.* **1995**, *15*, 929–940. [CrossRef] [PubMed]
5. Kakkar, S.; Bais, S. A review on protocatechuic Acid and its pharmacological potential. *ISRN Pharmacol.* **2014**, *2014*, 952943. [CrossRef] [PubMed]
6. Adefegha, S.A.; Oboh, G.; Omojokun, O.S.; Adefegha, O.M. Alterations of Na^+/K^+-ATPase, cholinergic and antioxidant enzymes activity by protocatechuic acid in cadmium-induced neurotoxicity and oxidative stress in Wistar rats. *Biomed. Pharmacother.* **2016**, *83*, 559–568. [CrossRef] [PubMed]
7. Yuksel, M.; Yildar, M.; Basbug, M.; Cavdar, F.; Cikman, O.; Aksit, H.; Aslan, F.; Aksit, D. Does protocatechuic acid, a natural antioxidant, reduce renal ischemia reperfusion injury in rats? *Ulus. Travma Acil. Cerrahi Derg.* **2017**, *23*, 1–6. [CrossRef] [PubMed]
8. Zhang, Z.; Li, G.; Szeto, S.S.W.; Chong, C.M.; Quan, Q.; Huang, C.; Cui, W.; Guo, B.; Wang, Y.; Han, Y.; et al. Examining the neuroprotective effects of protocatechuic acid and chrysin on in vitro and in vivo models of Parkinson disease. *Free Radic. Biol. Med.* **2015**, *84*, 331–343. [CrossRef] [PubMed]
9. Liu, C.L.; Wang, J.M.; Chu, C.Y.; Cheng, M.T.; Tseng, T.H. In vivo protective effect of protocatechuic acid on tert-butyl hydroperoxide-induced rat hepatotoxicity. *Food Chem. Toxicol.* **2002**, *40*, 635–641. [CrossRef]
10. Liu, W.H.; Lin, C.C.; Wang, Z.H.; Mong, M.C.; Yin, M.C. Effects of protocatechuic acid on trans fat induced hepatic steatosis in mice. *J. Agric. Food Chem.* **2010**, *58*, 10247–10252. [CrossRef] [PubMed]
11. Cueva, C.; Mingo, S.; Munoz-Gonzalez, I.; Bustos, I.; Requena, T.; del Campo, R.; Martin-Alvarez, P.J.; Bartolome, B.; Moreno-Arribas, M.V. Antibacterial activity of wine phenolic compounds and oenological extracts against potential respiratory pathogens. *Lett. Appl. Microbiol.* **2012**, *54*, 557–563. [CrossRef] [PubMed]
12. Kazlowska, K.; Hsu, T.; Hou, C.C.; Yang, W.C.; Tsai, G.J. Anti-inflammatory properties of phenolic compounds and crude extract from Porphyra dentata. *J. Ethnopharmacol.* **2010**, *128*, 123–130. [CrossRef] [PubMed]
13. Adefegha, S.A.; Omojokun, O.S.; Oboh, G. Modulatory effect of protocatechuic acid on cadmium induced nephrotoxicity and hepatoxicity in rats in vivo. *Springerplus* **2015**, *4*, 619. [CrossRef] [PubMed]
14. Hoane, M.R.; Kaplan, S.A.; Ellis, A.L. The effects of nicotinamide on apoptosis and blood-brain barrier breakdown following traumatic brain injury. *Brain Res.* **2006**, *1125*, 185–193. [CrossRef] [PubMed]
15. Tang, X.N.; Berman, A.E.; Swanson, R.A.; Yenari, M.A. Digitally quantifying cerebral hemorrhage using Photoshop and Image J. *J. Neurosci. Methods* **2010**, *190*, 240–243. [CrossRef] [PubMed]
16. Chen, Y.; Swanson, R.A. Astrocytes and brain injury. *J. Cereb. Blood Flow Metab.* **2003**, *23*, 137–149. [CrossRef] [PubMed]
17. Stoll, G.; Jander, S.; Schroeter, M. Inflammation and glial responses in ischemic brain lesions. *Prog. Neurobiol.* **1998**, *56*, 149–171. [CrossRef]

18. Ali, S.M.; Dunn, E.; Oostveen, J.A.; Hall, E.D.; Carter, D.B. Induction of apolipoprotein E mRNA in the hippocampus of the gerbil after transient global ischemia. *Brain Res. Mol. Brain Res.* **1996**, *38*, 37–44. [CrossRef]
19. Safonova, O.A.; Popova, T.N.; Kryl'skii, D.V. Glutathione System Activity in Rat Tissues under Phenylethyl Biguanide Action on the Background of Experimental Brain Ischemia/Reperfusion Development. *Eksp. Klin. Farmakol.* **2016**, *79*, 23–27. [PubMed]
20. Foster, M.; Samman, S. Zinc and redox signaling: Perturbations associated with cardiovascular disease and diabetes mellitus. *Antioxid. Redox Signal.* **2010**, *13*, 1549–1573. [CrossRef] [PubMed]
21. Freret, T.; Bouet, V.; Leconte, C.; Roussel, S.; Chazalviel, L.; Divoux, D.; Schumann-Bard, P.; Boulouard, M. Behavioral deficits after distal focal cerebral ischemia in mice: Usefulness of adhesive removal test. *Behav. Neurosci.* **2009**, *123*, 224–230. [CrossRef] [PubMed]
22. Aronowski, J.; Samways, E.; Strong, R.; Rhoades, H.M.; Grotta, J.C. An alternative method for the quantitation of neuronal damage after experimental middle cerebral artery occlusion in rats: Analysis of behavioral deficit. *J. Cereb. Blood Flow Metab.* **1996**, *16*, 705–713. [CrossRef] [PubMed]
23. Bouet, V.; Boulouard, M.; Toutain, J.; Divoux, D.; Bernaudin, M.; Schumann-Bard, P.; Freret, T. The adhesive removal test: A sensitive method to assess sensorimotor deficits in mice. *Nat. Protoc.* **2009**, *4*, 1560–1564. [CrossRef] [PubMed]
24. Bouet, V.; Freret, T.; Toutain, J.; Divoux, D.; Boulouard, M.; Schumann-Bard, P. Sensorimotor and cognitive deficits after transient middle cerebral artery occlusion in the mouse. *Exp. Neurol.* **2007**, *203*, 555–567. [CrossRef] [PubMed]
25. Freret, T.; Chazalviel, L.; Roussel, S.; Bernaudin, M.; Schumann-Bard, P.; Boulouard, M. Long-term functional outcome following transient middle cerebral artery occlusion in the rat: Correlation between brain damage and behavioral impairment. *Behav. Neurosci.* **2006**, *120*, 1285–1298. [CrossRef] [PubMed]
26. Zhang, L.; Chen, J.; Li, Y.; Zhang, Z.G.; Chopp, M. Quantitative measurement of motor and somatosensory impairments after mild (30 min) and severe (2 h) transient middle cerebral artery occlusion in rats. *J. Neurol. Sci.* **2000**, *174*, 141–146. [CrossRef]
27. Suh, S.W.; Shin, B.S.; Ma, H.; Van Hoecke, M.; Brennan, A.M.; Yenari, M.A.; Swanson, R.A. Glucose and NADPH oxidase drive neuronal superoxide formation in stroke. *Ann. Neurol.* **2008**, *64*, 654–663. [CrossRef] [PubMed]
28. Neumann, J.T.; Cohan, C.H.; Dave, K.R.; Wright, C.B.; Perez-Pinzon, M.A. Global cerebral ischemia: Synaptic and cognitive dysfunction. *Curr. Drug Targets* **2013**, *14*, 20–35. [CrossRef] [PubMed]
29. Muley, M.M.; Thakare, V.N.; Patil, R.R.; Bafna, P.A.; Naik, S.R. Amelioration of cognitive, motor and endogenous defense functions with silymarin, piracetam and protocatechuic acid in the cerebral global ischemic rat model. *Life Sci.* **2013**, *93*, 51–57. [CrossRef] [PubMed]
30. Lee, S.H.; Choi, B.Y.; Lee, S.H.; Kho, A.R.; Jeong, J.H.; Hong, D.K.; Suh, S.W. Administration of Protocatechuic Acid Reduces Traumatic Brain Injury-Induced Neuronal Death. *Int. J. Mol. Sci.* **2017**, *18*, 2510. [CrossRef] [PubMed]
31. Lee, S.H.; Choi, B.Y.; Kho, A.R.; Jeong, J.H.; Hong, D.K.; Lee, S.H.; Lee, S.Y.; Lee, M.W.; Song, H.K.; Choi, H.C.; et al. Protective Effects of Protocatechuic Acid on Seizure-Induced Neuronal Death. *Int. J. Mol. Sci.* **2018**, *19*, 187. [CrossRef] [PubMed]
32. Guan, S.; Ge, D.; Liu, T.Q.; Ma, X.H.; Cui, Z.F. Protocatechuic acid promotes cell proliferation and reduces basal apoptosis in cultured neural stem cells. *Toxicol. In Vitro* **2009**, *23*, 201–208. [CrossRef] [PubMed]
33. Zhang, H.N.; An, C.N.; Zhang, H.N.; Pu, X.P. Protocatechuic acid inhibits neurotoxicity induced by MPTP in vivo. *Neurosci. Lett.* **2010**, *474*, 99–103. [CrossRef] [PubMed]
34. Zhang, Y.J.; Wu, L.; Zhang, Q.L.; Li, J.; Yin, F.X.; Yuan, Y. Pharmacokinetics of phenolic compounds of Danshen extract in rat blood and brain by microdialysis sampling. *J. Ethnopharmacol.* **2011**, *136*, 129–136. [CrossRef] [PubMed]
35. Hua, J.S.; Li, L.P.; Zhu, X.M. Effects of moxibustion pretreating on SOD and MDA in the rat of global brain ischemia. *J. Tradit. Chin. Med.* **2008**, *28*, 289–292. [CrossRef]
36. An, L.J.; Guan, S.; Shi, G.F.; Bao, Y.M.; Duan, Y.L.; Jiang, B. Protocatechuic acid from Alpinia oxyphylla against MPP+-induced neurotoxicity in PC12 cells. *Food Chem. Toxicol.* **2006**, *44*, 436–443. [CrossRef] [PubMed]

37. Shi, G.F.; An, L.J.; Jiang, B.; Guan, S.; Bao, Y.M. Alpinia protocatechuic acid protects against oxidative damage in vitro and reduces oxidative stress in vivo. *Neurosci. Lett.* **2006**, *403*, 206–210. [CrossRef] [PubMed]
38. Kalgutkar, A.S.; Crews, B.C.; Rowlinson, S.W.; Marnett, A.B.; Kozak, K.R.; Remmel, R.P.; Marnett, L.J. Biochemically based design of cyclooxygenase-2 (COX-2) inhibitors: Facile conversion of nonsteroidal antiinflammatory drugs to potent and highly selective COX-2 inhibitors. *Proc. Natl. Acad. Sci. USA* **2000**, *97*, 925–930. [CrossRef] [PubMed]
39. Das, K.K.; Das, S.N.; DasGupta, S. The influence of ascorbic acid on nickel-induced hepatic lipid peroxidation in rats. *J. Basic Clin. Physiol. Pharmacol.* **2001**, *12*, 187–195. [CrossRef] [PubMed]
40. Khan, A.K.; Rashid, R.; Fatima, N.; Mahmood, S.; Mir, S.; Khan, S.; Jabeen, N.; Murtaza, G. Pharmacological Activities of Protocatechuic Acid. *Acta Pol. Pharm.* **2015**, *72*, 643–650. [PubMed]
41. Abbott, N.J.; Patabendige, A.A.; Dolman, D.E.; Yusof, S.R.; Begley, D.J. Structure and function of the blood-brain barrier. *Neurobiol. Dis.* **2010**, *37*, 13–25. [CrossRef] [PubMed]
42. Dalkara, T.; Gursoy-Ozdemir, Y.; Yemisci, M. Brain microvascular pericytes in health and disease. *Acta Neuropathol.* **2011**, *122*, 1–9. [CrossRef] [PubMed]
43. Yang, Y.; Rosenberg, G.A. Blood-brain barrier breakdown in acute and chronic cerebrovascular disease. *Stroke* **2011**, *42*, 3323–3328. [CrossRef] [PubMed]
44. Kumar, A.; Loane, D.J. Neuroinflammation after traumatic brain injury: Opportunities for therapeutic intervention. *Brain Behav. Immun.* **2012**, *26*, 1191–1201. [CrossRef] [PubMed]
45. Harrison, E.B.; Hochfelder, C.G.; Lamberty, B.G.; Meays, B.M.; Morsey, B.M.; Kelso, M.L.; Fox, H.S.; Yelamanchili, S.V. Traumatic brain injury increases levels of miR-21 in extracellular vesicles: Implications for neuroinflammation. *FEBS Open Bio* **2016**, *6*, 835–846. [CrossRef] [PubMed]
46. Britschgi, M.; Wyss-Coray, T. Systemic and acquired immune responses in Alzheimer's disease. *Int. Rev. Neurobiol.* **2007**, *82*, 205–233. [PubMed]
47. Woodruff, T.M.; Thundyil, J.; Tang, S.C.; Sobey, C.G.; Taylor, S.M.; Arumugam, T.V. Pathophysiology, treatment, and animal and cellular models of human ischemic stroke. *Mol. Neurodegener.* **2011**, *6*, 11. [CrossRef] [PubMed]
48. Miyamoto, N.; Pham, L.D.; Maki, T.; Liang, A.C.; Arai, K. A radical scavenger edaravone inhibits matrix metalloproteinase-9 upregulation and blood-brain barrier breakdown in a mouse model of prolonged cerebral hypoperfusion. *Neurosci. Lett.* **2014**, *573*, 40–45. [CrossRef] [PubMed]
49. Sifat, A.E.; Vaidya, B.; Abbruscato, T.J. Blood-Brain Barrier Protection as a Therapeutic Strategy for Acute Ischemic Stroke. *AAPS J.* **2017**, *19*, 957–972. [CrossRef] [PubMed]
50. Liu, W.; Wang, X.; Yang, S.; Huang, J.; Xue, X.; Zheng, Y.; Shang, G.; Tao, J.; Chen, L. Electroacupuncture improves motor impairment via inhibition of microglia-mediated neuroinflammation in the sensorimotor cortex after ischemic stroke. *Life Sci.* **2016**, *151*, 313–322. [CrossRef] [PubMed]
51. Dvoriantchikova, G.; Barakat, D.; Brambilla, R.; Agudelo, C.; Hernandez, E.; Bethea, J.R.; Shestopalov, V.I.; Ivanov, D. Inactivation of astroglial NF-kappa B promotes survival of retinal neurons following ischemic injury. *Eur. J. Neurosci.* **2009**, *30*, 175–185. [CrossRef] [PubMed]
52. Schafer, F.Q.; Buettner, G.R. Redox environment of the cell as viewed through the redox state of the glutathione disulfide/glutathione couple. *Free Radic. Biol. Med.* **2001**, *30*, 1191–1212. [CrossRef]
53. Sun, N.; Hao, J.R.; Li, X.Y.; Yin, X.H.; Zong, Y.Y.; Zhang, G.Y.; Gao, C. GluR6-FasL-Trx2 mediates denitrosylation and activation of procaspase-3 in cerebral ischemia/reperfusion in rats. *Cell Death Dis.* **2013**, *4*, e771. [CrossRef] [PubMed]
54. Aoyama, K.; Nakaki, T. Inhibition of GTRAP3-18 may increase neuroprotective glutathione (GSH) synthesis. *Int. J. Mol. Sci.* **2012**, *13*, 12017–12035. [CrossRef] [PubMed]
55. Ohana, E.; Hoch, E.; Keasar, C.; Kambe, T.; Yifrach, O.; Hershfinkel, M.; Sekler, I. Identification of the Zn^{2+} binding site and mode of operation of a mammalian Zn^{2+} transporter. *J. Biol. Chem.* **2009**, *284*, 17677–17686. [CrossRef] [PubMed]
56. Beyersmann, D.; Haase, H. Functions of zinc in signaling, proliferation and differentiation of mammalian cells. *Biometals* **2001**, *14*, 331–341. [CrossRef] [PubMed]
57. Yamashita, S.; Miyagi, C.; Fukada, T.; Kagara, N.; Che, Y.S.; Hirano, T. Zinc transporter LIVI controls epithelial-mesenchymal transition in zebrafish gastrula organizer. *Nature* **2004**, *429*, 298–302. [CrossRef] [PubMed]

58. Yamasaki, S.; Sakata-Sogawa, K.; Hasegawa, A.; Suzuki, T.; Kabu, K.; Sato, E.; Kurosaki, T.; Yamashita, S.; Tokunaga, M.; Nishida, K.; et al. Zinc is a novel intracellular second messenger. *J. Cell Biol.* **2007**, *177*, 637–645. [CrossRef] [PubMed]
59. Choi, B.Y.; Jung, J.W.; Suh, S.W. The Emerging Role of Zinc in the Pathogenesis of Multiple Sclerosis. *Int. J. Mol. Sci.* **2017**, *18*, 2070. [CrossRef] [PubMed]
60. Smith, M.L.; Auer, R.N.; Siesjo, B.K. The density and distribution of ischemic brain injury in the rat following 2–10 min of forebrain ischemia. *Acta Neuropathol.* **1984**, *64*, 319–332. [CrossRef] [PubMed]
61. Auer, R.N.; Olsson, Y.; Siesjo, B.K. Hypoglycemic brain injury in the rat. Correlation of density of brain damage with the EEG isoelectric time: A quantitative study. *Diabetes* **1984**, *33*, 1090–1098. [CrossRef] [PubMed]
62. Schmued, L.C.; Hopkins, K.J. Fluoro-Jade B: A high affinity fluorescent marker for the localization of neuronal degeneration. *Brain Res.* **2000**, *874*, 123–130. [CrossRef]
63. Kho, A.R.; Choi, B.Y.; Kim, J.H.; Lee, S.H.; Hong, D.K.; Lee, S.H.; Jeong, J.H.; Sohn, M.; Suh, S.W. Prevention of hypoglycemia-induced hippocampal neuronal death by N-acetyl-L-cysteine (NAC). *Amino Acids* **2017**, *49*, 367–378. [CrossRef] [PubMed]
64. Suh, S.W.; Gum, E.T.; Hamby, A.M.; Chan, P.H.; Swanson, R.A. Hypoglycemic neuronal death is triggered by glucose reperfusion and activation of neuronal NADPH oxidase. *J. Clin. Investig.* **2007**, *117*, 910–918. [CrossRef] [PubMed]
65. Ruth, R.E.; Feinerman, G.S. Foreign and endogenous serum protein extravasation during harmaline tremors or kainic acid seizures in the rat: A comparison. *Acta Neuropathol.* **1988**, *76*, 380–387. [CrossRef] [PubMed]
66. Hsu, S.M.; Raine, L.; Fanger, H. Use of avidin-biotin-peroxidase complex (ABC) in immunoperoxidase techniques: A comparison between ABC and unlabeled antibody (PAP) procedures. *J. Histochem. Cytochem.* **1981**, *29*, 577–580. [CrossRef] [PubMed]
67. Kauppinen, T.M.; Swanson, R.A. Poly(ADP-ribose) polymerase-1 promotes microglial activation, proliferation, and matrix metalloproteinase-9-mediated neuron death. *J. Immunol.* **2005**, *174*, 2288–2296. [CrossRef] [PubMed]
68. Kauppinen, T.M.; Higashi, Y.; Suh, S.W.; Escartin, C.; Nagasawa, K.; Swanson, R.A. Zinc triggers microglial activation. *J. Neurosci.* **2008**, *28*, 5827–5835. [CrossRef] [PubMed]
69. Frederickson, C.J.; Kasarskis, E.J.; Ringo, D.; Frederickson, R.E. A quinoline fluorescence method for visualizing and assaying the histochemically reactive zinc (bouton zinc) in the brain. *J. Neurosci. Methods* **1987**, *20*, 91–103. [CrossRef]

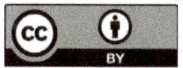

© 2018 by the authors. Licensee MDPI, Basel, Switzerland. This article is an open access article distributed under the terms and conditions of the Creative Commons Attribution (CC BY) license (http://creativecommons.org/licenses/by/4.0/).

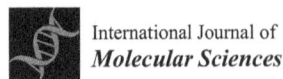

Review

Possible Molecular Targets of Novel Ruthenium Complexes in Antiplatelet Therapy

Thanasekaran Jayakumar [1,†], Chia-Yuan Hsu [1,2,†], Themmila Khamrang [3], Chih-Hsuan Hsia [1], Chih-Wei Hsia [1], Manjunath Manubolu [4] and Joen-Rong Sheu [1,5,*]

1. Graduate Institute of Medical Sciences, College of Medicine, Taipei Medical University, Taipei 110, Taiwan; tjaya_2002@yahoo.co.in (T.J.); gordanmilke1003@gmail.com (C.-Y.H); d119102013@tmu.edu.tw (C.-H.H.); d119106003@tmu.edu.tw (C.-W.H.)
2. Department of Life Sciences, National Chung Hsing University, Taichung 402, Taiwan
3. Department of Chemistry, North Eastern Hill University, Shillong 793022, India; themmilakhamrang@gmail.com
4. Department of Evolution, Ecology and Organismal Biology, Ohio State University, Columbus, OH 43212, USA; manubolu.1@osu.edu
5. Department of Pharmacology, School of Medicine, College of Medicine, Taipei Medical University, Taipei 110, Taiwan
* Correspondence: sheujr@tmu.edu.tw; Tel.: +886-2-2736-1661 (ext. 3199); Fax: +886-2-2739-0450
† These two authors contributed equally to this work.

Received: 1 June 2018; Accepted: 15 June 2018; Published: 20 June 2018

Abstract: In oncotherapy, ruthenium (Ru) complexes are reflected as potential alternatives for platinum compounds and have been proved as encouraging anticancer drugs with high efficacy and low side effects. Cardiovascular diseases (CVDs) are mutually considered as the number one killer globally, and thrombosis is liable for the majority of CVD-related deaths. Platelets, an anuclear and small circulating blood cell, play key roles in hemostasis by inhibiting unnecessary blood loss of vascular damage by making blood clot. Platelet activation also plays a role in cancer metastasis and progression. Nevertheless, abnormal activation of platelets results in thrombosis under pathological settings such as the rupture of atherosclerotic plaques. Thrombosis diminishes the blood supply to the heart and brain resulting in heart attacks and strokes, respectively. While currently used anti-platelet drugs such as aspirin and clopidogrel demonstrate efficacy in many patients, they exert undesirable side effects. Therefore, the development of effective therapeutic strategies for the prevention and treatment of thrombotic diseases is a demanding priority. Recently, precious metal drugs have conquered the subject of metal-based drugs, and several investigators have motivated their attention on the synthesis of various ruthenium (Ru) complexes due to their prospective therapeutic values. Similarly, our recent studies established that novel ruthenium-based compounds suppressed platelet aggregation via inhibiting several signaling cascades. Our study also described the structure antiplatelet-activity relationship (SAR) of three newly synthesized ruthenium-based compounds. This review summarizes the antiplatelet activity of newly synthesized ruthenium-based compounds with their potential molecular mechanisms.

Keywords: ruthenium complex; antiplatelet; antithrombosis; signaling cascades

1. Introduction

Platelets in atherosclerotic process and consequently in the pathophysiology of cardiovascular disease is essential, as platelets, in addition to their contribution to thrombosis and hemostasis, modulate inflammatory reactions and immune response. Platelet activation is considered to be highly associated with cancer progression. The impact of platelets in cancer development has been suggested to be an organized process that causes the pathobiology of cancer growth. Platelets play a critical role in cancer metastasis, counting tumor cell migration, and invasion [1]. Platelet contents are released into the peritumoral space after platelet activation and enhance tumor cell extravasation and metastases [2]. A potential obstruction that surrounds chronic administration of antiplatelet agents in the setting of active malignancy is directly related to the principal role that platelets play in maintaining hemostasis. An in vivo reduction of pulmonary metastases was found in a murine model of breast cancer by the platelet aggregation inhibitor cilostazol [3]. Wenzel et al. observed decreased ex vivo platelet aggregability and reduced platelet-tumor complex formation while administrating liposomal cilostazol [3]. The current antiplatelet agents permanently inhibit their target in inhibiting platelet aggregation; however, the bleeding risk is still difficult to mitigate. Therefore, the progress of harmless and potential therapeutic strategies for the prevention and treatment of thrombotic diseases is still required.

2. Ruthenium Metal Complexes

Inorganic medicinal chemistry is a rich area for controlling several diseases via the development of new therapeutic agents based on bioactive metal complexes. Cisplatin has been widely used as an antimetastatic drug for treating ovarian and testicular cancers for a long time [4]. The platinum diammolino compounds, cisplatin and carboplatin, have limitation due to their dose-limiting side effects and resistance after repeated use in treatment [5]. To solve these restrictions, the screening for anticancer activity among complexes of other metals has received much attention. Currently, ruthenium complexes are found to be striking alternatives for platinum because of several favorable properties suited to rational anticancer drug design and biological applications [6]. Therefore, ruthenium metal complexes are considered the most encouraging anticancer agents. Until now, two ruthenium complexes, NAMI-A and KP1019 have entered clinical trials. NAMI-A is effective against lung metastases [7]. In recent years, abundant progress has been made in the anticancer activity of ruthenium (II) polypyridyl complexes, as many Ru(II) polypyridyl complexes, show motivating anticancer activity [8,9]. A previous study shows [Ru(phen)$_2$(biim)](ClO$_4$)$_2$ inhibits the growth of HeLa cells via stimulating the apoptotic cell death [10]. Ruthenium polypyridyl complex [Ru(phen)$_2$(dbtcp)]$^{2+}$ found high mitochondria specificity, greater photostability, high resistance to the loss of mitochondrial membrane potential and considerable tolerance to environmental change [11]. To gather more insight into the bioactivity of Ru (II) complexes toward cancer cells, these compounds use various medical applications principally due efficient biological activity against some types of diseases. Recent studies found that ruthenium complexes possess potential antiplatelet and antithrombotic effects [12–14]. Some of the novel ruthenium complexes (TQ-1, TQ-2, TQ-3, TQ-5 and TQ-6) were prepared by following the reported methods [15]. Illustrative synthetic procedures of the ligands and complexes is shown in Figure 1A,B. The structures of ruthenium (II) methylimidazole complexes [Ru(MeIm)$_4$(4npip)]$^{2+}$ and [Ru(MeIm)$_4$(4mopip)]$^{2+}$ were given in Figure 1C. The molecular structures of some of the complexes were investigated by single-crystal X-ray studies.

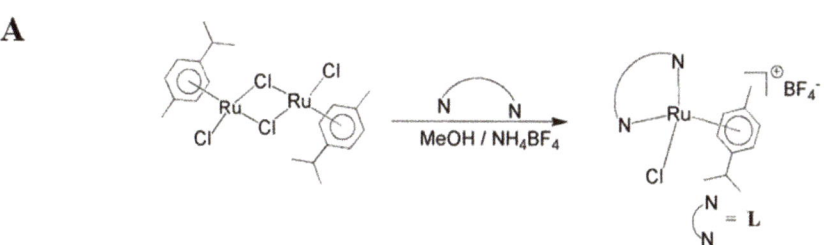

Figure 1. *Cont.*

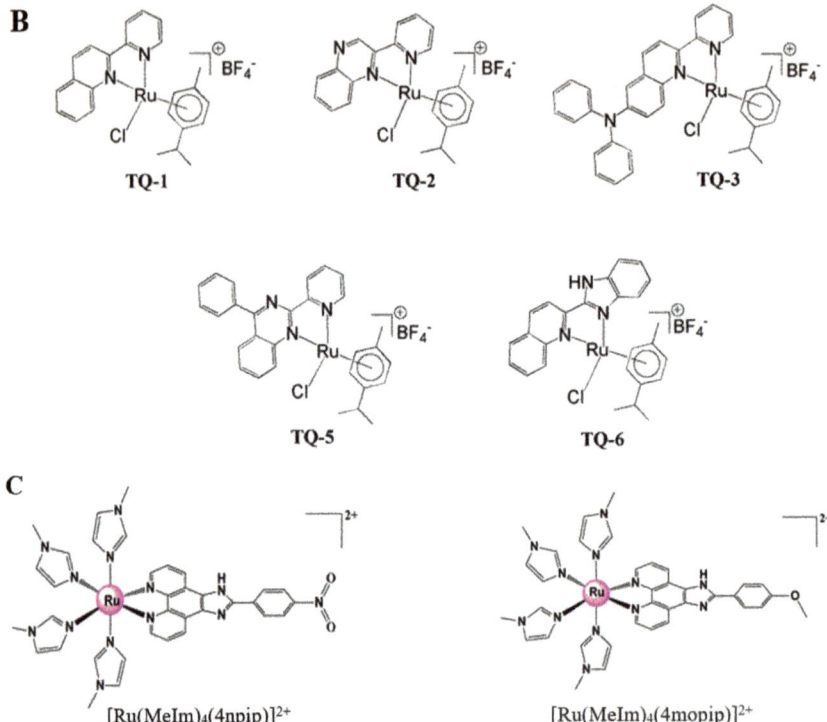

Figure 1. Synthetic procedure of the ligands (**A**) and its complexes (**B**) of TQ-1, TQ-2, TQ-3, TQ-5 and TQ-6; (**C**) Structures of ruthenium (II) methylimidazole complexes [Ru(MeIm)$_4$(4npip)]$^{2+}$ and [Ru(MeIm)$_4$(4mopip)]$^{2+}$.

3. Antiplatelet Effects of Ruthenium Compounds

Various chemical and biological properties displayed by ruthenium complexes make these molecules very interesting for developing new drugs. In vitro and in vivo studies established that numerous ruthenium-based compounds show high cytotoxicity towards a wide range of cancer cells with reduced side effects [16,17]. Fortunately, ruthenium-based complexes are not affected by platinum-induced resistance mechanisms. Although there are several in vitro and in vivo biological studies that have shown that ruthenium-based compounds have potent anticancer activity with condensed side effects, to date, no study exists that has investigated the effects of ruthenium compounds on platelet aggregation. Our recent study established that a novel ruthenium-based compound TQ-5 suppressed platelet aggregation in vitro in washed human platelets by inhibiting the phosphorylation of Akt and JNK1, and subsequently reducing the ATP release reaction and intracellular calcium mobilization [12]. Another interesting study from our group also showed ruthenium compound TQ-6 has a novel role in inhibiting platelet activation through the inhibition of the agonist receptor-mediated inside-out signaling such as Src-Syk-PLCγ2 cascade and subsequent suppression of granule secretion, leading to disturbance of integrin $α_{IIb}β_3$-mediated outside-in signaling, and ultimately inhibiting platelet aggregation [13]. Our recent SAR study also showed that among the three newly synthesized ruthenium-based compounds, TQ-3 has potently inhibited platelet aggregation in vitro, and this inhibitory effect was attributed to the suppression of Syk-Lyn-Fyn cascade and subsequent destruction of Akt, JNK and p38MAPKs activation [18]. Moreover, this study also found TQ-3 reduces the level of ATP, surface P-selectin expression and [Ca^{2+}]$_i$ and ultimately inhibits platelet aggregation. The incorporation of the additional nitrogen atom on the quinoline ring of TQ-1 ligand to obtain TQ-2 and TQ-5 respectively causing the change in electronic nature of ligand that enhances the electron density on the aromatic rings. Variation of ligands pK_a values tunes the aquation rate of the chloride ion by water molecule. Pyridine, 5.2 and Quinoline, 4.9 (TQ-1 and TQ-3); Quinoxaline, 0.60 (TQ-2); Benzimidazole, 5.3 (TQ-6); Quinazoline, 3.51 (TQ-5). TQ-3: The coordinated ligand containing freely rotating N-diphenyl amine group feasibly restricts the strong interaction between the complex and the biological systems. TQ-5: DNA binding affinity may be enhanced by the substitution of phenyl ring on the quinazoline core and improves the hydrophobic interaction and planarity of the molecule. TQ-6: NH functionality on the ligand modulates the lipophilicity/hydrophilicity. These characteristic features might be credited to the observed antiplatelet effects of TQ-3, TQ-5 and TQ-6 (Figure 2). This hypothesis can be further justified from the studies conducted by Giannini et al. [19] and Gorle et al. [20]. These authors proposed that the in vitro activity of anticancer drugs can regularly be associated in part, to their lipophilic character; higher hydrophobicity may contribute to an increased uptake of the complex by the cells, thereby enhancing the anticancer activity. These studies establish the importance of ruthenium-based organometallic complexes in the development of novel anti-platelet agents for the prevention and treatment of thrombotic diseases.

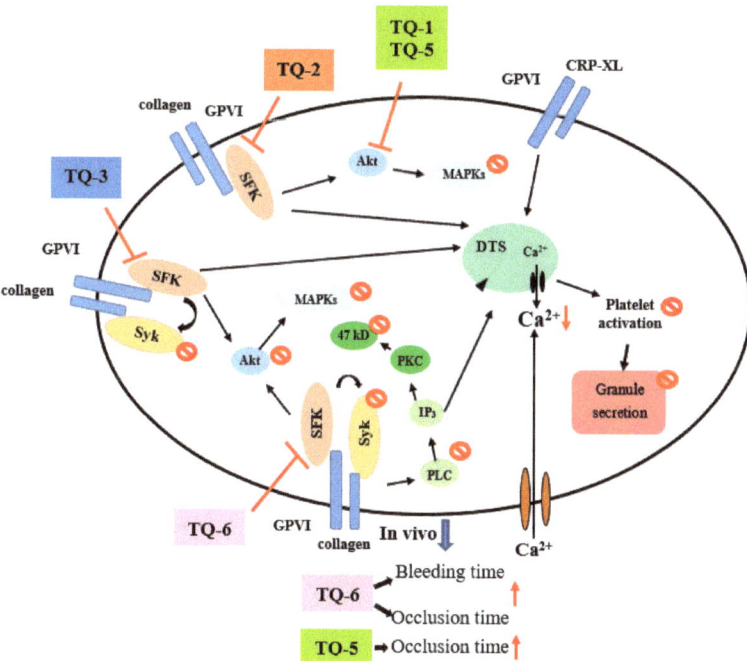

Figure 2. General representation of the main targets and proposed mechanisms of action of ruthenium compounds as antiplatelet drugs. ⊥ inhibits; ⊘ blocks; ↓ decrease; ↑ increase.

3.1. Ruthenium Compounds on ATP and $[Ca^{2+}]_i$ Mobilization in Antiplatelet Therapy

Secretion of platelets is an agonist-induced response, which is of importance for the enhancement of platelet activation and for the various effects of secreted platelet constituents in other tissues. The releasable substances are stored in dense granules, the a-granules and acid hydrolase-containing granules of platelets. Upon stimulation, the contents of these granules are rapidly emptied into the surrounding media by exocytosis. Human platelets are responsible for an ATP-dependent proteolysis of several regulatory proteins for cellular processes [21]. Protein degradation by 20S proteasomes in vivo requires ATP hydrolysis and the homologous ATPases in the eukaryotic 26S proteasome [22]. Therefore, the inhibition of 20S proteasome in platelets does not influence the collagen, epinephrine and thrombin dependent aggregating mechanisms. Interestingly, a previous study found that bortezomib, a first proteasome inhibitor entered to the clinical trials, holds antiproliferative and proapoptotic effects in patients with multiple myeloma [23]. These authors suggested that the anti-aggregating effects of bortezomib may be related to adenine nucleotide receptor dependent regulatory proteins which are essential for physiological and pathophysiological cellular processes.

Multiple studies revealed that ATP could stimulate its own release via P2Rs both in an autocrine and paracrine manner. This mechanism permits regenerative signal amplification via positive feedback and ATP-mediated propagation of the ATP-induced signal. Cell-to-cell spread of Ca^{2+} signals mediated through ATP receptors had observed early in rat basophilic leukemia cells and mast cells [24]. The authors suggested that extracellular ATP accelerates the release of secretory granules containing additional ATP by triggering intracellular Ca^{2+} in quiescent neighboring cells or in cells, which have begun to degranulate, thus amplifying the initial response. Another study showed that addition of ADP and a variety of nucleotide analogs stimulated ATP release through P2Y receptors from endothelial cells isolated from guinea pig heart [25]. Correspondingly, ATP induced the release of ATP in cultured human umbilical vein endothelial cells resulting in maintained extracellular ATP concentrations. This implicated a self-perpetuating mechanism of ATP-induced ATP release likely to play a role in local vascular control [26].

Thrombin, collagen, and ADP commonly generate numerous aggregation-inducing molecules, such as Ca^{2+}, thromboxane (TxA$_2$), etc. TxA$_2$ produces IP$_3$ to mobilize $[Ca^{2+}]_i$ through the G-protein-coupled receptor/PLC-β pathway, and constricts the blood vessel tract [27], which enforces thrombus formation. A lot of agonists such as collagen, thrombin, and ADP mobilize $[Ca^{2+}]_i$ to phosphorylate Ca^{2+}/calmodulin-dependent myosin light chain, which plays a role in secretion of granules such as serotonin and ATP [28], and platelet aggregation. Therefore, the inhibition of $[Ca^{2+}]_i$ mobilization and ATP production are very important for evaluating the antiplatelet effect of a substance. Our recent studies demonstrated that novel ruthenium complexes TQ-5 and TQ-6 potently inhibited collagen-induced $[Ca^{2+}]_i$ mobilization and ATP production in human platelets, representing that TQ-5 and TQ-6 inhibits platelet aggregation through suppressing $[Ca^{2+}]_i$ mobilization and ATP production (Figure 2). Another structural antiplatelet-activity relationship study of newly synthesized ruthenium (II) complexes, TQ-1, TQ-2 and TQ-3 in agonists-induced washed human platelets revealed that TQ-3 compound was effective at inhibition of collagen-induced ATP release, calcium mobilization ($[Ca^{2+}]_i$) without cytotoxicity [18]. A recent study from Ravisankar et al. [14] measured ATP in washed platelets activated by cross-linked collagen-related peptide (CRP-XL) in the presence and absence of different concentrations of chrysin and Ru-thio-chrysin. They found both chrysin and Ru-thio-chrysin significantly inhibited ATP (dense granule secretion). In addition, they found Ru-thio-chrysin exhibited significantly greater effects on inhibiting Ca^{2+} in platelet rich plasma compared to chrysin alone (Figure 3). These data demonstrate that ruthenium and its derivatives affect platelet granule secretion and calcium mobilization, which may influence the subsequent functions of platelets.

3.2. Ruthenium Compounds on MAPKs in Antiplatelet Effects

Mitogen-activated protein kinases (MAPKs) are serine/threonine kinases that regulate cellular proliferation and stimulators such as growth factors and hormones. MAPKs consist of four subgroups: p38, extracellular stimuli-responsive kinase (ERK), and c-Jun NH2-terminal kinase (JNK) and big mitogen-activated protein kinase 1 (BMK1; ERK5). Of these, ERK, JNK and p38 have been identified in platelets and regulated by an extensive range of receptors. In response to the platelet agonists, both p38 and ERK are activated, and the highest activity is demonstrable within minutes of agonist activation [29]. The agonist-induced activation of p38 and ERK seems temporary, possibly due to its negative regulation by integrin outside-in signaling. Ligand binding to integrin $\alpha_{IIb}\beta_3$ was found to down-regulate active p38 and ERK in platelets, ERK2 phosphorylation appears to regulate MEK 1/2 and PKC [30], and JNK was also recognized in platelets in a similar way to ERK2. The characters of JNK and ERK2 in physiopathology are uncertain and had been proposed as suppressors of $\alpha_{IIb}\beta_3$ activation or negative regulators of platelet activation [31]. Additionally, p38 provides a crucial signal that is necessary for aggregation induced by collagen or thrombin [32]. Among the numerous downstream targets of p38, cPLA2 is the most physiologically relevant in platelets, which catalyzes arachidonic acid (AA) release to produce TxA2 [33]. Therefore, p38 MAPK appears to provide a TxA2-dependent platelet aggregation pathway. Stimulation of platelets with various agonists resulted in Akt activation. It is known that Akt plays a role as one of the numerous downstream effectors of PI-3 kinase [34].

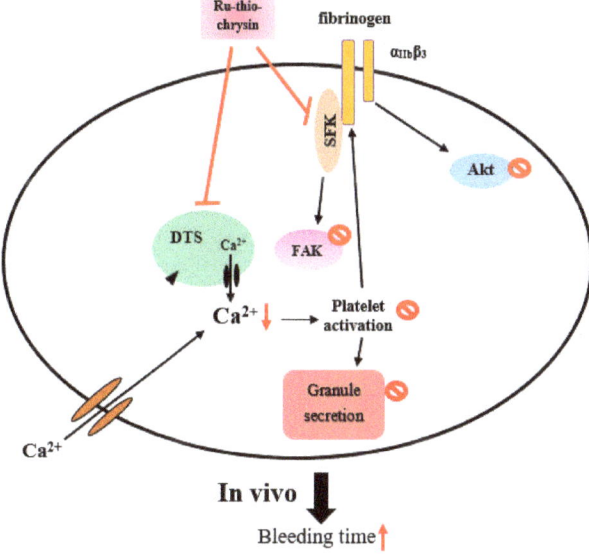

Figure 3. Molecular targets of Ru-thio-chrysin to its inhibitory effects on platelet function.

Studies have established that ERK2, JNK1, and p38MAPK play essential roles in ruthenium complex-mediated inhibition of platelet activation. In one study, the authors found that novel ruthenium compound TQ-5 dose-dependently suppressed collagen-induced Akt and JNK phosphorylation, whereas it does not affect the p38MAPK and ERK phosphorylation [12]. In that study, TQ-5 significantly demolished phosphorylation of Akt and JNK at a maximum concentration of 5 µM (Figure 2). These findings settled that Akt/JNK signaling implicate TQ-5's antiplatelet activity [12]. Another newly synthesized ruthenium compound TQ-6 was notably inhibited the phosphorylation of ERK2, JNK1, and p38 MAPK, representing that the inhibition of the MAPKs signaling pathways is crucial to the TQ-6-mediated inhibition of platelet activation [13]. A recent study was found where among the three novel synthesized ruthenium compounds TQ-1, TQ-2 and TQ-3, only TQ-3 inhibited Akt, JNK and p38 phosphorylation induced by collagen [18].

3.3. Ruthenium Compounds on Cyclic AMP and Cyclic GMP Signaling in Platelets

Cyclic nucleotides (cAMP- and cGMP) have long been accepted as potent inhibitors of platelet aggregation. Human platelet activation inhibited via intracellular cAMP- and cGMP-mediated pathways, and the importance of cyclic nucleotides in controlling platelet activation was confidently proven [35]. Cyclic GMP have been observed to inhibit platelet functions for several decades [36].

Abnormal cyclic nucleotide signaling in platelets might play a role in common diseases such as ischemic heart disease, heart failure, and diabetes [37]. Defects in prostacyclin signaling reduce cAMP levels, resulting in hyperactive platelets and a pro-thrombotic state [38]. cAMP and/or cGMP-elevating agents have shown clinical benefit as platelet inhibitors. For instance, dipyridamole in combination with low-dose aspirin is an approved therapy for stroke prevention [39]. Dipyridamole elevates cAMP levels in platelets by several mechanisms, including inhibition of phosphodiesterase (PDE)-mediated breakdown. Groups of compounds that activate cGMP production by soluble guanylyl cyclase have been shown to reduce thrombus formation [40]. cAMP and cGMP can block many aspects of platelet activation, including early activator signals such as release of Ca^{2+} from intracellular stores and G-protein activation, and adhesion, granule release, aggregation, and apoptosis [41]. Therefore, the adhesion, activation, and aggregation of platelets is a many stepped progression and pharmacological targeting of platelet activating factors and their receptors has become a main strategy in antithrombotic drug development.

Antiplatelets may inhibit platelet aggregation via increasing either cGMP or cAMP; therefore, these nucleotides can be measured in platelets stimulated in the presence of 9-(tetrahydro-2-furanyl)-9H-purin-6-amine (SQ22536), an adenylyl cyclase inhibitor and 1H-[1,2,4]oxadiazolo[4,3-a]quinoxalin-1-one (ODQ), a soluble guanylyl cyclase inhibitor. Our studies observed that neither SQ22536 nor ODQ significantly reversed the TQ-5 and TQ-6-mediated inhibition of collagen-induced platelet aggregation. Therefore, ruthenium complexes TQ-5 and TQ-6-mediated inhibition of platelet activation is independent of intracellular cyclic nucleotide formation [12,13].

3.4. Molecular Targets of Ruthenium Compounds in Antiplatelets Property

Different molecules have serious roles in defining cellular activity with distinct structures and function [42]. An understanding of how ruthenium complexes interact with specific targets within cells is therefore important for exploring the antiplatelet mechanism and choosing the most potent ruthenium complex for selective and effective therapy. In recent years, studies have been devoted to elucidating the signaling events downstream of GPVI and has described the role of signaling molecules that negatively regulate Syk activity [43,44]. A study explored the negative regulation of Syk by PKC in GPVI signaling. In human platelets, inhibition of PKC leads to Syk hyperphosphorylation on residues Tyr-525/526 whereas Tyr-323 and Tyr-352 phosphorylations are unaffected [45]. These authors have also found PKC negatively regulates Syk activity, since it induces hyperphosphorylation of downstream targets, PLCγ2 upon PKC inhibition. PLC activation results in IP_3 and DAG production, which triggers PKC, thus tempting p47 phosphorylation [46]. PLCs are characterized into six families, PLCβ, PLCγ, PLCδ, PLCε, PLCζ, and PLCη [47], and contain the isozymes of PLCγ1 and PLCγ2. PLCγ2 plays a role in collagen-dependent signaling in platelets [48].

Src family kinases (SFKs) contributed towards the regulation of several cellular events such as proliferation, differentiation, motility, and adhesion [49]. Studies have suggested that there are nine members of the Src family that include Src, Lck, Hck, Blk, Fyn, Lyn, Yes, Fgr, and Yrk [50,51]. Earlier studies designated that both human and rodent platelets contain high levels of Src as well as Fyn, Lyn, Hck, Yes, Lck, and Fgr [52]. Although platelets contain high levels of SFKs, their role in platelet function is not clarified yet. SFKs, principally Lyn and Fyn, play essential roles downstream of collagen receptors in platelets [53]. Studies have suggested that platelets from $Fyn^{-/-}$ mice exhibited delayed spreading on immobilized fibrinogen coated surfaces [54], whereas another study found platelets from $Lyn^{-/-}$ mice poorly spreading on von Willebrand factor [55]. Studies have also proven that SFKs play a role in thromboxane generation, shape change, as well as regulation of phosphorylation of Akt [56] and ERK [57]. Our recent studies established that ruthenium compound TQ-6 evidently diminished collagen-induced PLCγ2-PKC activation (Figure 2) but had no direct effects on PKC activation because it did not inhibit PDBu-induced platelet aggregation [13]. This result indicated that TQ-6-mediated inhibition of platelet activation involves PLCγ2 downstream signaling and clarifies how TQ-6 is more effective in inhibiting collagen-induced platelet aggregation than that induced by thrombin.

Another study found among the ruthenium complex, TQ-3 perceptibly reduced collagen-induced phosphorylation of Fyn, Lyn and Syk; however, TQ-1 and TQ-2 had no direct effects on these proteins, suggesting that TQ-3-mediated inhibition of platelet activation involves SFKs and Syk downstream signaling. Ru-thio-chrysin was found to inhibit Akt and FAK phosphorylation induced by CRP-XL (Figure 3), and this inhibitory effect may directly or indirectly influence other signaling pathways that render the inhibition of platelet function [14]. Ru-thio-chrysin was also found to have a significant impact on the dephosphorylation of Src at Y527, which is an essential phenomenon for the activation of platelets [14].

4. Antithrombotic Effect of Ruthenium Compounds

Platelets are vital to the progress of the pathological thrombus liable for cardiovascular disease [58]. Thrombosis can be described as the formation of a blood clot (thrombus) within a blood vessel [59]. This process is considered pathologic except in the case of traumatic injury, where thrombus formation may stop blood loss and protect against systemic infection. Aspirin, the most popular drug in the world, reduces platelet abnormal function by irreversibly inhibiting platelet cyclooxygenase (COX-1), responsible for the ultimate production of thromboxane A2, an activator of the coagulation cascade [60]. Although aspirin is effective on COX-1, it also affects COX-2. Aspirin therapy increases bleeding risk, particularly gastrointestinal. Small bowel bleeding with low dose aspirin therapy was found to be more common in patients. Clopidogrel permanently inhibits the P2Y12 purinergic receptor on platelets, preventing stimulation by adenosine diphosphate, thus inhibiting platelet aggregation [61].

In a previous study for thrombosis, the mesenteric venules were continuously irradiated by fluorescein sodium, resulting in considerable damage to the endothelial cells [62]. Despite aspirin being the most effective antiplatelet drug for preventing or treating cardiovascular diseases, it prolongs the bleeding time. For instance, in the tail transection model of mice, after 30 min of dosing 150 mg/kg aspirin through an intraperitoneal rout, the bleeding time was found to be considerably increased from 229.2 ± 20.5 s to 438.1 ± 22.6 s. In our recent ex vivo study, a shear-induced platelet plug formation in whole blood was analyzed [13]. The PFA-100 system was used to mimic the in vivo conditions of blood vessel injury, in which platelets were exposed to a high shear rate to record the time required for platelet aggregation to occlude an aperture in a collagen-coated membrane. The closure time (CT) of the collagen/epinephrine (CEPI)-coated membrane in whole blood treated with the solvent control (0.5% DMSO) was 93.2 ± 5.5 s. However, treatment with 1 µM TQ-6 significantly increased the CT of the CEPI-coated membranes (123.8 ± 5.7 s), indicating that the adherence of platelets to collagen was prolonged under flow conditions after 1 µM TQ-6 treatment. Similarly, the bleeding time in 0.4 mg/kg of the ruthenium compound TQ-6-treated mice was slightly longer than that of the solvent control (0.5% DMSO)-treated mice (Figure 2). Ru-thio-chrysin was reported to extend the bleeding time in mice (Figure 3). These results indicating that the prolongation of the bleeding time may at least partly be induced by the antiplatelet activity of TQ-6 and Ru-thio-chrysin.

5. Safety and Toxicity of Ruthenium Compounds in Platelets

The uptake of ruthenium complexes by cells is essential for effective antiplatelet therapy. To move into living cells, molecules and atoms must cross or enter the cell membrane. The cell membrane comprises different proteins and lipids, and its function is to control what substances enter the cells for the beneficial or toxic effects.

Previous studies had examined the toxic effects of ruthenium compounds in platelets by measuring extracellular activity of lactate dehydrogenase (LDH). In the most eukaryotic cells, LDH is present and released into the culture medium upon cell death due to the damage of plasma membrane. The LDH study revealed that ruthenium compound TQ-1 and TQ-2 (up to 250 µM), TQ-3 (5 µM), TQ-5 (3–10 µM) and TQ-6 (20–200 µM) incubated with platelets for 20 min did not significantly increase LDH activity in platelets [12,13,18], indicating that ruthenium compounds are safe and they do not affect platelet permeability or induce platelet cytolysis. The in vitro cytotoxic effects of ruthenium (II) methylimidazole complexes [Ru(MeIm)$_4$(4npip)]$^{2+}$ and [Ru(MeIm)$_4$(4mopip)]$^{2+}$ against four different human cancer cell lines (A549, NCI-H460, MCF-7, HepG2) and one normal cell line (HBE) was analyzed by 3-(4,5-dimethylthiazol-2-yl)-2,5-diphenyltetrazolium bromide (MTT) assay [63]. This study found that both complexes exhibit higher cytotoxicity in four cancer cell lines than in normal cells, suggesting that these complexes have high selectivity between tumor cells and normal cells [63]. Another important in vivo study established that the highest intraperitoneal dose (10 mg/kg) of ruthenium-II complex, cis-(Ru[phen]$_2$[ImH]$_2$)$^{2+}$ significantly reduced tumor volume and weight, induced oxidative stress in tumor tissue, reduced the respiration of tumor cells, and induced necrosis without inducing apoptosis in the tumor [64]. More importantly, there was no clinical signs of toxicity or death in tumor-bearing or healthy rats that were treated with cis-(Ru[phen]$_2$[ImH]$_2$)$^{2+}$ [64]. These results suggested that cis-(Ru[phen]$_2$[ImH]$_2$)$^{2+}$ has antitumor activity through the modulation of oxidative stress and impairment of oxidative phosphorylation, thus promoting cancer cell death without causing systemic toxicity.

Ruthenium complexes Δ-[Ru(bpy)$_2$(HPIP)](ClO$_4$)$_2$ bpy = 2,2′-bipyridine and HPIP = 2-(2-hydroxyphenyl)imidazo[4,5-f][1,10]phenanthroline presented high affinity for cancer cells in vitro [65], with no identified side effects on kidney, liver, peripheral nervous system, or the hematologic system, at the pharmacologically effective dose in vivo [66].

6. Conclusions

Despite current antiplatelet therapy preventing death and disability in patients with high risk of thrombotic disease by inhibiting thrombotic events, the lack of efficiency and inconsistent clinical procedures remains a problem. Therefore, a better understanding of platelet function is essential for discovering new antiplatelet approaches with improved clinical outcomes. Ruthenium compounds display fascinating anticancer activity in in vitro and in vivo models. Compared to platinum compounds, ruthenium is coordinated at two additional axial sites and it tends to form octahedral compounds. Commonly, the ligand arrangement and organization geometry between ruthenium and its ligands primarily regulate the activity of ruthenium compounds, especially to their reactivity, hydrophobicity, binding, cellular uptake and intracellular distribution. From this perspective, data presented in this review demonstrates that different classes of ruthenium compounds possess significant antiplatelet effects via multiple targets (Figures 2 and 3). The information of both platelet biology and the functions of ruthenium compounds used for antiplatelet therapy will provide new opportunities to develop therapeutic strategies aimed at promoting cerebro/cardiovascular health.

Author Contributions: T.J., C.-Y.H. and J.-R.S. prepared the manuscript. T.K., C.-H.H. and C.-W.H. collected the literature and aided to write the paper. M.M. contributed clarifications and assistance in drawing schematic diagram. All authors were involved in editing the manuscript.

Acknowledgments: This work was supported by grants (MOST103-2320-B-038-017, OST104-2622-B-038-003, and MOST 104-2320-B-038-045-MY2) from the National Science Council of Taiwan. One of the authors T.K. express her thanks to UGC, MRP-MAJOR-CHEM-2013-5144, (69/2014 F. No. 10-11/12) for financial assistance.

Conflicts of Interest: The authors declare no conflict of interest.

References

1. Belloc, C.; Lu, H.; Soria, C.; Fridman, R.; Legrand, Y.; Menashi, S. The effect of platelets on invasiveness and protease production of human mammary tumor cells. *Int. J. Cancer* **1995**, *60*, 413–417. [CrossRef] [PubMed]
2. Boucharaba, A.; Serre, C.M.; Gres, S.; Saulnier-Blache, J.S.; Bordet, J.C.; Guglielmi, J.; Clezardin, P.; Peyruchaud, O. Platelet-derived lysophosphatidic acid supports the progression of osteolytic bone metastases in breast cancer. *J. Clin. Investig.* **2004**, *114*, 1714–1725. [CrossRef] [PubMed]
3. Wenzel, J.; Zeisig, R.; Fichtner, I. Inhibition of metastasis in a murine 4T1 breast cancer model by liposomes preventing tumor cell-platelet interactions. *Clin. Exp. Metast.* **2010**, *27*, 25–34. [CrossRef] [PubMed]
4. Jamieson, E.R.; Lippard, S.J. Structure, recognition, and processing of cisplatin–DNA adducts. *Chem. Rev.* **1999**, *99*, 2467–2498. [CrossRef] [PubMed]

5. Siddik, Z.H. Cisplatin: Mode of cytotoxic action and molecular basis of resistance. *Oncogene* **2003**, *22*, 7265–7279. [CrossRef] [PubMed]
6. Levina, A.; Mitra, A.; Lay, P.A. Recent developments in ruthenium anticancer drugs. *Metallomics* **2009**, *1*, 458–470. [CrossRef] [PubMed]
7. Sava, G.; Bergamo, A.; Zorzet, S.B.; Gava, C.; Casarsa, M.; Cocchietto, A.; Furlani, V.; Scarcia, B.; Serli, B.; Iengo, E.; et al. Influence of chemical stability on the activity of the antimetastasis ruthenium compound NAMI-A. *Eur. J. Cancer* **2002**, *38*, 427–435. [CrossRef]
8. Li, W.; Han, B.J.; Yao, J.H.; Jiang, G.B.; Lin, G.J.; Xie, Y.Y.; Huang, H.L.; Liu, Y.J. Anticancer activity studies of a ruthenium(II) polypyridyl complex against human hepatocellular (BEL-7402) cells. *Spectrochim. Acta Part A* **2015**, *150*, 127–134. [CrossRef] [PubMed]
9. Peña, B.; David, A.; Pavani, C.; Baptista, M.S.; Pellois, J.P.; Turro, C.; Dunbar, K.M. Cytotoxicity studies of cyclometallated ruthenium (II) compounds: New applications for ruthenium dyes. *Organometallics* **2014**, *33*, 1100–1103. [CrossRef]
10. Xia, Y.; Chen, Q.C.; Qin, Y.Y.; Sun, D.D.; Zhang, J.N.; Liu, J. Studies of ruthenium(II)-2, 2′-bisimidazole complexes on binding to G-quadruplex DNA and inducing apoptosis in HeLa cells. *New J. Chem.* **2013**, *37*, 3706–3715. [CrossRef]
11. Xu, L.; Liu, Y.Y.; Chen, L.M.; Xie, Y.Y.; Liang, J.X.; Chao, H. Mitochondria-targeted ruthenium (II) polypyridyl complexes with benzofuran group for live cell imaging. *J. Inorg. Biochem.* **2016**, *15*, 982–988. [CrossRef] [PubMed]
12. Khamrang, T.; Hung, K.C.; Hsia, C.H.; Hsieh, C.Y.; Velusamy, M.; Jayakumar, T.; Sheu, J.R. Antiplatelet activity of a newly synthesized novel ruthenium (II): A potential role for Akt/JNK signaling. *Int. J. Mol. Sci.* **2017**, *18*, 916. [CrossRef] [PubMed]
13. Hsia, C.H.; Velusamy, M.; Sheu, J.R.; Khamrang, T.; Jayakumar, T.; Lu, W.J.; Lin, K.H.; Chang, C.C. A novel ruthenium (II)-derived organometallic compound, TQ-6, potently inhibits platelet aggregation: Ex vivo and in vivo studies. *Sci. Rep.* **2017**, *7*. [CrossRef] [PubMed]
14. Ravishankar, D.; Salamah, M.; Attina, A.; Pothi, R.; Vallance, T.M.; Javed, M.; Williams, H.F.; Alzahrani, E.M.S.; Kabova, E.; Vaiyapuri, R.; et al. Ruthenium-conjugated chrysin analogues modulate platelet activity, thrombus formation and haemostasis with enhanced efficacy. *Sci. Rep.* **2017**, *7*. [CrossRef] [PubMed]
15. Li, A.H.; Ahmed, E.; Chen, X.; Cox, M.; Crew, A.P.; Dong, H.O.; Jin, M.; Ma, L.; Panicker, B.; Siu, K.W.; et al. A highly effective one-pot synthesis of quinolines from o-nitroarylcarbaldehydes. *Org. Biomol. Chem.* **2007**, *5*, 61–64. [CrossRef] [PubMed]
16. Kelland, L. The resurgence of platinum-based cancer chemotherapy. *Nat. Rev. Cancer* **2007**, *7*, 573–584. [CrossRef] [PubMed]
17. Scolaro, C.; Bergamo, A.; Brescacin, L.; Delfino, R.; Cocchietto, M.; Laurenczy, G.; Geldbach, T.J.; Sava, G.; Dyson, P.J. In vitro and in vivo evaluation of ruthenium (II)-arene PTA c complexes. *J. Med. Chem.* **2005**, *48*, 4161–4171. [CrossRef] [PubMed]
18. Hsia, C.H.; Jayakumar, T.; Sheu, J.R.; Tsao, S.Y.; Velusamy, M.; Hsia, C.W.; Chou, D.S.; Chang, C.C.; Chung, C.L.; Khamrang, T.; et al. Structure-antiplatelet activity relationships of novel ruthenium (II) complexes: Investigation of its molecular targets. *Molecules* **2018**, *23*, 477. [CrossRef] [PubMed]
19. Giannini, F.; Paul, L.E.H.; Furrer, J.; Therrienb, B.; Suss-Fink, G. Highly cytotoxic diruthenium trithiolato complexes of the type [(h$_6$-p-MeC$_6$H$_4$Pri)$_2$Ru$_2$(m$_2$-SR)$_3$]t: Synthesis, characterization, molecular structure and in vitroanticancer activity. *New J. Chem.* **2013**, *37*, 3503–3511. [CrossRef]
20. Gorle, A.K.; Ammit, A.J.; Wallace, L.; Keene, F.R.; Collins, J.G. Multinuclear ruthenium (II) complexes as anticancer agents. *New J. Chem.* **2014**, *38*, 4049–4059. [CrossRef]
21. Coux, O.; Tanaka, K.; Goldberg, A.L. Structure and function of the 20S and 26S proteasomes. *Ann. Rev. Biochem.* **1996**, *65*, 801–847. [CrossRef] [PubMed]
22. Smith, D.M.; Benaroudj, N.; Gold berg, A. Proteasomes and their associated ATPases: A destructive combination. *J. Struct. Biol.* **2006**, *156*, 72–83. [CrossRef] [PubMed]
23. Avcu, F.; Ural, A.U.; Cetin, T.; Nevruz, O. Effects of bortezomib on platelet aggregation and ATP release in human platelets, in vitro. *Thromb. Res.* **2008**, *121*, 567–571. [CrossRef] [PubMed]
24. Osipchuk, Y.; Cahalan, M. Cell-to-cell spread of calcium signals mediated by ATP receptors in mast cells. *Nature* **1992**, *359*, 241–244. [CrossRef] [PubMed]
25. Yang, S.; Cheek, D.J.; Westfall, D.P. Purinergic axis in cardiac blood vessels. Agonist-mediated release of ATP from cardiac endothelial cells. *Circ. Res.* **1994**, *74*, 401–407. [CrossRef] [PubMed]

26. Bodin, P.; Burnstock, G. ATP-stimulated release of ATP by human endothelial cells. *J. Cardiovasc. Pharmacol.* **1996**, *27*, 872–875. [CrossRef] [PubMed]
27. Jennings, L.K. Role of platelets in atherothrombosis. *Am. J. Cardiol.* **2009**, *103*, 4A–10A. [CrossRef] [PubMed]
28. Kaibuchi, K.; Sano, K.; Hoshijima, M.; Takai, Y.; Nishizuka, Y. Phosphatidylinositol turnover in platelet activation: Calcium mobilization and protein phosphorylation. *Cell Calcium* **1982**, *3*, 323–335. [CrossRef]
29. Li, Z.; Xi, X.; Gu, M.; Feil, R.; Ye, R.D.; Eigenthaler, M.; Hofmann, F.; Du, X. A stimulatory role for cGMP-dependent protein kinase in platelet activation. *Cell* **2003**, *112*, 77–86. [CrossRef]
30. Rosado, J.A.; Sage, S.O. The ERK cascade, a new pathway involved in the activation of store-mediated calcium entry in human platelets. *Trends Cardiovasc. Med.* **2002**, *12*, 229–234. [CrossRef]
31. Hughes, P.E.; Renshaw, M.W.; Pfaff, M.; Forsyth, J.; Keivens, V.M.; Schwartz, M.A.; Ginsberg, M.H. Suppression of integrin activation: A novel function of a Ras/Raf-initiated MAP kinase pathway. *Cell* **1997**, *88*, 521–530. [CrossRef]
32. Saklatvala, J.; Rawlinson, L.; Waller, R.J.; Sarsfield, S.; Lee, J.C.; Morton, L.F.; Barnes, M.J.; Farndale, R.W. Role for p38 mitogen-activated protein kinase in platelet aggregation caused by collagen or a thromboxane analogue. *J. Biol. Chem.* **1996**, *271*, 6586–6589. [CrossRef] [PubMed]
33. Coulon, L.; Calzada, C.; Moulin, P.; Vericel, E.; Largarde, M. Activation of p38 mitogen-activated protein kinase/cytosolic phospholipase A2 cascade in hydroperoxide-stressed platelets. *Free Radic. Biol. Med.* **2003**, *35*, 616–625. [CrossRef]
34. Franke, T.F.; Yang, S.I.; Chan, T.O.; Datta, K.; Kazlauskas, A.; Morrison, D.K.; Kaplan, D.R.; Tsichlis, P.N. The protein kinase encoded by the Akt proto-oncogene is a target of the PDGF-activated phosphatidylinositol 3-kinase. *Cell* **1995**, *81*, 727–736. [CrossRef]
35. Walter, U.; Eigenthaler, M.; Geiger, J.; Reinhard, M. Role of cyclic nucleotide-dependent protein kinases and their common substrate VASP in the regulation of human platelets. *Adv. Exp. Med. Biol.* **1993**, *344*, 237–249. [PubMed]
36. Mellion, B.T.; Ignarro, L.J.; Ohlstein, E.H.; Pontecorvo, E.G.; Hyman, A.L.; Kadowitz, P.J. Evidence for the inhibitory role of guanosine 3′, 5′-monophosphate in ADP-induced human platelet aggregation in the presence of nitric oxide and related vasodilators. *Blood* **1981**, *57*, 946–955. [PubMed]
37. Chirkov, Y.Y.; Horowitz, J.D. Impaired tissue responsiveness to organic nitrates and nitric oxide: A new therapeutic frontier? *Pharmacol. Ther.* **2007**, *116*, 287–305. [CrossRef] [PubMed]
38. Van Geet, C.; Izzi, B.; Labarque, V.; Freson, K. Human platelet pathology related to defects in the G-protein signaling cascade. *J. Thromb. Haemost.* **2009**, *7*, 282–286. [CrossRef] [PubMed]
39. Shinohara, Y.; Katayama, Y.; Uchiyama, S. Cilostazol for prevention of secondary stroke (CSPS 2): An aspirin-controlled, double-blind, randomised non-inferiority trial. *Lancet Neurol.* **2010**, *9*, 959–968. [CrossRef]
40. Rukoyatkina, N.; Walter, U.; Friebe, A.; Gambaryan, S. Differentiation of cGMP-dependent and—Independent nitric oxide effects on platelet apoptosis and reactive oxygen species production using platelets lacking soluble guanylyl cyclase. *Thromb. Haemost.* **2011**, *106*, 922–933. [CrossRef] [PubMed]
41. Schwarz, U.R.; Walter, U.; Eigenthaler, M. Taming platelets with cyclic nucleotides. *Biochem. Pharmacol.* **2001**, *62*, 1153–1161. [CrossRef]
42. Komor, A.C.; Barton, J.K. The path for metal complexes to a DNA target. *Chem. Commun.* **2013**, *49*, 3617–3630. [CrossRef] [PubMed]
43. Dangelmaier, C.A.; Quinter, P.G.; Jin, J.; Tsygankov, A.Y.; Kunapuli, S.P.; Daniel, J.L. Rapid ubiquitination of Syk following GPVI activation in platelets. *Blood* **2005**, *105*, 3918–3924. [CrossRef] [PubMed]
44. Thomas, D.H.; Getz, T.M.; Newman, T.N.; Dangelmaier, C.A.; Carpino, N.; Kunapuli, S.P.; Tsygankov, A.Y.; Daniel, J.L. A novel histidine tyrosine phosphatase, TULA-2, associates with Syk and negatively regulates GPVI signaling in platelets. *Blood* **2010**, *116*, 2570–2578. [CrossRef] [PubMed]
45. Buitrago, L.; Bhavanasi, D.; Dangelmaier, C.; Manne, B.K.; Badolia, R.; Borgognone, A.; Tsygankov, A.Y.; McKenzie, S.E.; Kunapuli, S.P. Tyrosine phosphorylation on spleen tyrosine kinase (Syk) is differentially regulated in human and murine platelets by protein kinase C isoforms. *J. Biol. Chem.* **2013**, *288*, 29160–29169. [CrossRef] [PubMed]
46. Singer, W.D.; Brown, H.A.; Sternweis, P.C. Regulation of eukaryotic phosphatidylinositol-specific phospholipase C and phospholipase D. *Annu. Rev. Biochem.* **1997**, *66*, 475–509. [CrossRef] [PubMed]
47. Pascale, A.; Amadio, M.; Govoni, S.; Battaini, F. The aging brain, a key target for the future: The protein kinase C involvement. *Pharmacol. Res.* **2007**, *55*, 560–569. [CrossRef] [PubMed]

48. Ragab, A.; Severin, S.; Gratacap, M.P.; Aguado, E.; Malissen, M.; Jandrot-Perrus, M.; Malisses, B.; Ragab-Thomas, J.; Payrastre, B. Roles of the C-terminal tyrosine residues of LAT in GP VI-induced platelet activation: Insights into the mechanism of PLC gamma 2 activation. *Blood* **2007**, *110*, 2466–2474. [CrossRef] [PubMed]
49. Morris, R.E.; Aird, R.E.; Murdoch, P.S.; Chen, H.; Cummings, J.; Hughes, N.D.; Parsons, S.; Parkin, A.; Boyd Jodrell, D.I.; Sadler, P.J. Inhibition of cancer cell growth by ruthenium (II) arene complexes. *J. Med. Chem.* **2001**, *44*, 3616–3621. [CrossRef] [PubMed]
50. Thomas, S.M.; Brugge, J.S. Cellular functions regulated by Src family kinases. *Annu. Rev. Cell Dev. Biol.* **1997**, *13*, 513–609. [CrossRef] [PubMed]
51. Boggon, T.J.; Eck, M.J. Structure and regulation of Src family kinases. *Oncogene* **2004**, *23*, 7918–7927. [CrossRef] [PubMed]
52. Stenberg, P.E.; Pestina, T.I.; Barrie, R.J.; Jackson, C.W. The Src family kinases, Fgr, Fyn, Lck, and Lyn, colocalize with coated membranes in platelets. *Blood* **1997**, *89*, 2384–2393. [PubMed]
53. Quek, L.S.; Pasquet, J.M.; Hers, I.; Cornall, R.; Knight, G.; Barnes, M.; Hibbs, M.L.; Dunn, A.R.; Lowell, C.A.; Watson, S.P. Fyn and Lyn phosphorylate the Fc receptor gamma chain downstream of glycoprotein VI in murine platelets, and Lyn regulates a novel feedback pathway. *Blood* **2000**, *96*, 4246–4253. [PubMed]
54. Reddy, K.B.; Smith, D.M.; Plow, E.F. Analysis of Fyn function in hemostasis and alphaIIbbeta3-integrin signaling. *J. Cell Sci.* **2008**, *121*, 1641–1648. [CrossRef] [PubMed]
55. Yin, H.; Liu, J.; Li, Z.; Berndt, M.C.; Lowell, C.A.; Du, X. Src family tyrosine kinase Lyn mediates VWF/GPIb-IX-induced platelet activation via the cGMP signaling pathway. *Blood* **2008**, *112*, 1139–1146. [CrossRef] [PubMed]
56. Kim, S.; Jin, J.; Kunapuli, S.P. Relative contribution of G-protein-coupled pathways to protease-activated receptor-mediated Akt phosphorylation in platelets. *Blood* **2006**, *107*, 947–954. [CrossRef] [PubMed]
57. Garcia, A.; Shankar, H.; Murugappan, S.; Kim, S.; Kunapuli, S.P. Regulation and functional consequences of ADP receptor-mediated ERK2 activation in platelets. *Biochem. J.* **2007**, *404*, 299–308. [CrossRef] [PubMed]
58. Furie, B.; Furie, B.C. Mechanisms of thrombus formation. *N. Engl. J. Med.* **2008**, *359*, 938–949. [CrossRef] [PubMed]
59. Aird, W.C. Vascular bed-specific thrombosis. *J. Thromb. Haemost.* **2007**, *5*, 283–291. [CrossRef] [PubMed]
60. Suchon, P.; Al Frouh, F.; Ibrahim, M.; Sarlon, G.; Venton, G.; Alessi, M.C.; Tregouet, D.A.; Morange, P.E. Genetic risk factors for venous thrombosis in women using combined oral contraceptives: Update of the PILGRIM study. *Clin. Genet.* **2017**, *91*, 131–136. [CrossRef] [PubMed]
61. Amin, A.M.; Sheau Chin, L.; Azri Mohamed Noor, D.; Sk Abdul kader, M.A.; Kah hay, Y.; Ibrahim, B. The personalization of clopidogrel antiplatelet therapy: The role of integrative pharmacogenetics and pharmacometabolomics. *Cardiol. Res. Pract.* **2017**, *2017*. [CrossRef] [PubMed]
62. Sheu, J.R.; Lee, C.R.; Lin, C.H.; Hsiao, G.; Ko, W.C.; Chen, Y.C.; Yen, M.H. Mechanisms involved in the antiplatelet activity of Staphylococcus aureus lipoteichoic acid in human platelets. *Thromb. Haemost.* **2000**, *83*, 777–784. [PubMed]
63. Chen, J.; Zhang, Y.; Li, G.; Peng, F.; Jie, X.; She, J.; Dongye, G.; Zou, Z.; Rong, S.; Chen, L. Cytotoxicity in vitro, cellular uptake, localization and apoptotic mechanism studies induced by ruthenium (II) complex. *J. Biol. Inorg. Chem.* **2018**, *23*, 261–275. [CrossRef] [PubMed]
64. Alves de Souza, C.E.; Alves de Souza, H.M.; Stipp, M.C.; Corso, C.R.; Galindo, C.M.; Cardoso, C.R.; Dittrich, R.L.; de Souza Ramos, E.A.; Klassen, G.; Carlos, R.M.; et al. Ruthenium complex exerts antineoplastic effects that are mediated by oxidative stress without inducing toxicity in Walker-256 tumor-bearing rats. *Free Radic. Biol Med.* **2017**, *110*, 228–239. [CrossRef] [PubMed]
65. Wang, J.Q.; Zhang, P.Y.; Qian, C.; Hou, X.J.; Ji, L.N.; Chao, H. Mitochondria are the primary target in the induction of apoptosis by chiral ruthenium (II) polypyridyl complexes in cancer cells. *J. Biol. Inorg. Chem.* **2014**, *19*, 335–348. [CrossRef] [PubMed]
66. Wang, J.Q.; Zhang, P.Y.; Ji, L.N.; Chao, H. A ruthenium (II) complex inhibits tumor growth in vivo with fewer side-effects compared with cisplatin. *J. Inorg. Biochem.* **2015**, *146*, 89–96. [CrossRef] [PubMed]

© 2018 by the authors. Licensee MDPI, Basel, Switzerland. This article is an open access article distributed under the terms and conditions of the Creative Commons Attribution (CC BY) license (http://creativecommons.org/licenses/by/4.0/).

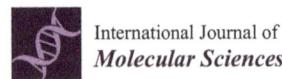

Article

Effect of Inhibition of DNA Methylation Combined with Task-Specific Training on Chronic Stroke Recovery

In-Ae Choi [1], Cheol Soon Lee [1], Hahn Young Kim [1], Dong-Hee Choi [1,2,*] and Jongmin Lee [1,3,*]

1. Center for Neuroscience Research, Institute of Biomedical Science and Technology, Konkuk University, Seoul 05029, Korea; adia86@naver.com (I.-A.C.); slaoa1428@naver.com (C.S.L.); hykimmd@gmail.com (H.Y.K.)
2. Department of Medical Science Konkuk University School of Medicine, Konkuk University, Seoul 05029, Korea
3. Department of Rehabilitation Medicine, Konkuk University School of Medicine, Konkuk University, Seoul 05029, Korea
* Correspondence: dchoi@kku.ac.kr (D.-H.C.); leej@kuh.ac.kr (J.L.); Tel.: +82-2-2049-6012 (D.-H.C.); +82-2-2030-5345 (J.L.)

Received: 23 May 2018; Accepted: 9 July 2018; Published: 11 July 2018

Abstract: To develop new rehabilitation therapies for chronic stroke, this study examined the effectiveness of task-specific training (TST) and TST combined with DNA methyltransferase inhibitor in chronic stroke recovery. Eight weeks after photothrombotic stroke, 5-Aza-2′-deoxycytidine (5-Aza-dC) infusion was done on the contralesional cortex for four weeks, with and without TST. Functional recovery was assessed using the staircase test, the cylinder test, and the modified neurological severity score (mNSS). Axonal plasticity and expression of brain-derived neurotrophic factor (BDNF) were determined in the contralateral motor cortex. TST and TST combined with 5-Aza-dC significantly improved the skilled reaching ability in the staircase test and ameliorated mNSS scores and cylinder test performance. TST and TST with 5-Aza-dC significantly increased the crossing fibers from the contralesional red nucleus, reticular formation in medullar oblongata, and dorsolateral spinal cord. Mature BDNF was significantly upregulated by TST and TST combined with 5-Azd-dC. Functional recovery after chronic stroke may involve axonal plasticity and increased mature BDNF by modulating DNA methylation in the contralesional cortex. Our results suggest that combined therapy to enhance axonal plasticity based on TST and 5-Aza-dC constitutes a promising approach for promoting the recovery of function in the chronic stage of stroke.

Keywords: stroke; chronic stage; task-specific training; DNA methylation; axonal plasticity; functional recovery; mature brain-derived neurotrophic factor

1. Introduction

Stroke is the most common cause of long-term adult disability [1]. There is currently no specific treatment for improving functional recovery after stroke, except during rehabilitation. It is well known that rehabilitation plays a pivotal role in the functional motor recovery of patients with stroke [2,3].

Neurological recovery culminates within 1–3 months after stroke. Most spontaneous recovery occurs up to six months after the condition [1–3]. The Copenhagen stroke study found that 80% of patients with stroke attain good neurological outcome within 4.5 weeks of stroke, with time profiles varying according to the initial post-stroke severity [4]. Therefore, an appropriate therapeutic period is very important for the restoration of function after stroke. Hence, there is a requirement for the improvement of effective therapeutic options that can enhance functional recovery in chronic stages after stroke.

One such promising therapy is specific behavioral experience (such as motor skill training after experimental brain injury), which provides functional benefits [5,6]. There is emerging evidence of the importance of task-specific training (TST) as a neuromotor intervention in neurological restoration [7,8]. TST can enhance experience-dependent motor skill learning and neural plastic changes in animal and human brain [7–9].

In addition, recent findings indicate a positive role of the contralesional hemisphere in the post-stroke recovery of upper extremity motor function [10]. Although motor cortex reorganization of the lesioned hemisphere is involved in post-stroke motor recovery and functions as a target of rehabilitation therapies, reorganization of the motor cortex in the contralateral hemisphere after stroke injury may represent an additional element of cortical reforming and related recovery [10]. Recent reports have demonstrated that the contralesional motor cortex plays an important role in functional recovery after stroke as a potential new target for rehabilitation in human and animal stroke models [5,11–13].

Ischemia leads to vast changes in gene expression [14–16]. The total levels of DNA methylation increase after ischemic damage and are strongly and directly related to the severity of brain injury [17,18]. Several researchers have expanded their investigations of the role of epigenetic mechanisms in ischemic stroke [19]. Epigenetic mechanisms, i.e., heritable changes in gene expression without changes in the DNA sequence [20], mainly include DNA methylation [14,21], histone modification [22], and microRNAs (miRNAs) [23,24], which specifically modulate the expression levels of single genes and functional gene networks [25,26].

Epigenetics is relevant for cellular response to ischemia. Epigenetic modifiers can influence diverse aspects of this response by altering transcriptional regulation in the ischemic disease process [14]. The transcriptional effects include diminution of cell damage, inhibition of inflammatory reactions, and advanced blood flow, as well as the restoration of mechanisms and enhancement of plasticity [14]. Neural-cell differentiation plasticity is regulated by cell-intrinsic epigenetic mechanisms and ischemic insults in the adult mammalian brain [19]. Furthermore, the targeting of epigenetic mechanisms may lead to the development of new therapeutic approaches for cerebral ischemia [19].

A recent study found that genes and proteins of brain-derived neurotrophic factor (BDNF), proBDNF and their processing enzymes such as tissue plasminogen activator (tPA), furin, and matrix metalloproteinases (MMPs) lead to up-regulation in cerebral ischemia [27]. Thus, this study has suggested that the stability of BDNF and proBDNF and their linked proteins may play a pivotal role in stroke recovery [27].

Therefore, the aims of this study were to implement a novel approach to chronic-phase stroke recovery. This study explored alterations in global DNA methylation from the acute to the chronic phase after stroke in the peri-infarct motor cortex and in the corresponding motor cortex region of the contralateral hemisphere. To develop a beneficial therapeutic protocol at late periods after stroke, task-specific training of the affected forelimb and regulation of DNA methylation were applied to ischemic injured rats. We examined the effects of these treatments on neuronal plasticity, stroke recovery, and neurotrophic factor production. This study will contribute to the development of a promising therapeutic strategy aimed at improving recovery from chronic stroke via TST and the control of DNA methylation in the contralesional cortex.

2. Results

2.1. Long-Term Post-Stroke Changes, Including Functional Outcome and Brain Injury

To confirm the effectiveness of rehabilitative therapies 2–3 months after a stroke, we assessed changes in infarction volume, motor function, and modified neurological severity score (mNSS) during the early-to-chronic phases after a severe stroke (post-stroke day 1 to week 12). Areas of infarction were noted in the striatum, motor cortex, and sensorimotor cortex. The infarct volumes are shown in Figure 1A. The mean values of the infarct volume in rats that received photothrombotic ischemia were

79.16 ± 5.16 mm³ (n = 6 per group) at day 1 and weeks 1, 2, 4, 6, 8, and 12 after a stroke. There was no significant difference in infarct volume between the time points ($p > 0.05$, Figure 1B). Motor outcome was evaluated in rats using modified neurological severity score (mNSS). A high score indicated that the rats suffered more neurological defects. Although the mNSS significantly decreased at 2 weeks after the stroke ($p < 0.01$, $n = 10$, Figure 1C), it remained unchanged thereafter (Figure 1C). Staircase tests showed that rats had a significantly impaired functional outcome at 12 weeks after stroke ($p < 0.001$, $n = 10$, Figure 1D). Ischemic injury resulted in a significant reduction in the number of pellets retrieved, when compared with control animals, there was no difference between the time points after stroke ($p > 0.05$, $n = 10$, Figure 1D).

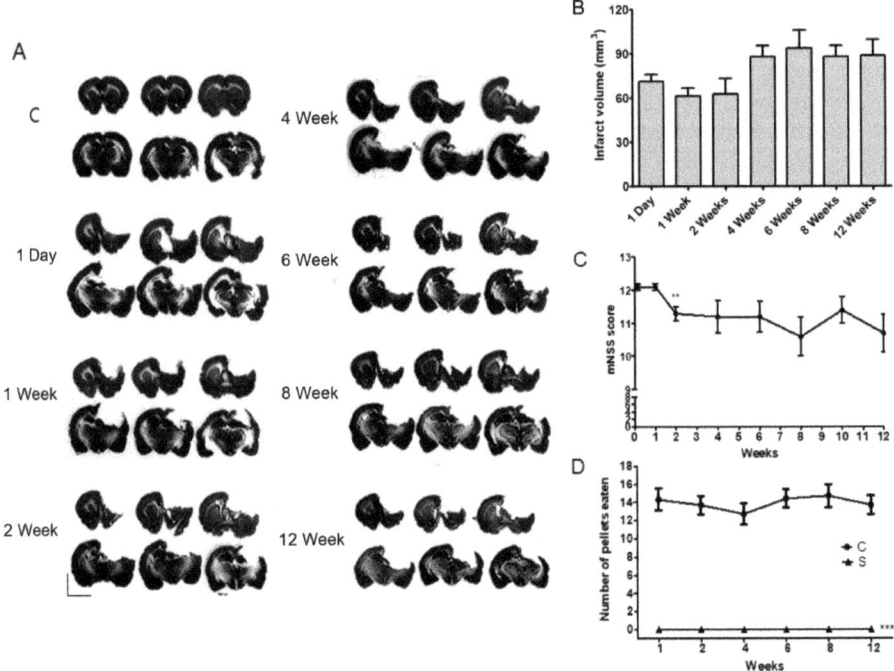

Figure 1. Evaluations of infarct volume and motor function from acute to chronic stages after a photothrombic ischemic stroke: (**A**) Representative photomicrography of Nissl-stained sections at several time points after a stroke; (**B**) Quantification of infarction size did not differ among time points after a photothrombic ischemic stroke (S). Results are presented as the mean ± SEM, $n = 6$; (**C**) while modified NSS levels were slightly improved at 2 weeks after a stroke, after then scores were continued until 12 weeks. Results are presented as the mean ± SEM, $n = 10$. ** $p < 0.01$ vs. 4 days after a stroke; (**D**) motor function impairment of the animals was maintained for 12 weeks after a stroke (S). Results of the staircase test are presented as the mean ± SEM, $n = 10$. *** $p < 0.001$ vs. sham control (C). Scale bars = 5 mm.

2.2. Increase in Contralateral and Ipsilateral DNA Methylation during the Chronic Phase after a Severe Stroke

Next, we confirmed the levels of global DNA methylation detected by 5-methylcytosine (5-mc) in the contralateral and ipsilateral cortices after a stroke. We found that the global DNA methylation levels were significantly increased 1 to 12 weeks (the chronic phase) after a stroke in both the contralateral cortex and the ipsilateral peri-infarct area, compared to the control ($p < 0.01$, $n = 6$, Figure 2). DNA methylation levels peaked at 1 week after a stroke in the contralateral and ipsilateral cerebral cortex. The DNA methylation levels, however, decreased at 2, 4, 8, and 12 weeks in the contralateral cortex and 4 and 8 weeks in the ipsilateral cortex compared with DNA methylation level of 1 week, respectively. The 5-mc level between the ipsilateral and the cortical cerebral cortex after a stroke was different 1 and 4 weeks after a stroke, but not significantly different between 8 and 12 weeks ($p < 0.05$, $n = 6$, Figure 2).

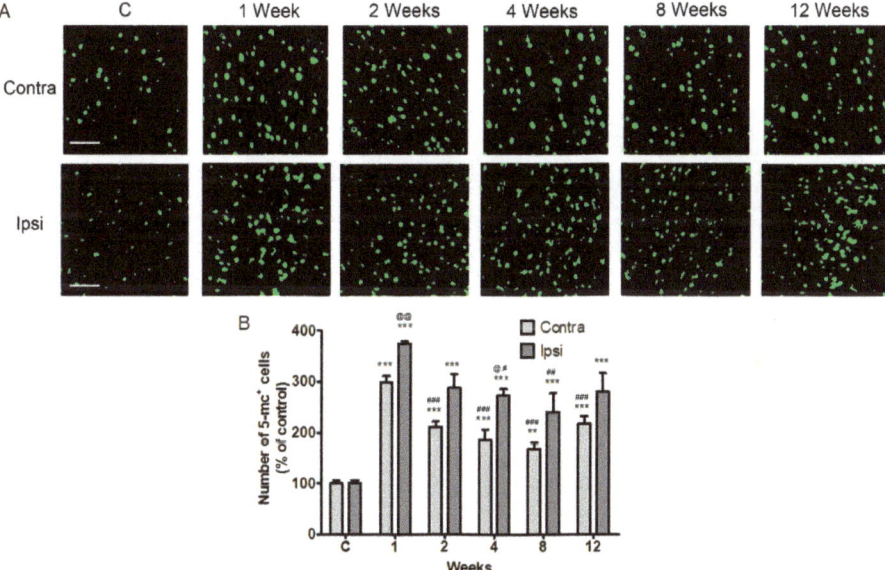

Figure 2. Localization of 5-methylcytosine (5-mc) in the contralesional and ipsilesional cortex after a stroke. (**A**) Fluorescent confocal microscopy shows that the 5-mc (green) is predominantly localized in the both the contralateral (contra) and ipsilateral (Ipsi) cortex from 1 week to 12 weeks after a stroke; (**B**) Quantification of 5-mc levels increased after a photothrombic ischemic stroke. Results are presented as the mean ± SEM, $n = 6$. ** $p < 0.01$; *** $p < 0.001$ vs sham control (**C**); # $p < 0.05$, ## $p < 0.01$, ### $p < 0.001$ vs. 1 day after stroke; @ $p < 0.05$, @@ $p < 0.01$ vs contralateral value at each time. Scale bars = 50 µm.

We hypothesized that regulation of contralateral DNA methylation levels and TST contributes to motor recovery in the chronic phase after a stroke. To assess the effects of TST and DNA methyltransferase (DNMT) inhibitor 5-Aza-2′-deoxycytidine (5-Aza-dC), we treated the contralesional cortex of rats, carrying a photothrombotic ischemic stroke unilateral lesion eight weeks after injury, with TST. A detailed timeline for the experiment is provided in Figure 3A. To address this hypothesis, we first confirmed the presence of changes in the levels of DNA methylation and in DNMT1, DNMT3a, and DNMT3b expression after 5-Aza-dC treatment of the contralateral cortex after a stroke. We found that the increased levels of 5-mc in neurons in the contralateral cortices of a stroke control group (S) and TST-treated stroke group (SR) decreased on 5-Aza-dC administration in 5-Aza-dC treated stroke group (SA) and TST and 5-AzadC treated stroke group (SAR) ($p < 0.001$, $n = 6$, Figure 3B,C). The levels of DNMT3a, DNMT3b, and DNMT1 in the contralesional cortex after a stroke ($p < 0.001$, $n = 6$, Figure 3D–G) significantly increased. These increased levels were downregulated in the SA and SAR groups ($p < 0.05$, $n = 6$, Figure 3D–G).

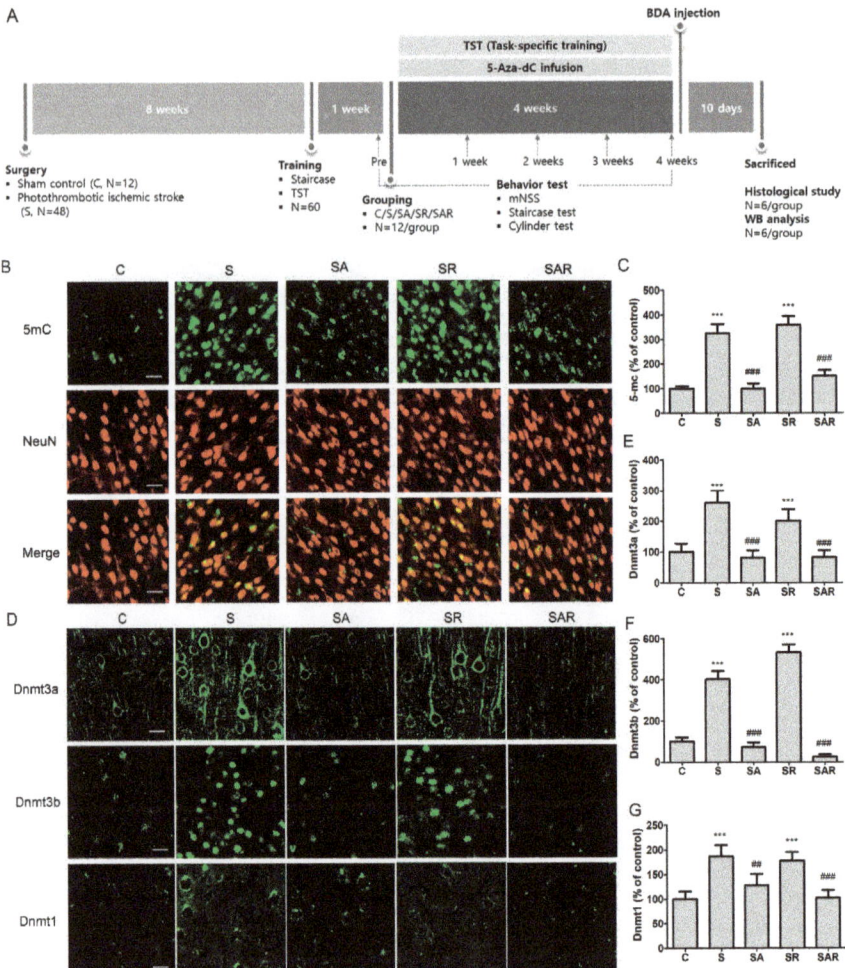

Figure 3. The timeline of the experiment and expressions of 5 mc, Dnmt3a, Dnmt3b, and Dnmt1 in the contralesional cortex after a stroke. (**A**) In a study on the effect of TST and DNMT inhibition on the functional recovery of chronic stroke, sham control (C) and stroke rats (S) with or without TST (SR) and with or without 5-Aza-dC (SA or SAR) were used for behavior test, neural plasticity, protein expression studies, and immunohistochemical analysis; (**B**) representative photomicrograph of 5-mc (green), NeuN (red) and co-localized merged cells (yellow) and (**D**) Dnmt3a, Dnmt3b, or Dnmt1 immunostaining in the contralesional cortex after stroke; (**C,E–G**) Counts of 5-mc, Dnmt3a, Dnmt3b, or Dnmt1 positive cells. Results are presented as the mean ± SEM, $n = 6$/group. *** $p < 0.001$ vs. C, ## $p < 0.01$; ### $p < 0.001$ vs. S, Scale bars = 20 µm.

2.3. Infarct Volume Was Not Altered by TST with or without 5-Aza-dc in the Chronic Phase after Severe Stroke

To determine the effects of TST and 5-Aza-dC on ischemic injury, we examined infarction volume using Nissl staining. Infarct volume in the SR, SA, and SAR groups did not differ from that observed in the stroke control group (S) ($p = 0.895$, $n = 6$, Figure 4A,B).

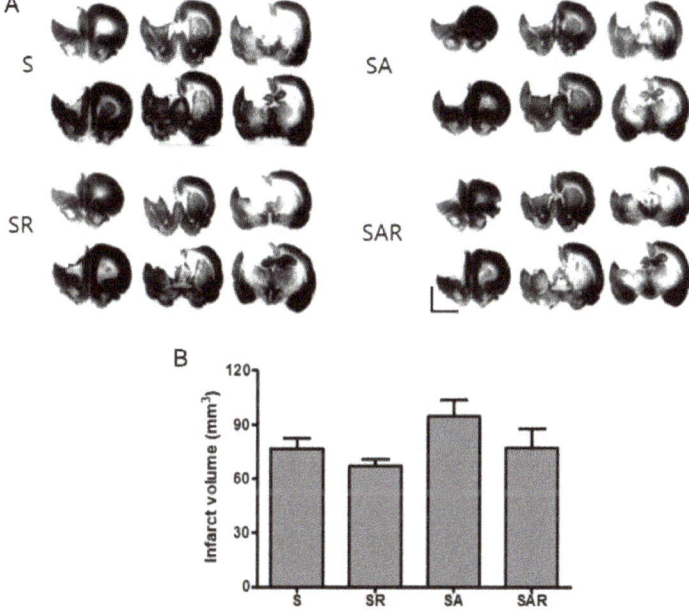

Figure 4. Effects of TST and 5-Aza-dC treatment on infarct volume after photothrombic ischemic stroke (**A**) Representative photomicrography of Nissl-stained sections four weeks after post-stroke treatment; (**B**) Quantification of infarction size did not differ in treatment groups after photothrombic ischemic stroke. Results are presented as the mean ± SEM, $n = 6$. Scale bars = 5 mm.

2.4. 5-Aza-dC Combined with TST Treatment Improved the Recovery of Motor Function on the Chronic Phase after Severe Stroke

To determine the effects of TST and 5-Aza-dC on functional recovery after a chronic stroke, we examined motor recovery and neurological function using the Montoya staircase test, mNSS, and cylinder test (Figure 5).

2.4.1. Montoya Staircase Test

The Montoya staircase test is used to assess the recovery of reaching and grasping skills, impaired by severe stroke. The lab animals were given 18 food pellets, and the number of pellets consumed was determined. Figure 5A shows the results of successful reaches throughout the course of the experiment. The reaching success was measured as the number of pellets retrieved and eaten by the paw contralateral to the lesion. A repeated-measures two-way ANOVA detected significant effects of group ($F_{4,55} = 140.8$; $p < 0.001$) and time ($F_{2,55} = 17.45$; $p < 0.001$), and a significant interaction between group and time ($F_{8,112} = 7.097$; $p < 0.001$). The stroke control group (S) exhibited profound impairment in reaching success ($p < 0.001$, $n = 12$, Figure 5A). The SR group, which received TST after stroke, and the SAR group, which received TST and 5-Aza-dC after stroke, exhibited significant improvement, compared to the S group ($p < 0.001$, $n = 12$, Figure 5A). The SAR group exhibited a more-pronounced improvement in performance compared to the SR group ($p < 0.01$, $n = 12$, Figure 5A). No differences were observed between the S and the SA group, which only received 5-Aza-dC.

2.4.2. mNSS

The SR and SAR groups exhibited significant amelioration in mNSS, compared to the S group at four weeks after a stroke. A repeated-measures two-way ANOVA detected significant effects of time ($F_{3,44} = 33.38$; $p < 0.001$) and interaction between group and time ($F_{6,88} = 2.944$; $p < 0.05$). At four weeks after a stroke, there was a pronounced improvement in the groups that underwent TST (SR) and TST combined with 5-Aza-dC (SAR) ($p < 0.05$, $n = 12$) (Figure 5B).

2.4.3. Cylinder Test

The decreased usage of the impaired paw ameliorated in the SR and SAR groups at four weeks after a stroke (Figure 5C). ANOVA detected a significant main effect of group ($F_{4,55} = 9.228$; $p < 0.001$).

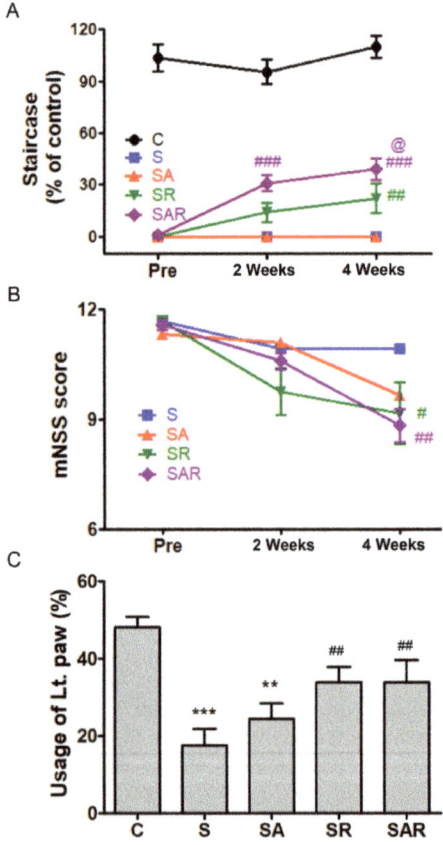

Figure 5. Recovery of motor function on treatment with TST and 5-Azd-dC after a photothrombotic chronic stroke. TST and TST combined with 5-Aza-dC treatment helped improve recovery of motor function after stroke; the staircase test (**A**) and mNSS (**B**), usage scores of damaged limb (**C**). TST combined with 5-Aza-dC enhanced motor recovery in the treated group, as shown in the staircase test performance (**A**). Pre-indicated 1 day before rehabilitation after a stroke. ** $p < 0.01$; *** $p < 0.001$ vs. C (sham control), # $p < 0.05$; ## $p < 0.01$, ### $p < 0.001$ vs. S (Stroke). @ $p < 0.05$ vs. SR (TST treated stroke). Results are presented as the mean ± SEM, $n = 12$/group. Lt. paw: impaired left paw.

2.5. Aza-dC Treatment with TST Enhanced the Neuronal Plasticity of Motor Pathways

The corticospinal tract (CST) was labeled with biotinylated dextran amine tracer (BDA) via injection into the contralesional side of the motor cortex, and labeled CST axon fibers sprouting from descending fibers in the non-ischemic side of the red nucleus (RN), medullary reticular formation (RF), pyramid, and cervical spinal cord were examined [28]. The location of the BDA injections produced no major differences between groups and the density of CST fibers showed no differences between groups before stroke in our previous study [5]. First, we examined whether TST and 5-Aza-dC treatment in stroke rats influenced the formation of CST fibers. Tracing of the CST revealed that the number of crossing fibers from the contralesional RN was significantly increased in the SR and SAR groups (Figure 6B). The quantitative data showed the presence of significant increases in the mean number of crossing fibers in the RN of the SR and SAR groups after stroke, by 251.32% ± 8.37% and 288.93% ± 24.69% compared with the stroke (S) group, respectively ($p < 0.05$, $n = 6$, Figure 6B); in contrast, significant decrease was observed in the SA group after stroke ($p < 0.05$, $n = 6$, Figure 6B). The SAR group showed an enhancement in the number of crossing fibers compared with the SR group ($p < 0.001$, $n = 6$, Figure 6B). Next, we quantified the number of BDA-labeled CST fibers that crossed the midline toward the ischemic side in the RF (Figure 6C). The crossing fibers from the pyramidal to RF in the medulla were increased. Regarding the crossing fibers, a statistical analysis using one-way ANOVA revealed that BDA-labeled fibers significantly increased after treatment with TST and 5-Aza-dC combined with TST, by 146.18% ± 9.20% and 197.84% ± 7.45% compared with the stroke (S) group, respectively ($p < 0.001$, $n = 6$, Figure 6C). The number of these fibers in the SAR group was significantly higher than that observed in the SR group after stroke ($p < 0.001$, $n = 6$, Figure 6C). The fibers in the dorsolateral parts of the spinal cord (dlCST) was increased in the SR and SAR group after stroke, by 166.68% ± 9.30% and 221.68% ± 9.83% compared with the stroke (S) group, respectively ($p < 0.01$, $n = 6$, Figure 6D). The CST fibers in ipsilateral gray matter that came from dorsal CST were enhanced in the SR and SAR groups, by 150.60% ± 16.22% and 225.08% ± 9.78% compared with the stroke (S) group, respectively ($p < 0.01$, $n = 6$, Figure 6E).

2.6. The Level of Mature Brain-Derived Neurotrophic Factor (BDNF) in the Contralateral Cortex Was Increased by 5-Aza-dc Combined with TST Treatment

To determine whether the expression and maturation of BDNF were affected by TST and 5-Aza-dC treatment and enhanced contralateral neuronal plasticity after stroke, we immunoblotted protein extracts from contralesional cortical tissues. The pro-brain-derived neurotrophic factor (proBDNF) levels in the contralesional side were increased in the S and SR groups compared with the control ($p < 0.001$, Figure 7A,B). However, mature BDNF (mBDNF) levels were higher in the S, SR, SA, and SAR groups compared with the control ($p < 0.001$, $n = 6$, Figure 7A,C). The SR and SAR groups exhibited an enhancement in mBDNF expression compared with the S group (Figure 7A,C). Mature BDNF levels were significantly higher in the SAR vs. the SR group (Figure 7A,C). Next, we examined the effects of TST and 5-Aza-dC on the expression of intracellular (furin) and extracellular tissue plasminogen activator (tPA) proteases that are involved in proBDNF processing in the brain. Furin and tPA expression in the contralesional cortex was significantly increased in the S, SR, SA, and SAR groups ($p < 0.05$, $n = 6$, Figure 7A,D,E) after stroke. We also measured and compared the ratios of furin or tPA and proBDNF among the groups. The ratio of furin to proBDNF was significantly increased in the S, SR, SA, and SAR groups. The ratio observed in the SAR group was higher than that detected in the S or SR groups ($p < 0.001$, $n = 6$, Figure 7F). The ratio of tPA to proBDNF was higher in the SR, SA, and SAR groups compared to the control group. The SA and SAR groups exhibited a significant increase in the ratio vs the SR group ($p < 0.01$; $p < 0.001$, $n = 6$, Figure 7G).

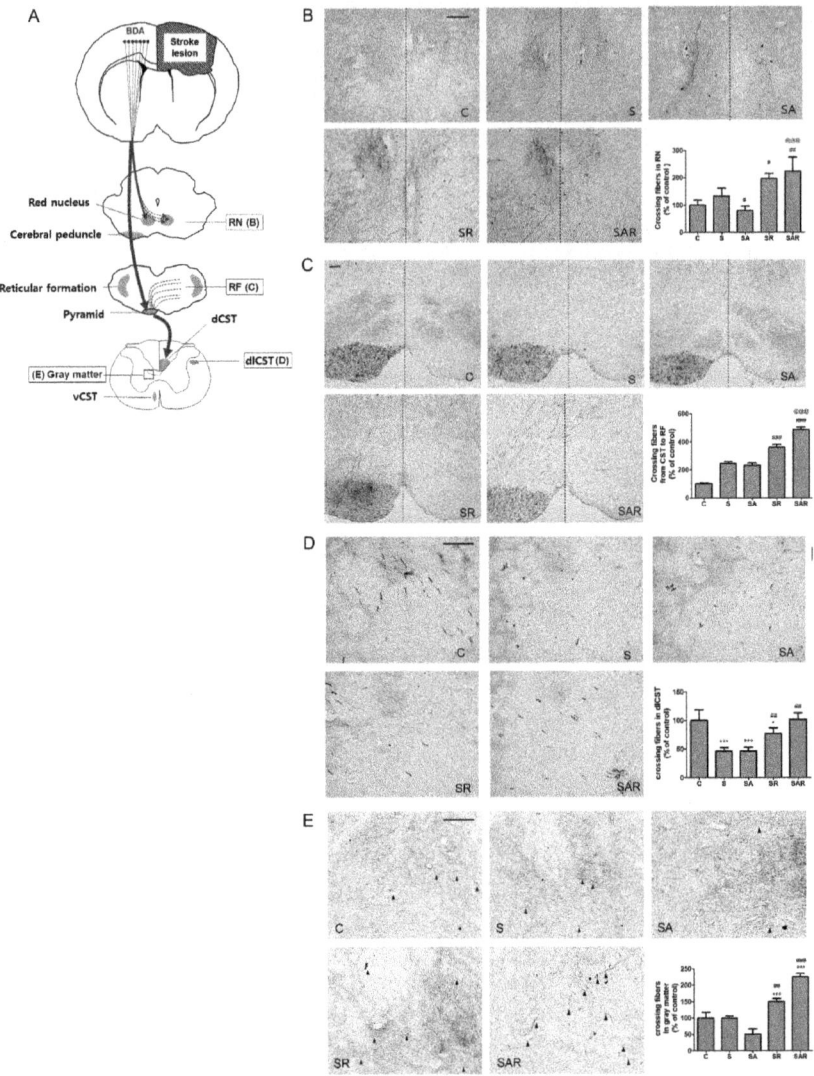

Figure 6. Task-specific training (TST) and TST combined with 5-Aza-C treatment promote contralesional CST plasticity in chronic stroke. (**A**) Schematic illustration of CST including contralesional red nucleus (RN), reticular formation (RF) in medullar oblongata, dorsolateral spinal tract (dlCST) and ipsilesional gray matter in the spinal cord. Solid square boxes indicate analysis area for CST plasticity in this study; (**B**–**E**) photomicrographs of BDA staining in the contralesional RN, RF in medullar oblongata, dlCST and ipsilesional gray matter in spinal cord sections. (**B**,**C**) Broken lines in RN and RF indicate the midline of the midbrain; (**E**) midline-crossing fibers indicate black arrowheads. dCST: dorsal CST; dlCST: dorsolateral CST; vCST: ventral CST. Scale bars = 50 μm. Mean density of BDA-positive axonal crossing fibers in the RN (**B**), RF (**C**), dlCST (**D**), and gray matter of spinal cord (**E**) shown as% increase of sham control (**C**). Results are presented as the mean ± SEM in the graphs. $n = 6$. Significance is indicated by * $p < 0.05$; *** $p < 0.001$ vs. sham control (C), # $p < 0.05$; ## $p<0.01$; ### $p < 0.001$ vs. Stroke (S), @@@ $p < 0.001$ vs. SR.

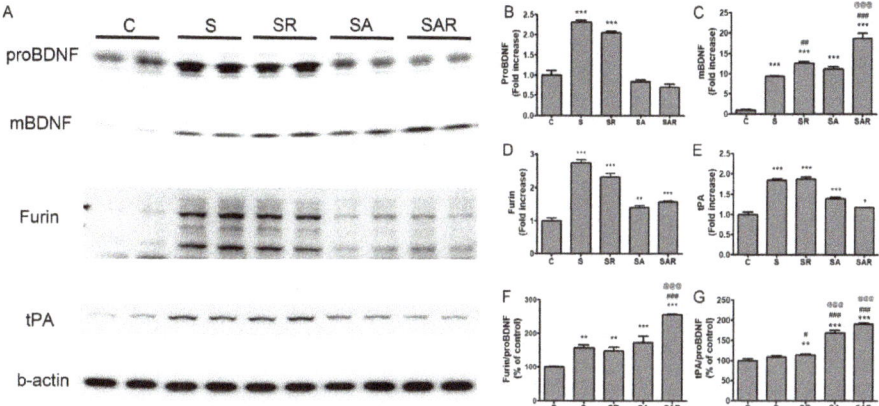

Figure 7. Effect of TST and TST combined with 5-Aza-dC treatment on the expression of mature BDNF in protein extracts of contralesional cortex after stroke. (**A**) Representative photomicrographs of western blots for pro-brain-derived neurotrophic factor (proBDNF), mature BDNF (mBDNF), furin, tissue plasminogen activator (tPA), and β-actin in total lysates of the contralesional cortex at 4 w after post-stroke treatment. (**B–E**) Signal intensities of proBDNF, mBDNF, furin and tPA were measured using Quantity One software and are shown as a percentage of control. (**F,G**) Signal intensities of the ratio of furin to proBDNF and tPA to proBDNF are shown as a percentage of control. Beta-actin, internal control. Results are presented as the mean ± SE, $n = 6$. * $p < 0.05$; ** $p < 0.01$; *** $p < 0.001$ vs. C, # $p < 0.05$; ## $p < 0.01$; ### $p < 0.001$ vs. S, @@@ $p < 0.001$ vs. SR.

3. Discussion

In the present study, we confirmed the effects of TST and inhibition of contralesional DNA methylation on functional outcome, neuronal plasticity, and expression of axonal-growth-enhancing molecules (such as BDNF) in the chronic stage after stroke in a rat model. Although the beneficial effects of TST with affected forelimb and inhibition of ipsilateral DNA methylation have been suggested for the acute stage of stroke, it is uncertain whether TST and the regulation of contralesional DNA methylation have any positive effects on the chronic stage of ischemic stroke. Several studies have demonstrated that rehabilitative training, such as TST, plays beneficial roles in improving motor performance at the acute or subacute stage after stroke [5,7,8,29]. Roles of epigenetics in cerebral ischemia have also been reported, as inhibiting histone deacetylase 2 (HDAC2) promotes functional recovery [30,31] and protection against ischemic insult by inhibiting DNA methylation after treatment with a DNA methyltransferase (DNMT) inhibitor, 5-aza-2′-deoxycytidine (5-Aza-dC) [17,18,20].

Our results demonstrated that TST and TST combined with 5-Aza-dC treatment enhanced behavioral performance, as assessed using the modified neurological severity score, the staircase test, and the cylinder test. In particular, significant differences were observed in the staircase test after stroke between the TST-treated group and the TST combined with 5-Aza-dC-treated group. These findings suggest that motor recovery is enhanced to a greater extent by the inhibition of DNA methylation combined with TST than it is by TST alone. Therefore, epigenetic regulation after stroke may enhance improvement in motor function provided by TST at the chronic stage.

Neuronal network reorganization is a major mechanism that is used to maintain neuronal functions after brain injury [28]. The reorganization of the neural network after a stroke leads to recovery from functional deficits in the remaining areas [32,33]. The motor cortex of the undamaged side may have a supplementary function that restores lost motor functions [33,34].

Axonal sprouting occurs mainly after stroke in the peri-infarct cortex, near the site of stroke. Furthermore, axonal sprouting appears to arise from the contralateral cortex to the ipsilateral RN and the cervical spinal cord [33,35,36]. After severe strokes, plastic alterations are observed from the unaffected cortex to subcortical efferent projections of the corticospinal tract (CST) [33,35]. New CST axons sprout into the lesional subcortical areas at multiple levels of the brain and spinal cord [37]. The process of enhanced axonal sprouting involves axonal growth and promotes functional recovery after stroke [33,37].

TST is normally used in patients with chronic stroke [7]. Axonal remodeling is accepted as one of the components of TST-induced functional recovery and has been detected in parts of the CST [7]. Several studies of the beneficial effect of TST on functional recovery after injury have reported that rehabilitative training induces the growth of saved CST axons and the projection of new axons into the damaged spinal cord, subsequently contributing to motor recovery [8,29,38,39]. Our previous research demonstrated that early TST after stroke enhanced the contralesional plasticity of the CSTs in motor cortical and sensorimotor cortical lesions at the acute stage after stroke [5]. A recent report showed that the number of CST axonal fibers sprouting from the non-ischemic hemisphere was increased in the ipsilateral medullary reticular formation and cervical spinal cord after middle cerebral artery occlusion in rats [28].

In this study, the data showed that the number of crossing fibers from the unaffected side to the RN and medullary reticular formation in the affected side was significantly increased by TST and TST combined with 5-Aza-dC treatment after stroke. The number of spinal cord fibers located in the dlCST and the number of crossing fibers in the gray matter was increased by TST combined with 5-Aza-dC treatment after stroke. Taken together with previous reports, our data suggest that regulation of DNA methylation in the contralesional cortex positively contributes to the enhancement of neuronal plasticity afforded by TST of the affected forelimb in motor recovery at the chronic phase after stroke.

Post-stroke motor recovery involves regaining and relearning skills and is related to neural plasticity [40]. Although various molecular signaling pathways are engaged in neural plasticity and recovery after stroke, BDNF signaling has emerged as a key player in these processes [40]. The activity-dependent upregulation of BDNF contributes to the minimization of the extent of cell death during both the acute phase (hours to days) and the subacute phase (days to weeks), thus promoting plasticity and improving function [41]. Previous reports have demonstrated that exercise [40,42,43], environment enrichment [44,45], and neuronal pharmacotherapy [46–48] after stroke mediate neuroplastic changes through the expression of BDNF in the contralateral and ipsilateral hemispheres [49]. Cerebral ischemia in rats led to the upregulation of the BDNF precursor protein (proBDNF), mature BDNF (mBDNF), and their processing enzymes, such as furin and prohormone convertases, in the intracellular milieu, and matrix metalloproteinases (MMPs) or plasmin in the extracellular milieu [27,50]. The mBDNF protein (converted from proBDNF) is mainly involved in the promotion of functional recovery after ischemia [27,51–53].

Our data showed that the expression of mBDNF was significantly increased by TST and TST combined with 5-Aza-dC treatment after stroke. The expression of proBDNF-converting enzymes, such as tPA and furin, was also increased by TST combined with 5-Aza-dC treatment. These results suggest that the inhibition of DNA methylation by 5-Aza-dC treatment might alter the production of mBDNF via the regulation of the expression of tPA or furin.

On the other hand, 5-Aza-dC treatment alone after stroke did not show protective effects. Effect of 5-Aza-dC may be different between control-contralateral cortex and TST-treated contralateral cortex. TST-induced microenvironmental status after stroke may differ from stroke without TST. 5-Aza-dC treatment in the contralateral cortex after an ischemic stroke may provide a supportive microenvironment for the repairing process promoted by TST [54].

Therefore, the overall data generated in this study suggest that TST with an affected forelimb at the chronic phase after severe stroke plays a beneficial role in functional recovery via neuronal plastic changes, enhanced proBDNF expression, and mBDNF production in the contralesional cortex. Those effects were significantly enhanced by additional inhibition of DNA methylation in the contralateral motor cortex after a stroke, and were mediated by increased CST plasticity and mBDNF products (via the upregulation of tPA and furin enzymes).

4. Materials and Methods

4.1. Animals

A total of 142 male Wistar rats (8 weeks of age, weighing 283.88 ± 2.06 g; Orent Bio Inc., Seongnam, Korea; 24 sham control rats (C) and 118 photothrombotic-stroke rats, Stroke) were used. The study animals were exposed to a temperature-controlled room (23 ± 0.5 °C) with 12-h light/dark cycle. All experimental procedures were approved by the Animal Experiment Review Board of Institutional Animal Care and Use Committee (IACUC) of Konkuk University (Permit Number: KU17042, licensed on 21 March 2017). Animal care, including anesthesia and euthanasia, was performed in accordance with the Principle of Laboratory Animal Care (NIH publication No. 85-23, revised 1985). The authors also followed the criteria for Stroke Therapy Academic Industry Roundtable (STAIR) for preclinical stroke investigations [55].

4.2. Photothrombotic Ischemia Surgery

The cerebral cortical infarct was made by projecting light onto the sensory motor and motor cortex after Rose Bengal treatment. To briefly summarize the method, the rats were anesthetized with a mixture of ketamine (50 mg/kg) and xylazine (5 mg/kg) After intraperitoneal (ip) injection, the animals were anesthetized and placed in a fixed bed frame (Stoelting Co., Wood Dale, IL, USA). The skull was exposed and a fiber bundle of 4 mm caliber KL1500 LCD cold light source (Carl Zeiss, Jena, Germany) was placed in the bregma of the skull and placed 4.0 mm lateral to the midline of the right sensory motor. Photochemical dye Rose Bengal (Sigma-Aldrich, St. Louis, MO, USA) was infused via i.p. injection. After injection for 5 min (20 mg/kg), the light was switched on for 30 min. Sham control animals were exposed to light for 30 min without the injection of Rose Bengal.

4.3. Animal Grouping

In the temporal change study conducted on 80 rats, 70 underwent photothrombotic ischemic stroke surgery and 70 survivors were equally distributed to 1 day, 1 week, 2, 4, 6, 8, and 12 weeks after stroke (n = 10 rats/group). Ten sham control rats were treated similarly to the operated rats, except for exposure to light source. In the rehabilitation therapy study, 48 rats were subjected to photothrombic stroke. After 4 weeks, 24 rats were injected with 5-Aza-dC (10 μg/day, Sigma-Aldrich, St. Louis, MO, USA) using osmotic minipump. After 3 days, 12 rats of the 24 stroke rats and 12 rats of 5-Aza-dC treated stroke rats were provided task-specific training (TST). Twelve stroke rats and 12 sham control rats were not treated with 5-Azd-dC or TST. All experimental groups were randomly allocated to the following treatment groups: sham control (C, n = 12), stroke control (S, n = 12), TST-treated stroke rats (SR, n = 12), 5-Aza-d-C treated stroke rats (SA, n = 12), TST and 5-Aza-dC cotreated stroke rats (SAR, n = 12). Animals were number-coded and investigators were blinded to the treatment groups until the end of data analysis.

4.4. Infusion of 5-Aza-dC in Contralateral Motor Cortex

5-Aza-dC (10 μg/day) was delivered to the contralesional hemisphere sensorimotor cortex using osmotic pump system for 28 days. Osmotic minipumps (0.25 μg/h, 200 μL volume, model 2004, Alzet, Cupertino, CA, USA) filled with 10 mg 5-Aza-dC in 3% DMSO solution 200 μL placed into 15 mL conical tubes containing 0.9% saline were primed at 37 °C incubator 2 days before the implantation surgery. Animals were anesthetized with ketamine (50 mg/kg) and xylazine (5 mg/kg) mixed cocktail through intraperitoneal (i.p.) injection then their head were fixed at a stereotaxic frame (Stoelting Co., Wood Dale, IL, USA). The skull was exposed and the cannula (Brain infusion kit3, Alzet, Cupertino, CA, USA), which is connected to osmotic pump through tube, was implanted on the sensorimotor cortex of the contralesional hemisphere (ML 2, AP 0.5, DV-2). Screws (2 mm diameter) were anchored onto the skull to secure the implantation; dental cement (Poly-F standard kit, Dentsply, York, PA, USA) then covered the skull. Osmotic minipumps were placed subcutaneously on the back of each rat.

4.5. Task-Specific Training

Nine weeks after induction of photo-thrombotic stroke, animals were implanted with osmotic pump delivering 5-Aza-dC. It took 3 days to recover from the surgery; rehabilitation training then begun. Animals were randomized to the following treatment groups: sham control (C, $n = 12$), stroke control (S, $n = 12$), stroke with task-specific training (TST) (SR, $n = 12$), stroke with 5-aza-d-C (SA, $n = 12$), stroke with TST combined with 5-aza-dC (SAR, $n = 12$). The task-specific training was performed as described previously for 4 weeks [55].

4.6. Staircase Test

The training began from 8 weeks after surgery and the animals received daily handling for 1 week. They were feed restricted for 2 weeks during staircase training (two trials per day, 15 min each) and their weight was checked every day; body weight was not under 85% of start weight. Animals were trained to reach for feed pellets in the modified staircase apparatus (three pellets per step with 6 steps on each side) according to previously published research [55]. The total number of pellets eaten was counted. The performance score was calculated using the following formula: the number of pellets eaten/total number of pellets.

4.7. Modified Neurological Severity Score

Animals were examined with modified neurological severity score (mNSS) one day prior to rehabilitation, and 1, 2, 3 and 4 weeks after rehabilitation. This evaluation was performed by a blinded tester. mNSS consists of motor, sensory, reflex and balance test. Scores ranged from 0 to maximum 14. mNSS was performed as described previously.

4.8. Cylinder Test (Asymmetrical Forelimb Use)

The animals were placed in a transparent Plexiglas cylinder (diameter 20 mm) placed on a glass plate and videotaped with a camcorder from below. Single (ipsilateral and contralateral) and bilateral forelimb wall contacts were recorded for 5 min (or until more than 15 wall contacts were observed). Contralateral forelimb use was expressed as follows: ([contralateral forelimb contacts + 0.5 × bilateral forelimb contacts]/total number of forelimb contacts) × 100 [5]. Animals were tested several times before and after recovery therapy.

4.9. Video Recording

Filming was performed 1 day before rehabilitation after photothrombotic ischemia, and 1, 2, 3, and 4 weeks of training or 5-Aza-dC treatment using a Sony HDR-CX350 Handycam (Tokyo, Japan). The animals were filmed from frontal and ventral viewpoints. The tapes were viewed on a Sony DV cam HDR-CX350 player. Representative movements were captured by GOM Player v2.3 (Seoul, South Korea) using a Windows 10 computer.

4.10. Nissle Staining

The rats ($n = 6$/group) were deeply anesthetized with a mixture of ketamine (50 mg/kg) and xylazine (5 mg/kg) (ip) followed by saline containing 0.5% sodium nitrite and 10 U/mL heparin sulfate. After perfusion, the brains were perfused with cold fixative solution of 0.1 M PBS (pH 7.2) containing 4% formaldehyde, and the brains were postfixed overnight in the same solution and infiltrated with 30% sucrose. Using a cryostat, a floating section (40 μm) from bregma −5.2 to 2.2 mm was obtained and the section was mounted on a glass slide and stained with Nissl [56].

4.11. Measurement of Infarct Volume

Using Nissl stained sections, the infarct volume (total cortex and posterior cortex) was quantified using image analysis software (Image J v1.3 (Bethesda, MD, USA), NIH) to calibrate cerebral edema according to the following formula: CIV = (LHA − RHA − RIA) × Thickness, CIV is the corrected infarct volume, LHA is the left hemisphere, RHA is the right hemisphere, RIA is the right hemisphere infarct area. The total infarct size was estimated using the corrected infarct area and the width between individual brain slices [56].

4.12. CST Projections Using Biotinylated Dextran Amine

The anterograde tract tracer biotinylated dextran amine (BDA) was used to evaluate pyramidal tract plasticity contralateral of stroke in rats subjected to permanent focal cerebral ischemia [55]. One percent of BDA was stereotaxically injected into the motor cortex at 4 weeks after post-rehabilitation treatment in photothrombotic ischemic rats ($n = 6$/group). Ten days after BDA injection (at 4 weeks after rehabilitation), the rats were deeply anesthetized (ketamine and xylazine mixture 30 mg/kg, i.p.) and placed in a rat stereotaxic apparatus. BDA was then injected into contralateral site in the motor cortex (coordinate: AP, −1.5, 0, 0.5, 1, 1.5, 2, 2.5 mm; ML 1.5, 2.0, 1.8, 2.5, 2.5, 2.5, 3 mm; dorsoventral (DV), −1.5 mm). Each injection of BDA in 1 μL ice-cold sterilized phosphate buffered saline was used in every animal. The injection rate was 0.2 μL/min, and the syringe was kept in place for an additional 5 min before being retracted slowly. Thus, BDA was visualized by immunohistostaining.

4.13. Immunohistochemistry

Forty-μm-thick coronal cryosections of the brain were selected, each comprising six sections, including the red nucleus (RN) and pyramid (−8.72 to −11.60 mm at AP), and the spinal cord (SP) to detect BDA labeling. Briefly, free-floating sections were incubated with 0.3% H_2O_2 in 0.1 M phosphate-buffered saline (PBS, pH 7.4) for 20 min, washed with 0.1 M PBS, then incubated in 0.1 M PBS containing 5% normal horse serum and 0.3% Triton X-100 for 1 h. The sections were incubated with avidin–biotin–peroxidase complex (Vector Laboratories, Burlingame, CA, USA) in PBS/Triton X-100 at 4 °C for 3 days and BDA labeling was achieved with 0.05% 3,3′-diaminobenzidine and 0.003% H_2O_2 (Vector Laboratories) before light microscopy examination [5].

4.14. Western Blot Analysis

The contralesional cortices washed with PBS was lysed with RIPA buffer (50 mM Tris-HCl pH 7.4, 150 mM NaCl, 1% NP40, 0.25% Na-deoxycholate, and 0.1% SDS) containing a protease inhibitor mixture and phosphatase inhibitors (Sigma-Aldrich, St. Louis, MO, USA). (BDNF, tPA, furin: Santa Cruz (R)) was added to SDS-PAGE and electroporated into Polyvinylidene fluoride membrane. Thirty micrograms of soluble protein were subjected to SDS–PAGE and electrotransferred onto a PVDF membrane. Specific protein bands were detected using specific antibodies (BDNF, tPA, furin: Santa Cruz biotechnology, Inc., Dallas, TX, USA, and β-actin: Sigma-Aldrich, St. Louis, MO, USA) and enhanced chemiluminescence (Pierce, Rockford, IL, USA) [55].

4.15. Double-Fluorescence Immunostaining of Tissues

Free-floating sections (40 μm) were incubated in 0.1 M PBS containing 5% normal donkey serum and 0.3% Triton X-100 for 1 h, and subsequently incubated overnight with specific primary antibodies (NeuN: Millipore, Burlington, MA, USA, 5-mc: Active Motif, Carlsbad, CA, USA, Dnmt3a, Dnmt3b, and Dnmt 1: Santa Cruz biotechnology, Inc., Dallas, TX, USA) in 2% normal donkey serum (Vector Laboratories, Burlingame, CA, USA) in PBS at 4 °C and incubated with a 1:200 dilution of Alexa Fluor-conjugated donkey anti-rabbit (488) or donkey anti-mouse (546) antibodies (Invitrogen, Grand Island, NY, USA) for 1 h at room temperature and mounted on glass slides using Vectashield

(Vector Laboratories, Burlingame, CA, USA). Fluorescent signals were evaluated on a confocal microscope (LSM 710, Carl Zeiss, Oberkochen, Germany) [55].

4.16. Quantitative Analysis

The cortex sections from 6 rats per group were subjected to analysis. Five regions of interest (ROIs) of 0.1 mm^2 per one section were selected. The number of NeuN, 5 mc, DNMT1, DNMT3a, and DNMT3b-positive cells was counted in each ROI and averaged. Data are represented as the percentage of total cells. All quantitative analyses were carried out in a blind manner [55].

4.17. Analysis of CST Projections

Images were captured and analyzed with Axio Vision using a CCD camera (Jena, Germany) attached to an inverted light microscope with 10× or 20× objectives (Carl Zeiss, Jena, Germany). The mean account of the axonal fibers was quantified by an observer who was blind to the grouping using an automated program wizard, i.e., the "measurement" plug-in of Axio Vision. Objects of interest (fibers) were selected using the segmentation command. Artifacts were deleted manually from the selected group of objects. The number of crossing axonal fiber (μm^2) was measured based on the total area of a captured image. Five captured images were analyzed for each group.

4.18. Data Analysis and Statistics

The staircase test and mNSS was analyzed using a two-way repeated-measures analysis of variance (ANOVA), followed by a post hoc least significant differences multiple comparisons test. A one-way ANOVA was used to compare the infarct volume, cylinder test, intensity of Western blot results, cell counts after immunostaining, and counts of crossing fibers among groups. This statistical analysis comprised a one-way ANOVA followed by a Newman–Keuls multiple comparisons test. All data were expressed as the mean ± standard error. Null hypotheses of no differences were rejected if $p < 0.05$. All data analyses were performed using the SPSS version 22.0 software (IBM Corporation, New York, NY, USA).

5. Conclusions

This study demonstrated the beneficial role of TST in motor recovery in the chronic stage after stroke. Moreover, it showed that inhibition of DNA methylation in the contralesional cortex combined with TST enhanced motor function. The combination of contralesional inhibition of DNA methylation and TST with an affected limb may be especially effective for improving motor function after stroke, even if the initiation of rehabilitation occurs during a late phase. Enhanced axonal plasticity in the contralesional corticospinal tract, including the RN, pyramid, and spinal cord, is involved in motor recovery. The molecular mechanism underlying this axonal remodeling may rely on mature BDNF production induced by TST combined with inhibition of DNA methylation after stroke. Further studies are needed to elucidate the changes in molecule-specific DNA methylation induced by treatment with 5-Aza-dC in the contralateral motor cortex after stroke. Therefore, combined therapy of TST and 5-Aza-dC after stroke may constitute a promising therapy for promoting the recovery of function in the chronic stage of stroke.

Author Contributions: D.-H.C., H.Y.K. and J.L. conceived and designed the experiments; I.-A.C. and C.S.L. performed the experiments; D.-H.C. analyzed the data; I.-A.C., C.S.L. and D.-H.C. contributed reagents/materials/analysis tools; I.-A.C. and D.-H.C. wrote the paper.

Acknowledgments: This research was supported by the Basic Science Research Program through the National Research Foundation of Korea (NRF) funded by the Ministry of Science, Information and Communications Technology (ICT) and Future Planning (NRF-2014R1A2A1A11050236 grant to DHC, NRF-2014R1A2A1A11050248 and NRF-2017R1A2B4004837 grant to JL); and the National Research Foundation of Korea (NRF) grant funded by the Korean government (NRF-2016R1A5A2012284).

Conflicts of Interest: The authors declare no conflict of interest.

Abbreviations

TST	Task specific training
DNMTs	DNA methyltransferases
5-mc	5-methylcytosine
mNSS	Modified neurological severity score
5-Aza-dC	5-aza-2′-deoxycytidine
C	Sham Control group
S	Stroke group
SA	5-Aza-dC treated stroke group
SR	TST treated stroke group
SAR	5-Aza-dC combined with TST treated stroke group
ANOVA	Analysis of variance
RN	Red nucleus
RF	Reticular formation
CST	Corticospinal tract
BDA	Biotinylated dextran amine
dlCST	Dorsolateral parts of the spinal cord
Pro-BDNF	Pro-brain-derived neurotrophic factor
mBDNF	Mature BDNF
t-PA	Tissue plasminogen activator

References

1. Ovbiagele, B.; Nguyen-Huynh, M.N. Stroke epidemiology: Advancing our understanding of disease mechanism and therapy. *Neurotherapeutics* **2011**, *8*, 319–329. [CrossRef] [PubMed]
2. Maulden, S.A.; Gassaway, J.; Horn, S.D.; Smout, R.J.; DeJong, G. Timing of initiation of rehabilitation after stroke. *Arch. Phys. Med. Rehabil.* **2005**, *86*, S34–S40. [CrossRef] [PubMed]
3. Langhorne, P.; Bernhardt, J.; Kwakkel, G. Stroke rehabilitation. *Lancet* **2011**, *377*, 1693–1702. [CrossRef]
4. Jorgensen, H.S.; Kammersgaard, L.P.; Houth, J.; Nakayama, H.; Raaschou, H.O.; Larsen, K.; Hubbe, P.; Olsen, T.S. Who benefits from treatment and rehabilitation in a stroke unit? A community-based study. *Stroke* **2000**, *31*, 434–439. [CrossRef] [PubMed]
5. Lee, K.H.; Kim, J.H.; Choi, D.H.; Lee, J. Effect of task-specific training on functional recovery and corticospinal tract plasticity after stroke. *Restor. Neurol. Neurosci.* **2013**, *31*, 773–785. [PubMed]
6. Petrosyan, T. Initial training facilitates posttraumatic motor recovery in rats after pyramidal tract lesion and in conditions of induced regeneration. *Somatosens. Mot. Res.* **2015**, *32*, 21–24. [CrossRef] [PubMed]
7. Okabe, N.; Himi, N.; Maruyama-Nakamura, E.; Hayashi, N.; Narita, K.; Miyamoto, O. Rehabilitative skilled forelimb training enhances axonal remodeling in the corticospinal pathway but not the brainstem-spinal pathways after photothrombotic stroke in the primary motor cortex. *PLoS ONE* **2017**, *12*, e0187413. [CrossRef] [PubMed]
8. Higo, N. Effects of rehabilitative training on recovery of hand motor function: A review of animal studies. *Neurosci. Res.* **2014**, *78*, 9–15. [CrossRef] [PubMed]
9. Hubbard, I.J.; Parsons, M.W.; Neilson, C.; Carey, L.M. Task-specific training: Evidence for and translation to clinical practice. *Occup. Ther. Int.* **2009**, *16*, 175–189. [CrossRef] [PubMed]
10. Buetefisch, C.M. Role of the contralesional hemisphere in post-stroke recovery of upper extremity motor function. *Front. Neurol.* **2015**, *6*, 214. [CrossRef] [PubMed]
11. Dancause, N.; Touvykine, B.; Mansoori, B.K. Inhibition of the contralesional hemisphere after stroke: Reviewing a few of the building blocks with a focus on animal models. *Prog. Brain Res.* **2015**, *218*, 361–387. [PubMed]
12. Classen, J.; Liepert, J.; Wise, S.P.; Hallett, M.; Cohen, L.G. Rapid plasticity of human cortical movement representation induced by practice. *J. Neurophysiol.* **1998**, *79*, 1117–1123. [CrossRef] [PubMed]
13. Buga, A.M.; Sascau, M.; Pisoschi, C.; Herndon, J.G.; Kessler, C.; Popa-Wagner, A. The genomic response of the ipsilateral and contralateral cortex to stroke in aged rats. *J. Cell. Mol. Med.* **2008**, *12*, 2731–2753. [CrossRef] [PubMed]

14. Schweizer, S.; Meisel, A.; Marschenz, S. Epigenetic mechanisms in cerebral ischemia. *J. Cereb. Blood Flow Metab.* **2013**, *33*, 1335–1346. [CrossRef] [PubMed]
15. Kogure, K.; Kato, H. Altered gene expression in cerebral ischemia. *Stroke* **1993**, *24*, 2121–2127. [CrossRef] [PubMed]
16. Papadopoulos, M.C.; Giffard, R.G.; Bell, B.A. An introduction to the changes in gene expression that occur after cerebral ischaemia. *Br. J. Neurosurg.* **2000**, *14*, 305–312. [CrossRef] [PubMed]
17. Endres, M.; Meisel, A.; Biniszkiewicz, D.; Namura, S.; Prass, K.; Ruscher, K.; Lipski, A.; Jaenisch, R.; Moskowitz, M.A.; Dirnagl, U. DNA methyltransferase contributes to delayed ischemic brain injury. *J. Neurosci.* **2000**, *20*, 3175–3181. [CrossRef] [PubMed]
18. Endres, M.; Fan, G.; Meisel, A.; Dirnagl, U.; Jaenisch, R. Effects of cerebral ischemia in mice lacking DNA methyltransferase 1 in post-mitotic neurons. *Neuroreport* **2001**, *12*, 3763–3766. [CrossRef] [PubMed]
19. Hu, Z.; Zhong, B.; Tan, J.; Chen, C.; Lei, Q.; Zeng, L. The emerging role of epigenetics in cerebral ischemia. *Mol. Neurobiol.* **2017**, *54*, 1887–1905. [CrossRef] [PubMed]
20. Kong, M.; Ba, M.; Liang, H.; Ma, L.; Yu, Q.; Yu, T.; Wang, Y. 5′-Aza-dc sensitizes paraquat toxic effects on PC12 cell. *Neurosci. Lett.* **2012**, *524*, 35–39. [CrossRef] [PubMed]
21. Doerfler, W. In pursuit of the first recognized epigenetic signal–DNA methylation: A 1976 to 2008 synopsis. *Epigenetics* **2008**, *3*, 125–133. [CrossRef] [PubMed]
22. Narlikar, G.J.; Fan, H.Y.; Kingston, R.E. Cooperation between complexes that regulate chromatin structure and transcription. *Cell* **2002**, *108*, 475–487. [CrossRef]
23. Yin, K.J.; Deng, Z.; Hamblin, M.; Xiang, Y.; Huang, H.; Zhang, J.; Jiang, X.; Wang, Y.; Chen, Y.E. Peroxisome proliferator-activated receptor delta regulation of miR-15a in ischemia-induced cerebral vascular endothelial injury. *J. Neurosci.* **2010**, *30*, 6398–6408. [CrossRef] [PubMed]
24. Wang, P.; Liang, J.; Li, Y.; Li, J.; Yang, X.; Zhang, X.; Han, S.; Li, S.; Li, J. Down-regulation of miRNA-30a alleviates cerebral ischemic injury through enhancing beclin 1-mediated autophagy. *Neurochem. Res.* **2014**, *39*, 1279–1291. [CrossRef] [PubMed]
25. Zhao, H.; Han, Z.; Ji, X.; Luo, Y. Epigenetic regulation of oxidative stress in ischemic stroke. *Aging Dis.* **2016**, *7*, 295–306. [PubMed]
26. Moore, L.D.; Le, T.; Fan, G. DNA methylation and its basic function. *Neuropsychopharmacology* **2013**, *38*, 23–38. [CrossRef] [PubMed]
27. Rahman, M.; Luo, H.; Sims, N.R.; Bobrovskaya, L.; Zhou, X.F. Investigation of mature BDNF and proBDNF signaling in a rat photothrombotic ischemic model. *Neurochem. Res.* **2018**, *43*, 637–649. [CrossRef] [PubMed]
28. Takase, H.; Kurihara, Y.; Yokoyama, T.A.; Kawahara, N.; Takei, K. Lotus overexpression accelerates neuronal plasticity after focal brain ischemia in mice. *PLoS ONE* **2017**, *12*, e0184258. [CrossRef] [PubMed]
29. Wiersma, A.M.; Fouad, K.; Winship, I.R. Enhancing spinal plasticity amplifies the benefits of rehabilitative training and improves recovery from stroke. *J. Neurosci.* **2017**, *37*, 10983–10997. [CrossRef] [PubMed]
30. Lin, Y.H.; Dong, J.; Tang, Y.; Ni, H.Y.; Zhang, Y.; Su, P.; Liang, H.Y.; Yao, M.C.; Yuan, H.J.; Wang, D.L.; et al. Opening a new time window for treatment of stroke by targeting HDAC2. *J. Neurosci.* **2017**, *37*, 6712–6728. [CrossRef] [PubMed]
31. Tang, Y.; Lin, Y.H.; Ni, H.Y.; Dong, J.; Yuan, H.J.; Zhang, Y.; Liang, H.Y.; Yao, M.C.; Zhou, Q.G.; Wu, H.Y.; et al. Inhibiting histone deacetylase 2 (HDAC2) promotes functional recovery from stroke. *J. Am. Heart Assoc.* **2017**, *6*, e007236. [CrossRef] [PubMed]
32. Cramer, S.C.; Crafton, K.R. Somatotopy and movement representation sites following cortical stroke. *Exp. Brain Res.* **2006**, *168*, 25–32. [CrossRef] [PubMed]
33. Lee, S.; Ueno, M.; Yamashita, T. Axonal remodeling for motor recovery after traumatic brain injury requires downregulation of gamma-aminobutyric acid signaling. *Cell Death Dis.* **2011**, *2*, e133. [CrossRef] [PubMed]
34. Murphy, T.H.; Corbett, D. Plasticity during stroke recovery: From synapse to behaviour. *Nat. Rev. Neurosci.* **2009**, *10*, 861–872. [CrossRef] [PubMed]
35. Benowitz, L.I.; Carmichael, S.T. Promoting axonal rewiring to improve outcome after stroke. *Neurobiol. Dis.* **2010**, *37*, 259–266. [CrossRef] [PubMed]
36. Carmichael, S.T.; Wei, L.; Rovainen, C.M.; Woolsey, T.A. New patterns of intracortical projections after focal cortical stroke. *Neurobiol. Dis.* **2001**, *8*, 910–922. [CrossRef] [PubMed]
37. Lee, J.K.; Kim, J.E.; Sivula, M.; Strittmatter, S.M. Nogo receptor antagonism promotes stroke recovery by enhancing axonal plasticity. *J. Neurosci.* **2004**, *24*, 6209–6217. [CrossRef] [PubMed]

38. Okabe, N.; Shiromoto, T.; Himi, N.; Lu, F.; Maruyama-Nakamura, E.; Narita, K.; Iwachidou, N.; Yagita, Y.; Miyamoto, O. Neural network remodeling underlying motor map reorganization induced by rehabilitative training after ischemic stroke. *Neuroscience* **2016**, *339*, 338–362. [CrossRef] [PubMed]
39. Nakagawa, H.; Ueno, M.; Itokazu, T.; Yamashita, T. Bilateral movement training promotes axonal remodeling of the corticospinal tract and recovery of motor function following traumatic brain injury in mice. *Cell Death Dis.* **2013**, *4*, e534. [CrossRef] [PubMed]
40. Mang, C.S.; Campbell, K.L.; Ross, C.J.; Boyd, L.A. Promoting neuroplasticity for motor rehabilitation after stroke: Considering the effects of aerobic exercise and genetic variation on brain-derived neurotrophic factor. *Phys. Ther.* **2013**, *93*, 1707–1716. [CrossRef] [PubMed]
41. Berretta, A.; Tzeng, Y.C.; Clarkson, A.N. Post-stroke recovery: The role of activity-dependent release of brain-derived neurotrophic factor. *Expert Rev. Neurother.* **2014**, *14*, 1335–1344. [CrossRef] [PubMed]
42. Ploughman, M.; Granter-Button, S.; Chernenko, G.; Attwood, Z.; Tucker, B.A.; Mearow, K.M.; Corbett, D. Exercise intensity influences the temporal profile of growth factors involved in neuronal plasticity following focal ischemia. *Brain Res.* **2007**, *1150*, 207–216. [CrossRef] [PubMed]
43. Gomez-Pinilla, F.; Zhuang, Y.; Feng, J.; Ying, Z.; Fan, G. Exercise impacts brain-derived neurotrophic factor plasticity by engaging mechanisms of epigenetic regulation. *Eur. J. Neurosci.* **2011**, *33*, 383–390. [CrossRef] [PubMed]
44. MacLellan, C.L.; Keough, M.B.; Granter-Button, S.; Chernenko, G.A.; Butt, S.; Corbett, D. A critical threshold of rehabilitation involving brain-derived neurotrophic factor is required for poststroke recovery. *Neurorehabil. Neural Repair* **2011**, *25*, 740–748. [CrossRef] [PubMed]
45. Hirata, K.; Kuge, Y.; Yokota, C.; Harada, A.; Kokame, K.; Inoue, H.; Kawashima, H.; Hanzawa, H.; Shono, Y.; Saji, H.; et al. Gene and protein analysis of brain derived neurotrophic factor expression in relation to neurological recovery induced by an enriched environment in a rat stroke model. *Neurosci. Lett.* **2011**, *495*, 210–215. [CrossRef] [PubMed]
46. Wang, Y.C.; Sanchez-Mendoza, E.H.; Doeppner, T.R.; Hermann, D.M. Post-acute delivery of memantine promotes post-ischemic neurological recovery, peri-infarct tissue remodeling, and contralesional brain plasticity. *J. Cereb. Blood Flow Metab.* **2017**, *37*, 980–993. [CrossRef] [PubMed]
47. Ploughman, M.; Windle, V.; MacLellan, C.L.; White, N.; Dore, J.J.; Corbett, D. Brain-derived neurotrophic factor contributes to recovery of skilled reaching after focal ischemia in rats. *Stroke* **2009**, *40*, 1490–1495. [CrossRef] [PubMed]
48. Clarkson, A.N.; Overman, J.J.; Zhong, S.; Mueller, R.; Lynch, G.; Carmichael, S.T. Ampa receptor-induced local brain-derived neurotrophic factor signaling mediates motor recovery after stroke. *J. Neurosci.* **2011**, *31*, 3766–3775. [CrossRef] [PubMed]
49. Madinier, A.; Bertrand, N.; Rodier, M.; Quirie, A.; Mossiat, C.; Prigent-Tessier, A.; Marie, C.; Garnier, P. Ipsilateral versus contralateral spontaneous post-stroke neuroplastic changes: Involvement of BDNF? *Neuroscience* **2013**, *231*, 169–181. [CrossRef] [PubMed]
50. Mowla, S.J.; Farhadi, H.F.; Pareek, S.; Atwal, J.K.; Morris, S.J.; Seidah, N.G.; Murphy, R.A. Biosynthesis and post-translational processing of the precursor to brain-derived neurotrophic factor. *J. Biol. Chem.* **2001**, *276*, 12660–12666. [CrossRef] [PubMed]
51. Pak, M.E.; Jung, D.H.; Lee, H.J.; Shin, M.J.; Kim, S.Y.; Shin, Y.B.; Yun, Y.J.; Shin, H.K.; Choi, B.T. Combined therapy involving electroacupuncture and treadmill exercise attenuates demyelination in the corpus callosum by stimulating oligodendrogenesis in a rat model of neonatal hypoxia-ischemia. *Exp. Neurol.* **2018**, *300*, 222–231. [CrossRef] [PubMed]
52. Han, J.; Pollak, J.; Yang, T.; Siddiqui, M.R.; Doyle, K.P.; Taravosh-Lahn, K.; Cekanaviciute, E.; Han, A.; Goodman, J.Z.; Jones, B.; et al. Delayed administration of a small molecule tropomyosin-related kinase B ligand promotes recovery after hypoxic-ischemic stroke. *Stroke* **2012**, *43*, 1918–1924. [CrossRef] [PubMed]
53. Zhu, J.M.; Zhao, Y.Y.; Chen, S.D.; Zhang, W.H.; Lou, L.; Jin, X. Functional recovery after transplantation of neural stem cells modified by brain-derived neurotrophic factor in rats with cerebral ischaemia. *J. Int. Med. Res.* **2011**, *39*, 488–498. [CrossRef] [PubMed]
54. Qureshi, I.A.; Mehler, M.F. The emerging role of epigenetics in stroke: III. Neural stem cell biology and regenerative medicine. *Arch. Neurol.* **2011**, *68*, 294–302. [CrossRef] [PubMed]

55. Choi, D.H.; Ahn, J.H.; Choi, I.A.; Kim, J.H.; Kim, B.R.; Lee, J. Effect of task-specific training on Eph/ephrin expression after stroke. *BMB Rep.* **2016**, *49*, 635–640. [CrossRef] [PubMed]
56. Choi, D.H.; Kim, J.H.; Lee, K.H.; Kim, H.Y.; Kim, Y.S.; Choi, W.S.; Lee, J. Role of neuronal nadph oxidase 1 in the peri-infarct regions after stroke. *PLoS ONE* **2015**, *10*, e0116814. [CrossRef] [PubMed]

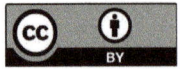

© 2018 by the authors. Licensee MDPI, Basel, Switzerland. This article is an open access article distributed under the terms and conditions of the Creative Commons Attribution (CC BY) license (http://creativecommons.org/licenses/by/4.0/).

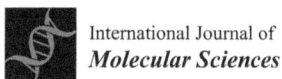

Article

Whole Body Vibration Therapy after Ischemia Reduces Brain Damage in Reproductively Senescent Female Rats

Ami P. Raval [1,*], Marc Schatz [1], Pallab Bhattacharya [1,†], Nathan d'Adesky [1], Tatjana Rundek [2], W. Dalton Dietrich [3] and Helen M. Bramlett [3,4,*]

1. Cerebral Vascular Disease Research Laboratories, Department of Neurology, Leonard M. Miller School of Medicine, University of Miami, Miami, FL 33136, USA; marc.schatz@med.miami.edu (M.S.); pallab.bhu@gmail.com (P.B.); nathandadesky@gmail.com (N.d.)
2. Department of Neurology, University of Miami School of Medicine, Miami, FL 33136, USA; TRundek@med.miami.edu
3. Department of Neurological Surgery, Leonard M. Miller School of Medicine, University of Miami, Miami, FL 33136, USA; ddietrich@med.miami.edu
4. Bruce W. Carter Department of Veterans Affairs Medical Center, Miami, FL 33125, USA
* Correspondence: Araval@med.miami.edu (A.P.R.); Hbramlett@med.miami.edu (H.M.B.); Tel.: +1-305-243-7491 (A.P.R.); +1-305-243-8926 (H.M.B.)
† Current affiliation: Department or Pharmacology and Toxicology, National Institute of Pharmaceutical Education and Research, Ahmedabad (NIPER-A), Gandhinagar 382355, Gujarat, India

Received: 23 August 2018; Accepted: 5 September 2018; Published: 13 September 2018

Abstract: A risk of ischemic stroke increases exponentially after menopause. Even a mild-ischemic stroke can result in increased frailty. Frailty is a state of increased vulnerability to adverse outcomes, which subsequently increases risk of cerebrovascular events and severe cognitive decline, particularly after menopause. Several interventions to reduce frailty and subsequent risk of stroke and cognitive decline have been proposed in laboratory animals and patients. One of them is whole body vibration (WBV). WBV improves cerebral function and cognitive ability that deteriorates with increased frailty. The goal of the current study is to test the efficacy of WBV in reducing post-ischemic stroke frailty and brain damage in reproductively senescent female rats. Reproductively senescent Sprague-Dawley female rats were exposed to transient middle cerebral artery occlusion (tMCAO) and were randomly assigned to either WBV or no-WBV groups. Animals placed in the WBV group underwent 30 days of WBV (40 Hz) treatment performed twice daily for 15 min each session, 5 days each week. The motor functions of animals belonging to both groups were tested intermittently and at the end of the treatment period. Brains were then harvested for inflammatory markers and histopathological analysis. The results demonstrate a significant reduction in inflammatory markers and infarct volume with significant increases in brain-derived neurotrophic factor and improvement in functional activity after tMCAO in middle-aged female rats that were treated with WBV as compared to the no-WBV group. Our results may facilitate a faster translation of the WBV intervention for improved outcome after stroke, particularly among frail women.

Keywords: brain-derived neurotrophic factor; frailty; inflammasome proteins; interleukin-1β; peri-infarct area

1. Introduction

A woman's risk of a stroke increases exponentially following the onset of menopause, and even a mild-ischemic episode can result in a woman becoming increasingly frail with age. Frailty is characterized by an increased vulnerability to acute stressors and the reduced capacity of various bodily systems due to age-associated physiological deterioration [1]. Therefore, older women are more likely to experience decreased energy and strength, weight loss, increased susceptibility to disease and physical injury, increased hospitalization, and reduced daily living activities. Our understanding of the link between frailty and cerebrovascular diseases is limited [1]. Thus, understanding the factors that contribute to frailty in women could potentially allow for preventative measures that could decrease or slow down its onset, reduce risk of stroke and provide the basis for new treatment options.

Exercise is a powerful behavioral intervention that has the potential to improve health outcomes in elderly stroke survivors. Multiple studies using human and animal models have shown that pre-ischemic physical activity reduces stroke impact on functional motor outcomes, edema, and infarct volume. The same studies also attributed these benefits to the mechanism of decreasing inflammation, and increasing brain-derived neurotrophic factor (BDNF) expression [2–6]. In many cases, however, stroke patients are unable to adhere to the physical activity regimen following their ischemic episodes due to a wide range of individual factors such as stroke severity, preexisting and comorbid conditions, motivation, fatigue, and depression. As a result, whole body vibration, a procedure mimicking exercise, has been proposed as an alternative to physical therapy [7]. Whole body vibration (WBV) is a novel rehabilitative exercise that uses low amplitude, low frequency vibration administered through a platform or Power Plate. WBV shows potential as an effective therapeutic approach and has been studied in a variety of clinical settings that include rehabilitation of patients with chronic stroke [8], spinal cord injury [9], lumbar disk disease and lower back pain syndromes [10], Parkinson's disease [11], elderly with sarcopenia [12,13], chronic obstructive pulmonary disease (COPD) [14], multiple sclerosis [15], obesity, osteoporosis, osteoarthritis and fibromyalgia [16] and children with cerebral palsy [17]. A growing body of evidence in laboratory animals and patients with chronic stroke has shown that WBV reduces or reverses pathological remodeling of bone and such a treatment could also help reduce frailty-related physiological deterioration [18–20]. Although WBV has shown to be an effective therapy under many different conditions, its specific application in stroke remains unclear. Several studies of WBV in stroke patients [21,22], of which none were specifically screened for frailty or pre-frailty, have produced inconclusive results [23]. Also, WBV has not yet been systematically studied specifically in women who are often more critically affected by stroke than men. Therefore, the goal of our current study is to investigate the effect of WBV on ischemic outcome in the reproductively senescent (RS) female rat model. Our selection of using a RS female rat model in this study is also adhering to Stroke Therapy Academic and Industry Roundtable (STAIR) guidelines that recommend more relevant animal models to better correlate with the aged population. Based on the currently available literature, we hypothesize that the benefit observed from WBV will be similar in mechanism to the one followed by physical therapy—reducing inflammation and increasing BDNF—resulting in reduced post-ischemic injury, improved activity and neurobehavior in reproductively senescent female rats. These results would serve as preliminary translational data for adoption in a clinical trial of pre-frail and frail women after stroke.

2. Results

2.1. Post-Ischemic WBV Reduced Infarct Volume in Middle-Aged Female Rats

Our first hypothesis was that post-ischemic WBV reduced infarct volume. Rats exposed to transient middle cerebral artery occlusion (tMCAO) were treated with WBV or no-WBV and a month later, brain tissue was collected for histopathological assessment (Figure 1A). The results demonstrate a significant reduction in infarct volume in a mild stroke model following WBV treatment as compared to no-WBV rats (Figure 1B,C). We observed a 41% reduction in infarct volume of WBV treated rats as compared to no-WBV. Histological analysis of WBV or no-WBV-treated rat brains that underwent sham surgery did not show any infarct. In parallel, we also monitored neurological deficit of rats that were exposed to WBV/no-WBV treatment after tMCAO (Figure 1D). Results demonstrated a significant improvement in the neurological score following WBV as compared to no-WBV rats.

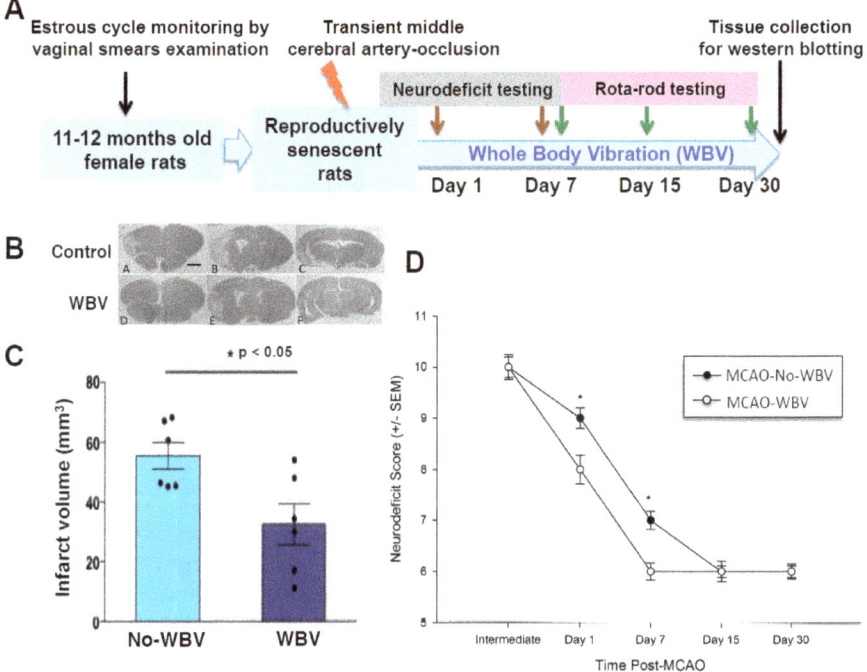

Figure 1. (**A**) Experimental design. (**B**) Representative histological images of the brain (Bregma levels 1.2, −3.8, −5, 10X). (**C**) Geometric mean infarct volumes are compared between whole body vibration WBV and no-WBV groups. Post-ischemic WBV treatment shows reduced infarct volume as compared to the no-WBV group (* $p < 0.05$ as compared to no-WBV using student *t*-test). (**D**) Neurological deficit (ND) assessment scores were significantly improved in the WBV treated group as compared to no-WBV (* $p < 0.05$ as compared to no-WBV using Student Newman-Keuls).

2.2. Post-Ischemic WBV Improved Neuro-Deficit Score and Motor Function in Middle-Aged Female Rats

Secondly, we tested the hypothesis that post-tMCAO WBV treatment improves neurodeficit and motor coordination along with an observed reduction in ischemic damage. The neurodeficit score in each group was more than 9 at baseline when tested at 1 h after tMCAO. Over the period of 7 days, the neurodeficit score was reduced significantly in rats that were treated with WBV ($p < 0.05$) after tMCAO as compared with corresponding no-WBV-treated groups. The rotarod test scores from rats receiving WBV treatment as compared to no-WBV group were significantly higher on day 30 ($p < 0.05$) at 10, 30, and 40 rotations per minute (rpm) speed. These results demonstrate a significant improvement in functional activity after tMCAO in animals that were treated with WBV as compared to the no-WBV group (Figure 2).

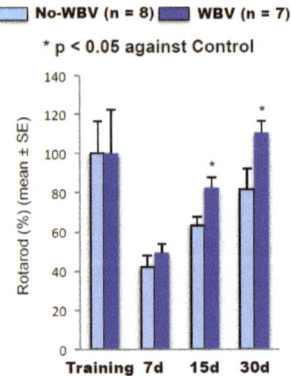

Figure 2. Post-ischemic WBV improves motor coordination (* $p < 0.05$ as compared to no-WBV using student t-test).

2.3. Post-Ischemic WBV Decreased Inflammasome Activation in the Brain of Middle-Aged Female Rats

Western blot results demonstrated a two-fold decrease in the inflammasome proteins caspase-1, caspase recruitment domain (ASC), and interleukin-1β in the peri-infarct area of WBV treated rats. Since the peri-infarct area is salvageable tissue after stroke, for this study, we focused on investigating alterations in inflammasome proteins in the peri-infarct area of WBV treated versus the no-WBV rats (Figure 3). Post-ischemic WBV decreased protein levels of caspase-1, ASC and IL-1β by 88% ($p < 0.05$), 57% ($p < 0.05$) and 148% ($p < 0.05$) in peri-infarct area as compared to no-WBV-treated group.

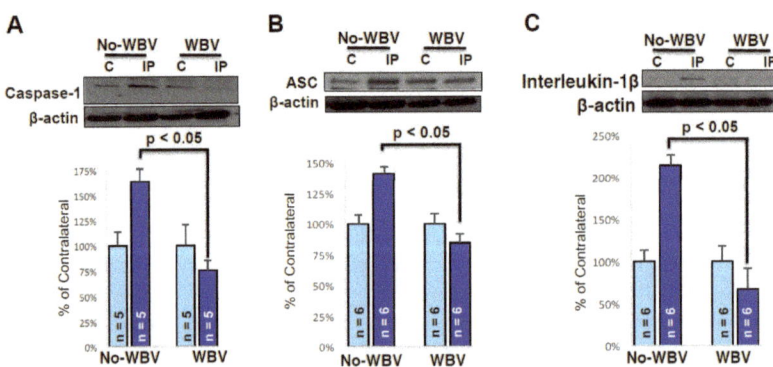

Figure 3. Representative immunoblots showing the protein levels of caspase 1 (**A**-Top), ASC (**B**-Top), and IL-1β (**C**-Top), in the contra-lateral and ipsilateral peri-infarct region of the brain, respectively. Post-ischemic WBV decreases inflammasome proteins caspase 1 (**A**-Bottom), ASC (**B**-Bottom), and IL-1β (**C**-Bottom), in the contra-lateral and ipsilateral peri-infarct region of the brain, respectively (* $p < 0.05$ as compared to no-WBV using student t-test).

2.4. Post-Ischemic WBV Increased Brain-Derived Growth Factor (BDNF) and Trk-B Protein Levels in the Peri-Infarct Area

Studies from various laboratories demonstrate that growth factors play an important role in preserving brain function after ischemia. Therefore, we tested whether WBV treatment after tMCAO increases BDNF release and tyrosine kinase receptor subtype B (Trk-B) signaling in the female brain. We observed significant increases in levels of BDNF and pTrK-B in the peri-infarct region of WBV treated group as compared to the no-WBV (Figure 4). Post-ischemic WBV increased protein levels of BDNF and pTrk-B by 58% ($p < 0.05$) and 59% ($p < 0.05$) in peri-infarct area as compared to no-WBV-treated group.

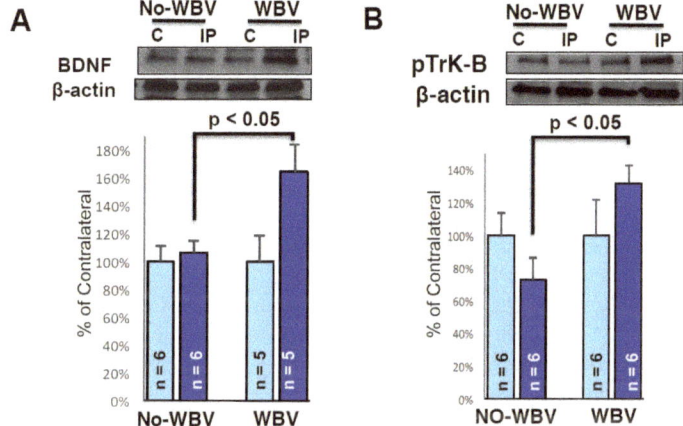

Figure 4. Representative immunoblots showing the protein levels of BDNF and phosphorylated Trk-B in the peri-infarct area. β-actin (cytoskeletal), was used as a loading control. Densitometric analysis of scanned Western blots and expressed as percent of contralateral, showed baseline expression of BDNF (**A**) and phosphorylated Trk-B (**B**) proteins. Note the WBV treatment significantly increased BDNF and phosphorylated Trk-B in the peri-infarct area as compared to no-WBV (* $p < 0.05$ as compared to no-WBV using student *t*-test).

3. Discussion

The current study demonstrates that the post-stroke WBV intervention reduces brain injury in reproductively senescent female rats. Our study also demonstrated that the post-stroke WBV intervention significantly improved neurological and motor capabilities in female rats. The mechanism by which the WBV intervention improved outcomes after stroke is likely multi-factorial, similar to that of exercise. The benefits of post-stroke exercise go beyond reduced infarct volume and have shown to improve motor and cognitive functions. Studies in recent years demonstrate that physical exercise has a profound effect on the normal functioning of the immune system [24–26]. Moderate intensity exercise was shown to be beneficial for immunity, which could be the result of reduced inflammation, thymic mass maintenance, changes in immune cells' compositions, increased immunosurveillance, and/or amelioration of psychological stress [24–26]. It is well known that exercise is an important intervention that can improve immunity and health outcomes in elderly stroke survivors. However, after stroke, patients are unable to exercise or less likely to adhere to the physical activity regimen following their ischemic episodes. A wide range of individual factors may affect stroke patient participation in physical therapy including stroke severity, preexisting and comorbid conditions, motivation, fatigue, and depression. Therefore, the current approach to reduce post-stroke inflammation and frailty using WBV has important translational value.

The current study demonstrated that post-stroke WBV reduces pro-inflammatory cytokine IL-1β and inflammasome proteins in the brain in middle-aged female rats. The importance of inflammasome as a key component of the innate immune response in brain injury has been recently emphasized and targeted for therapeutic interventions [27–30]. Specifically, the inflammasome was shown to activate caspase-1 and initiate the processing of the inflammatory cytokines IL-1β and IL-18 [31]. In models of brain ischemia, evidence for inflammasome activation has been reported with elevations in inflammatory proteins such as ASC, and caspase-1. Our previously published studies demonstrated elevations in inflammasome proteins in the hippocampus of aged rats [32,33]. Consistent with our findings, others have demonstrated increased pro-inflammatory cytokine levels in middle-aged female rats [34]. It is now well documented that the depletion of estrogens at menopause/reproductive senescence elevates pro-inflammatory cytokines, which may increase the chances of inflammatory diseases in the body, including the brain. This decline in estrogen is also associated with a loss of muscle mass, bone, and strength that represent the core of the frailty syndrome [35,36]. Our use of reproductively senescent female rats closely mimics the age group of peri-menopausal women and the population that is likely to suffer frailty following stroke. Therefore, showing benefits of post-stroke WBV in reducing inflammation in the brain is of a translational value.

Since post-ischemic inflammation eventually subsides while injured tissue undergoes structural and functional reconstruction, this process may further require the release/presence of variety of growth factors such as BDNF [37]. In our current study, we observed significant increases in levels of BDNF and pTrK-B in the peri-infarct region after WBV. BDNF, a member of the neurotrophic factor family, is one of the most powerful neuroprotective agents [38–40]. BDNF expression is regulated in an activity-dependent manner by physiological stimuli, and its biological effects are mediated through the high-affinity receptor, tyrosine kinase receptor subtype B (Trk-B) [41]. Since BDNF expression is augmented in neurons by various stressors (e.g., ischemia, epilepsy, hypoglycemia, and trauma [42]), chronic exposure to BDNF confers neuroprotection. In addition to pro-survival mechanism(s), BDNF also modulates synaptic plasticity and neurogenesis [43–46]. A direct application of BDNF is neuroprotective in focal and global cerebral ischemia models [47,48]. Importantly, continuous intraventricular administration of BDNF was required for mitigating ischemic brain damage in the aforementioned in vivo studies. Despite BDNF's neuroprotective ability against ischemic damage, treating patients with BDNF remains challenging because BDNF is unable to cross the blood-brain barrier [49,50]. Due to the difficulty of administering BDNF directly to the brain, a model in which BDNF is increased intrinsically has been proposed. Several studies have shown a strong correlation between increased levels of circulating BDNF and exercises, yet no studies have shown an increase in BDNF levels with WBV. One study has shown that exercise in mice is effective at preventing a decrease in BDNF levels in the CA1 and dentate gyrus that would otherwise be caused by exposure to Arsenic [51]. It is proposed that training to volatile fatigue is the optimal way to increase circulating BDNF levels in elderly participants [52]. Intravenous BDNF delivery enhances post-stroke sensorimotor recovery and stimulates neurogenesis [53]. It has also been demonstrated that BDNF up-regulation following exercise is associated with a robust activation of survival pathways that enhance adult neurogenesis in experimental animals [54,55]. Currently, it is unknown whether WBV leads to increases in hippocampal BDNF and whether this response promotes neurogenesis associated with improved cognitive outcome after stroke, but we suspect that this may be the missing link between WBV and exercise.

The caveats of the current study are that (1) it lacks a mechanistic approach to prove the role of either inflammation or BDNF in WBV-mediated ischemic protection, and (2) the effects of post-stroke WBV are only tested on RS female rats. Therefore, the observed improvement in motor function and reduced infarct volume could not be generalizable to both rat sexes.

In conclusion, the results of our study demonstrated that the post-ischemic WBV intervention reduces brain injury and frailty in reproductively senescent female rats, suggesting WBV may be a potential therapy to reduce post-ischemic frailty and improve functional and cognitive outcomes in women after stroke. Our use of reproductively senescent female rats closely mimics the age group of peri-menopausal women and is clinically relevant as it is estimated that 7 million American adults are living with a stroke and the majority of them are post-menopausal women. This is particularly important because we now know that stroke disproportionately kills more women than men. Although women are naturally protected against stroke in their pre-menopausal life, a woman's risk of stroke increases exponentially after menopause. The decline in ovarian hormones, especially estrogen, at menopause is associated with loss of muscle mass, bone and strength that represents the core of the frailty syndrome [35,36]. Whole body vibration as a simple and an inexpensive intervention that can be administered at homes has a great potential to aid in prevention and treatment of post-stroke frailty. Future pre-clinical studies investigating the specific mechanism of post-stroke frailty and efficacy of WBV in improving post-stroke frailty and other stroke outcomes can lead to its clinical translation.

4. Materials and Methods

All animal procedures were carried out in accordance with the Guide for the Care and Use of Laboratory Animals published by the U.S. National Institutes of Health and were approved (protocol # 17-034; 03-08-2017) by the Animal Care and Use Committee of the University of Miami, University of Miami, Florida, USA. Retired breeder (9–12 months) Sprague-Dawley female rats (280–350 g) were purchased, and their estrous cycles were checked for 14–20 days before experimentation by daily vaginal smears [56]. Rats that persisted in a single stage for 7 days were considered acyclic. The acyclic rats and rats that remained in constant diestrous were considered reproductively senescent (RS) and were used in the study [57].

Reproductively senescent rats were randomly exposed to 60 min of transient middle cerebral artery occlusion (tMCAO) or sham surgery. Transient MCAO was adapted from previous publications [58,59]. tMCAO was achieved by intraluminal suture. A 30-mm-long 3-0 nylon monofilament suture coated with silicone (Doccol) and was placed 19–20 mm into the internal carotid artery to occlude the ostium of the MCA. The suture was placed in the MCA for 60 min and the drop in cerebral blood pressure was confirmed using laser Doppler (LDF, Perimed Inc., Ardmore, PA, USA). For sham surgical procedure, rats were exposed to anesthesia for a period similar to that of the tMCAO group. Physiological parameters including, pCO_2, pO_2, and pH were maintained within normal limits through the surgery or sham-surgery. Mean arterial blood pressure (MABP) was continuously monitored and head and body temperatures were maintained at 37 °C.

One day after the tMCAO, animals were randomly assigned to (1) a WBV intervention group or to (2) a no-WBV group. Animals randomized to the WBV group underwent 30 days of treatment performed twice daily for 15 min each session, 5 days each week. The vibration device was programmed in order to achieve a frequency of vibration within a range of about 40 Hz (0.3 g) similar to those used in clinical studies [9,60,61]. The duration and frequency of sessions were selected based on our recent publication [18], where we demonstrated an ability of WBV to improve selected biomarkers of bone turnover and gene expression and to reduce osteoclastogenesis after spinal cord injury. The no-WBV animals post tMCAO were also placed on the platform with no activation. To provide WBV intervention, animals were placed in a plexiglass box that contained four chambers. One rat was placed into each chamber in a random order from one session to the next to avoid any bias due to chamber placement. The vibration parameters were measured in each chamber and differences in these parameters between the chambers were negligible.

Rats exposed to WBV or no-WBV treatment after tMCAO were allowed to survive for a month for histopathological assessment. At one month, rats were anesthetized and perfused via the ascending aorta with FAM (a mixture of 40% formaldehyde, glacial acetic acid, and methanol, 1:1:8 by volume) for 20 min after first being perfused for 2 min with saline. The rat heads were immersed in FAM for 1 day before the brains were removed. The brains were kept in FAM at 4 °C for at least 1 additional day, and then coronal brain blocks were fixed in paraffin. All brains were cut into 10-µm thick sections from 5.5 mm to −7.5 mm from bregma at 9 standard levels to span the entire infarcted area. Sections of the 9 levels were stained with hematoxylin and eosin to visualize the infarcted areas and to calculate infarct volumes. The electronic images of the tissue sections were obtained using a CCD camera and infarct volume was quantified using an MCID image analysis system [62].

4.1. Neurodeficit Sscoring and Motor Deficit Test

A standardized neurobehavioral test battery was conducted as described previously [62]. This test consists of quantifications of postural reflex, sensorimotor integration and proprioception. Total neurodeficit score ranged from a score of 0, indicating normal results, to a maximal possible score of 12, indicating a severe deficit.

To further test motor function, we performed the rotarod test as described in our previous publication [63]. In this test, the rats were placed on the rotarod cylinder, and the time that animals remained on the rotarod was measured. The speed was slowly increased from 10 to 40 rpm over 5 min. The trial ended if a rat fell off of the device or spun around for 2 consecutive revolutions without the rat attempting to walk. The rats were trained for 3 consecutive days before undergoing the MCAO procedure. The average duration (in seconds) on the machine was recorded from 3 different rotarod measurements 1 day prior to surgery. Motor function data are presented as percentage of mean duration (3 trials) on the rotarod compared to the internal baseline control (before surgery). The rats were tested at 1, 15, and 30 days after MCAO.

4.2. Immunoblot Analysis

Brain tissue was harvested 30 days after WBV or no-WBV. We isolated the peri-infarct and corresponding contralateral region of the brain for the analysis of the WBV or no-WBV groups and tissues were stored at −80 °C. At the time of immunoblotting, tissues were homogenized; protein content was analyzed and proteins were separated by 12% SDS-PAGE as described [56]. Proteins were transferred to Immobilon-P (Millipore, Burlington, MA, USA) membrane and incubated with primary antibodies against caspase-1 (mouse monoclonal; 1:1000; Novus Biologicals, Littleton, CO, USA), ASC (mouse monoclonal; 1:1000; Santa Cruz Biotechnology, Santa Cruz, CA, USA), IL-1β (1:1000, Cell Signaling, Danvers, MA, USA), BDNF (rabbit polyclonal; 1:500; Santa Cruz Biotechnology, Santa Cruz, CA, USA) and Trk-B (rabbit polyclonal; 1:500; Santa Cruz Biotechnology, Santa Cruz, CA, USA). All data were normalized to β-actin (monoclonal; 1:1000; Sigma, St. Louis, MO, USA). Immunoblot images were digitized and subjected to densitometric analysis [56].

4.3. Statistical Analysis

The data are shown as the mean value ± SEM or median ± SEM, and the results from the densitometric analysis were analyzed by a two-tailed Student's t-test. The neurodeficit score was analyzed with a two-way repeated measures ANOVA followed by Student Newman Keuls test. A $p < 0.05$ was considered statistically significant.

Author Contributions: A.P.R., H.M.B., T.R. and D.D. conceived and designed the experiments; A.P.R., P.B., M.S. and N.d. performed the experiments; H.M.B. analyzed the data; A.P.R. and M.S. wrote the paper; and H.M.B., T.R. and D.D. edited the paper.

Acknowledgments: We thank Bonnie Levin (Department of Neurology, University of Miami, Miami, FL, USA) and Juan Pablo de Rivero Vaccari (Department of Neurological Surgery, The Miami Project to Cure Paralysis, University of Miami School of Medicine, Miami, FL, USA) for their suggestions during design of this study. This work was supported by an Endowment from Chantal and Peritz Scheinberg (Ami P. Raval), Florida Department of Heath#7JK01 funds (Helen M. Bramlett & Ami P. Raval), the American Heart Association Grant-in-aid #16GRNT31300011 (Ami P. Raval), and The Miami Project to Cure Paralysis (Helen M. Bramlett). Helen M. Bramlett and Dalton Dietrich are co-founders and managing members of InflamaCORE, LLC, a company dedicated to developing therapies and diagnostic tools focusing on the inflammasome.

Conflicts of Interest: The authors declare no conflict of interest.

References

1. Xue, Q.L. The frailty syndrome: Definition and natural history. *Clin. Geriatr. Med.* **2011**, *27*, 1–15. [CrossRef] [PubMed]
2. Deplanque, D.; Masse, I.; Lefebvre, C.; Libersa, C.; Leys, D.; Bordet, R. Prior TIA, lipid-lowering drug use, and physical activity decrease ischemic stroke severity. *Neurology* **2006**, *67*, 1403–1410. [CrossRef] [PubMed]
3. Ding, Y.; Li, J.; Luan, X.; Ding, Y.H.; Lai, Q.; Rafols, J.A.; Phillis, J.W.; Clark, J.C.; Diaz, F.G. Exercise pre-conditioning reduces brain damage in ischemic rats that may be associated with regional angiogenesis and cellular overexpression of neurotrophin. *Neuroscience* **2004**, *124*, 583–591. [CrossRef] [PubMed]

4. Ding, Y.H.; Young, C.N.; Luan, X.; Li, J.; Rafols, J.A.; Clark, J.C.; James, P.; McAllister, J.P., II; Ding, Y. Exercise preconditioning ameliorates inflammatory injury in ischemic rats during reperfusion. *Acta Neuropathol.* **2005**, *109*, 237–246. [CrossRef] [PubMed]
5. Krarup, L.H.; Truelsen, T.; Gluud, C.; Andersen, G.; Zeng, X.; Korv, J.; Oskedra, A.; Boysen, G.; ExStroke Pilot Trial Group. Prestroke physical activity is associated with severity and long-term outcome from first-ever stroke. *Neurology* **2008**, *71*, 1313–1318. [CrossRef] [PubMed]
6. Rist, P.M.; Lee, I.M.; Kase, C.S.; Gaziano, J.M.; Kurth, T. Physical activity and functional outcomes from cerebral vascular events in men. *Stroke* **2011**, *42*, 3352–3356. [CrossRef] [PubMed]
7. Rees, S.S.; Murphy, A.J.; Watsford, M.L. Effects of whole body vibration on postural steadiness in an older population. *J. Sci. Med. Sport* **2009**, *12*, 440–444. [CrossRef] [PubMed]
8. Lee, G. Does whole-body vibration training in the horizontal direction have effects on motor function and balance of chronic stroke survivors? A preliminary study. *J. Phys. Ther. Sci.* **2015**, *27*, 1133–1136. [CrossRef] [PubMed]
9. Herrero, A.J.; Menendez, H.; Gil, L.; Martin, J.; Martin, T.; Garcia-Lopez, D.; Gil-Agudo, Á.; Marin, P.J. Effects of whole-body vibration on blood flow and neuromuscular activity in spinal cord injury. *Spinal Cord* **2011**, *49*, 554–559. [CrossRef] [PubMed]
10. Bovenzi, M. The hand-arm vibration syndrome: (II). The diagnostic aspects and fitness criteria. *Med. Lav.* **1999**, *90*, 643–649. [PubMed]
11. Kalbe, E.; Calabrese, P.; Kohn, N.; Hilker, R.; Riedel, O.; Wittchen, H.U.; Dodel, R.; Otto, J.; Ebersbach, G.; Kessler, J. Screening for cognitive deficits in Parkinson's disease with the Parkinson neuropsychometric dementia assessment (PANDA) instrument. *Parkinsonism Relat. Disord.* **2008**, *14*, 93–101. [CrossRef] [PubMed]
12. Bautmans, I.; Van Hees, E.; Lemper, J.C.; Mets, T. The feasibility of Whole Body Vibration in institutionalised elderly persons and its influence on muscle performance, balance and mobility: A randomised controlled trial [ISRCTN62535013]. *BMC Geriatr.* **2005**, *5*, 17. [CrossRef] [PubMed]
13. Roelants, M.; Delecluse, C.; Goris, M.; Verschueren, S. Effects of 24 weeks of whole body vibration training on body composition and muscle strength in untrained females. *Int. J. Sports Med.* **2004**, *25*, 1–5. [PubMed]
14. Gloeckl, S.; Tyndall, J.D.; Stansfield, S.H.; Timms, P.; Huston, W.M. The active site residue V266 of Chlamydial HtrA is critical for substrate binding during both in vitro and in vivo conditions. *J. Mol. Microbiol. Biotechnol.* **2012**, *22*, 10–16. [CrossRef] [PubMed]
15. Jackson, K.J.; Merriman, H.L.; Vanderburgh, P.M.; Brahler, C.J. Acute effects of whole-body vibration on lower extremity muscle performance in persons with multiple sclerosis. *J. Neurol. Phys. Ther.* **2008**, *32*, 171–176. [CrossRef] [PubMed]
16. Verschueren, S.M.; Roelants, M.; Delecluse, C.; Swinnen, S.; Vanderschueren, D.; Boonen, S. Effect of 6-month whole body vibration training on hip density, muscle strength, and postural control in postmenopausal women: A randomized controlled pilot study. *J. Bone Miner. Res.* **2004**, *19*, 352–359. [CrossRef] [PubMed]
17. Semler, O.; Fricke, O.; Vezyroglou, K.; Stark, C.; Schoenau, E. Preliminary results on the mobility after whole body vibration in immobilized children and adolescents. *J. Musculoskelet. Neuronal Interact.* **2007**, *7*, 77–81. [PubMed]
18. Bramlett, H.M.; Dietrich, W.D.; Marcillo, A.; Mawhinney, L.J.; Furones-Alonso, O.; Bregy, A.; Peng, Y.; Wu, Y.; Pan, J.; Wang, J. Effects of low intensity vibration on bone and muscle in rats with spinal cord injury. *Osteoporos. Int.* **2014**, *25*, 2209–2219. [CrossRef] [PubMed]
19. Rubin, C.; Turner, A.S.; Bain, S.; Mallinckrodt, C.; McLeod, K. Anabolism: Low mechanical signals strengthen long bones. *Nature* **2001**, *412*, 603–604. [CrossRef] [PubMed]
20. Xie, L.; Rubin, C.; Judex, S. Enhancement of the adolescent murine musculoskeletal system using low-level mechanical vibrations. *J. Appl. Physiol.* **2008**, *104*, 1056–1062. [CrossRef] [PubMed]
21. Van Nes, I.J.; Latour, I.J.; Schils, H.; Meijer, F.; van Kuijk, R.A.; Geurts, A.C. Long-term effects of 6-week whole-body vibration on balance recovery and activities of daily living in the postacute phase of stroke: A randomized, controlled trial. *Stroke* **2006**, *37*, 2331–2335. [CrossRef] [PubMed]
22. Tihanyi, T.K.; Horváth, M.; Fazekas, G.; Hortobágyi, T.; Tihanyi, J. One session of whole body vibration increases voluntary muscle strength transiently in patients with stroke. *Clin. Rehabil.* **2007**, *21*, 782–793. [CrossRef] [PubMed]

23. Del Pozo-Cruz, B.; Hernández Mocholí, M.A.; Adsuar, J.C.; Parraca, J.A.; Muro, I.; Gusi, N. Effects of whole body vibration therapy on main outcome measures for chronic non-specific low back pain: A single-blind randomized controlled trial. *J. Rehabil. Med.* **2011**, *43*, 689–694. [PubMed]
24. Simpson, R.J.; Kunz, H.; Agha, N.; Graff, R. Exercise and the Regulation of Immune Functions. *Prog. Mol. Biol. Transl. Sci.* **2015**, *135*, 355–380. [PubMed]
25. Nieman, D.C. Exercise immunology: Practical applications. *Int. J. Sports Med.* **1997**, *18*, 91–100. [CrossRef] [PubMed]
26. Mackinnon, L.T. Immunity in athletes. *Int. J. Sports Med.* **1997**, *18*, S62–S68. [CrossRef] [PubMed]
27. Gertz, K.; Kronenberg, G.; Kälin, R.E.; Baldinger, T.; Werner, C.; Balkaya, M.; Eom, G.D.; Regen, J.H.; Kröber, J.; Miller, K.R. Essential role of interleukin-6 in post-stroke angiogenesis. *Brain* **2012**, *135*, 1964–1980. [CrossRef] [PubMed]
28. Kamel, H.; Iadecola, C. Brain-immune interactions and ischemic stroke: Clinical implications. *Arch. Neurol.* **2012**, *69*, 576–581. [PubMed]
29. Eltzschig, H.K.; Eckle, T. Ischemia and reperfusion–from mechanism to translation. *Nat. Med.* **2011**, *17*, 1391–1401. [CrossRef] [PubMed]
30. Mulcahy, N.J.; Ross, J.; Rothwell, N.J.; Loddick, S.A. Delayed administration of interleukin-1 receptor antagonist protects against transient cerebral ischaemia in the rat. *Br. J. Pharmacol.* **2003**, *140*, 471–476. [CrossRef] [PubMed]
31. Lotocki, G.; de Rivero Vaccari, J.P.; Perez, E.R.; Sanchez-Molano, J.; Furones-Alonso, O.; Bramlett, H.M.; Dietrich, W.D. Alterations in blood-brain barrier permeability to large and small molecules and leukocyte accumulation after traumatic brain injury: Effects of post-traumatic hypothermia. *J. Neurotrauma* **2009**, *26*, 1123–1134. [CrossRef] [PubMed]
32. Mawhinney, L.J.; de Rivero Vaccari, J.P.; Dale, G.A.; Keane, R.W.; Bramlett, H.M. Heightened inflammasome activation is linked to age-related cognitive impairment in Fischer 344 rats. *BMC Neurosci.* **2011**, *12*, 123. [CrossRef] [PubMed]
33. De Rivero Vaccari, J.P.; Patel, H.H.; Brand, F.J., III; Perez-Pinzon, M.A.; Bramlett, H.M.; Raval, A.P. Estrogen receptor β signaling alters cellular inflammasomes activity after global cerebral ischemia in reproductively senescence female rats. *J. Neurochem.* **2016**, *136*, 492–496. [CrossRef] [PubMed]
34. Sarvari, M.; Kalló, I.; Hrabovszky, E.; Solymosi, N.; Liposits, Z. Ovariectomy and subsequent treatment with estrogen receptor agonists tune the innate immune system of the hippocampus in middle-aged female rats. *PLoS ONE* **2014**, *9*, e88540. [CrossRef] [PubMed]
35. Colson, B.A.; Petersen, K.J.; Collins, B.C.; Lowe, D.A.; Thomas, D.D. The myosin super-relaxed state is disrupted by estradiol deficiency. *Biochem. Biophys. Res. Commun.* **2015**, *456*, 151–155. [CrossRef] [PubMed]
36. Nedergaard, A.; Henriksen, K.; Karsdal, M.A.; Christiansen, C. Menopause, estrogens and frailty. *Gynecol. Endocrinol.* **2013**, *29*, 418–423. [CrossRef] [PubMed]
37. Iadecola, C.; Anrather, J. The immunology of stroke: From mechanisms to translation. *Nat. Med.* **2011**, *17*, 796–808. [CrossRef] [PubMed]
38. Barbacid, M. Neurotrophic factors and their receptors. *Curr. Opin. Cell Biol.* **1995**, *7*, 148–155. [CrossRef]
39. Thoenen, H. Neurotrophins and neuronal plasticity. *Science* **1995**, *270*, 593–598. [CrossRef] [PubMed]
40. Greenberg, M.E.; Xu, B.; Lu, B.; Hempstead, B.L. New insights in the biology of BDNF synthesis and release: Implications in CNS function. *J. Neurosci.* **2009**, *29*, 12764–12767. [CrossRef] [PubMed]
41. Binder, D.K.; Scharfman, H.E. Brain-derived neurotrophic factor. *Growth Factors* **2004**, *22*, 123–131. [CrossRef] [PubMed]
42. Lindvall, O.; Kokaia, Z.; Bengzon, J.; Elme, E.; Kokaia, M. Neurotrophins and brain insults. *Trends Neurosci.* **1994**, *17*, 490–496. [CrossRef]
43. Kramar, E.A.; Lin, B.; Lin, C.Y.; Arai, A.C.; Gall, C.M.; Lynch, G. A novel mechanism for the facilitation of theta-induced long-term potentiation by brain-derived neurotrophic factor. *J. Neurosci.* **2004**, *24*, 5151–5161. [CrossRef] [PubMed]
44. Rex, C.S.; Lin, C.Y.; Kramár, E.A.; Chen, L.Y.; Gall, C.M.; Lynch, G. Brain-derived neurotrophic factor promotes long-term potentiation-related cytoskeletal changes in adult hippocampus. *J. Neurosci.* **2007**, *27*, 3017–3029. [CrossRef] [PubMed]
45. Bramham, C.R.; Messaoudi, E. BDNF function in adult synaptic plasticity: The synaptic consolidation hypothesis. *Prog. Neurobiol.* **2005**, *76*, 99–125. [CrossRef] [PubMed]

46. Bath, K.G.; Akins, M.R.; Lee, F.S. BDNF control of adult SVZ neurogenesis. *Dev. Psychobiol.* **2012**, *54*, 78–89. [CrossRef] [PubMed]
47. Beck, T.; Lindholm, D.; Castren, E.; Wree, A. Brain-derived neurotrophic factor protects against ischemic cell damage in rat hippocampus. *J. Cereb. Blood Flow Metab.* **1994**, *14*, 689–692. [CrossRef] [PubMed]
48. Schabitz, W.R.; Schwab, S.; Spranger, M.; Hacke, W. Intraventricular brain-derived neurotrophic factor reduces infarct size after focal cerebral ischemia in rats. *J. Cereb. Blood Flow Metab.* **1997**, *17*, 500–506. [CrossRef] [PubMed]
49. Pardridge, W.M. Blood-brain barrier delivery. *Drug Discov. Today* **2007**, *12*, 54–61. [CrossRef] [PubMed]
50. Pardridge, W.M.; Wu, D.; Sakane, T. Combined use of carboxyl-directed protein pegylation and vector-mediated blood-brain barrier drug delivery system optimizes brain uptake of brain-derived neurotrophic factor following intravenous administration. *Pharm. Res.* **1998**, *15*, 576–582. [CrossRef] [PubMed]
51. Sun, B.F.; Wang, Q.Q.; Yu, Z.J.; Yu, Y.; Xiao, C.L.; Kang, C.S.; Ge, G.; Linghu, Y.; Zhu, J.D.; Li, Y.M. Exercise Prevents Memory Impairment Induced by Arsenic Exposure in Mice: Implication of Hippocampal BDNF and CREB. *PLoS ONE* **2015**, *10*, e0137810. [CrossRef] [PubMed]
52. Forti, L.N.; Van Roie, E.; Njemini, R.; Coudyzer, W.; Beyer, I.; Delecluse, C.; Bautmans, I. Dose-and gender-specific effects of resistance training on circulating levels of brain derived neurotrophic factor (BDNF) in community-dwelling older adults. *Exp. Gerontol.* **2015**, *70*, 144–149. [CrossRef] [PubMed]
53. Schabitz, W.R.; Steigleder, T.; Cooper-Kuhn, C.M.; Schwab, S.; Sommer, C.; Schneider, A.; Kuhn, H.G. Intravenous brain-derived neurotrophic factor enhances poststroke sensorimotor recovery and stimulates neurogenesis. *Stroke* **2007**, *38*, 2165–2171. [CrossRef] [PubMed]
54. Li, Y.; Luikart, B.W.; Birnbaum, S.; Chen, J.; Kwon, C.H.; Kernie, S.G.; Bassel-Dub, R.; Parada, L.F. TrkB regulates hippocampal neurogenesis and governs sensitivity to antidepressive treatment. *Neuron* **2008**, *59*, 399–412. [CrossRef] [PubMed]
55. Marlatt, M.W.; Potter, M.C.; Lucassen, P.J.; van Praag, H. Running throughout middle-age improves memory function, hippocampal neurogenesis, and BDNF levels in female C57BL/6J mice. *Dev. Neurobiol.* **2012**, *72*, 943–952. [CrossRef] [PubMed]
56. Raval, A.P.; Saul, I.; Dave, K.R.; DeFazio, R.A.; Perez-Pinzon, M.A.; Bramlett, H. Pretreatment with a single estradiol-17β bolus activates cyclic-AMP response element binding protein and protects CA1 neurons against global cerebral ischemia. *Neuroscience* **2009**, *160*, 307–318. [CrossRef] [PubMed]
57. Selvamani, A.; Sohrabji, F. The neurotoxic effects of estrogen on ischemic stroke in older female rats is associated with age-dependent loss of insulin-like growth factor-1. *J. Neurosci.* **2010**, *30*, 6852–6861. [CrossRef] [PubMed]
58. Belayev, L.; Alonso, O.F.; Busto, R.; Zhao, W.; Ginsberg, M.D. Middle cerebral artery occlusion in the rat by intraluminal suture. Neurological and pathological evaluation of an improved model. *Stroke* **1996**, *27*, 1616–1623. [CrossRef] [PubMed]
59. Lin, H.W.; Saul, I.; Gresia, V.L.; Neumann, J.T.; Dave, K.R.; Perez-Pinzon, M.A. Fatty acid methyl esters and Solutol HS 15 confer neuroprotection after focal and global cerebral ischemia. *Transl. Stroke Res.* **2014**, *5*, 109–117. [CrossRef] [PubMed]
60. Xie, L.; Jacobson, J.M.; Choi, E.S.; Busa, B.; Donahue, L.R.; Miller, L.M.; Rubin, C.T.; Judex, S. Low-level mechanical vibrations can influence bone resorption and bone formation in the growing skeleton. *Bone* **2006**, *39*, 1059–1066. [CrossRef] [PubMed]
61. Wysocki, A.; Butler, M.; Shamliyan, T.; Kane, R.L. Whole-Body Vibration Therapy for Osteoporosis. In Proceedings of the Agency for Healthcare Research and Quality, Rockville, MD, USA, 15 November 2011.

62. Ley, J.J.; Vigdorchik, A.; Belayev, L.; Zhao, W.; Busto, R.; Khoutorova, L.; Becker, D.A.; Ginsberg, M.D. Stilbazulenyl nitrone, a second-generation azulenyl nitrone antioxidant, confers enduring neuroprotection in experimental focal cerebral ischemia in the rat: Neurobehavior, histopathology, and pharmacokinetics. *J. Pharmacol. Exp. Ther.* **2005**, *313*, 1090–1100. [CrossRef] [PubMed]
63. Abulafia, D.P.; de Rivero Vaccari, J.P.; Lozano, J.D.; Lotocki, G.; Keane, R.W.; Dietrich, W.D. Inhibition of the inflammasome complex reduces the inflammatory response after thromboembolic stroke in mice. *J. Cereb. Blood Flow Metab.* **2009**, *29*, 534–544. [CrossRef] [PubMed]

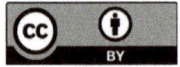

© 2018 by the authors. Licensee MDPI, Basel, Switzerland. This article is an open access article distributed under the terms and conditions of the Creative Commons Attribution (CC BY) license (http://creativecommons.org/licenses/by/4.0/).

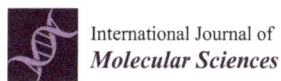

Article

Structure–Activity Relationship Study of Newly Synthesized Iridium-III Complexes as Potential Series for Treating Thrombotic Diseases

Chih-Hao Yang [1,†], Chih-Wei Hsia [2], Thanasekaran Jayakumar [2,†], Joen-Rong Sheu [1,2,†], Chih-Hsuan Hsia [2], Themmila Khamrang [3], Yen-Jen Chen [1,2], Manjunath Manubolu [4] and Yi Chang [2,5,6,*]

[1] Department of Pharmacology, Schools of Medicine, College of Medicine, Taipei Medical University, No. 250, Wu Hsing St., Taipei 110, Taiwan; chyang@tmu.edu.tw (C.-H.Y.); sheujr@tmu.edu.tw (J.-R.S.); m120104004@tmu.edu.tw (Y.-J.C.)

[2] Graduate Institute of Medical Sciences, College of Medicine, Taipei Medical University, No. 250, Wu Hsing St., Taipei 110, Taiwan; d119106003@tmu.edu.tw (C.-W.H.); jayakumar@tmu.edu.tw (T.J.); d119102013@tmu.edu.tw (C.-H.H.)

[3] Department of Chemistry, North Eastern Hill University, Shillong 793022, India; themmilakhamrang@gmail.com

[4] Department of Evolution, Ecology and Organismal Biology, Ohio State University, Columbus, OH 43212, USA; manubolu.1@osu.edu

[5] Department of Anesthesiology, Shin Kong Wu Ho-Su Memorial Hospital, No. 95, Wen Chang Rd., Taipei 111, Taiwan

[6] School of Medicine, Fu-Jen Catholic University, No. 510, Zhong Zheng Rd, Xin Zhuang Dist., New Taipei City 242, Taiwan

* Correspondence: m004003@ms.skh.org.tw; Tel.: +886-984-160920; Fax: +886-2-2832-6912

† These authors contributed equally to this work.

Received: 20 September 2018; Accepted: 15 November 2018; Published: 19 November 2018

Abstract: Platelets play a major role in hemostatic events and are associated with various pathological events, such as arterial thrombosis and atherosclerosis. Iridium (Ir) compounds are potential alternatives to platinum compounds, since they exert promising anticancer effects without cellular toxicity. Our recent studies found that Ir compounds show potent antiplatelet properties. In this study, we evaluated the in vitro antiplatelet, in vivo antithrombotic and structure–activity relationship (SAR) of newly synthesized Ir complexes, Ir-1, Ir-2 and Ir-4, in agonists-induced human platelets. Among the tested compounds, Ir-1 was active in inhibiting platelet aggregation induced by collagen; however, Ir-2 and Ir-4 had no effects even at their maximum concentrations of 50 µM against collagen and 500 µM against U46619-induced aggregation. Similarly, Ir-1 was potently inhibiting of adenosine triphosphate (ATP) release, calcium mobilization ($[Ca^{2+}]i$) and P-selectin expression induced by collagen-induced without cytotoxicity. Likewise, Ir-1 expressively suppressed collagen-induced Akt, PKC, p38MAPKs and JNK phosphorylation. Interestingly, Ir-2 and Ir-4 had no effect on platelet function analyzer (PFA-100) collagen-adenosine diphosphate (C-ADP) and collagen-epinephrine (C-EPI) induced closure times in mice, but Ir-1 caused a significant increase when using C-ADP stimulation. Other in vivo studies revealed that Ir-1 significantly prolonged the platelet plug formation, increased tail bleeding times and reduced the mortality of adenosine diphosphate (ADP)-induced acute pulmonary thromboembolism in mice. Ir-1 has no substitution on its phenyl group, a water molecule (like cisplatin) can replace its chloride ion and, hence, the rate of hydrolysis might be tuned by the substituent on the ligand system. These features might have played a role for the observed effects of Ir-1. These results indicate that Ir-1 may be a lead compound to design new antiplatelet drugs for the treatment of thromboembolic diseases.

Keywords: iridium complexes; platelets; ATP; $[Ca^{2+}]i$; signaling cascades; SAR

1. Introduction

Platelets form a plug after their interaction with endothelial matrix proteins to stop excessive bleeding during vascular injury. However, platelet aggregation contributes to thrombotic events, initiating acute coronary syndrome, heart attacks, and strokes [1,2]. After vessel injury, the exposed subendothelial surface makes platelet adhere. Platelet activation and secretion of soluble mediators, such as adenosine 5′-diphosphate (ADP), thromboxane A2 (TXA2), and thrombin, are all involved in the recruitment of other circulating platelets. Currently, numerous antiplatelet drugs are clinically accepted for the treatment and prevention of thrombotic complications. These drugs include acetylsalicylic acid, clopidogrel, eptifibatide, triflusal and tirofiban; however, some have several indemnity effects and battle in long term therapy, such as the known clinical aspirin resistance [3]. Several studies also have reported inter-individual variability in platelet reaction to aspirin and clopidogrel, the well-known oral antiplatelet drugs [4]. The possibility of using antiplatelet agents to substitute oral anticoagulant treatment has been reported in the literature for secondary prevention of further vascular events after limited ischemic stroke due to their lower risk [5].

Platelets also play a serious role in cancer metastasis, including tumor cell migration and invasion [6]. When platelets are activated, they release into the peritumoral space and enhance tumor cell extravasation and metastases [7]. Chronic administration of antiplatelet agents during active malignancy clearly shows the principal role platelets play in maintaining hemostasis. A platelet aggregation inhibitor, cilostazol, reduced pulmonary metastases in a murine model of breast cancer [8]. The authors also observed that liposomal cilostazol decreased ex vivo platelet aggregation and reduced platelet–tumor complex formation in vivo. The existing antiplatelet agents permanently inhibit their target by inhibiting platelet aggregation, however the bleeding risk is still difficult to alleviate. Therefore, efforts are being taken globally to develop new antiplatelet agents with low side effects [9,10].

Organometallic iridium complexes (Ir) have attracted abundant consideration recently due to their unique properties of having rich synthetic chemistry, having variable oxidation states that are prevailing under physiological conditions and being kinetically constant [11]. Furthermore, several organometallic iridium compounds were reported to bind DNA through intercalation [12]. Remarkably, the ligands of most organometallic iridium anticancer complexes are metallocenes, half-sandwich, carbene, CO, or π-ligands [13,14]. We have recently developed some novel Ir-III complexes (Ir-3, Ir-6 and Ir-11) and found they have strong antiplatelet effects with different molecular mechanisms [15–17]. From these studies, Shyu et al. found that Ir-3 inhibits platelet activation through the inhibition of signaling pathways, such as the PLCγ2-PKC cascade, and the subsequent suppression of Akt and JNK1 activation, ultimately inhibiting platelet aggregation. In another study, this author found that this compound evidently prolonged the bleeding time in experimental mice, and that this compound plays a crucial role by inhibiting platelet activation via the inhibiting PLCγ2–PKC cascade and the subsequent suppression of Akt and MAPK activation. Recently, our study also demonstrated that Ir-11 increased the bleeding time and reduced mortality related with acute pulmonary thromboembolism [15]. These results encouraged us to work further on Ir complexes on antiplatelet effects. Thus, here we report the synthesis, in vitro antiplatelet, in vivo antithrombotic, and cytotoxicity properties of complexes [Ir(Cp*)(1-(2-pyridyl)-3-phenylimidazo[1,5-α]pyridine)Cl]BF$_4$ (Ir-1), [Ir(Cp*)(1-(2-pyridyl)-3-(3-nitrophenyl)imidazo [1,5-α]pyridine) Cl]BF$_4$ (Ir-2) and [Ir(Cp*)(9-[4-(1-pyridin-2-yl-imidazo[1,5-α]pyridin-3-yl)-phenyl]-9H-carbazole) Cl]BF$_4$ (Ir-4). The structure–antiplatelet activity (SAR) of these compounds have also been analyzed in this paper.

2. Results

2.1. Effects of Synthetic Ir-III Compounds on Platelet Aggregation In Vitro

The synthetic Ir-III compounds (Figure 1) were tested for their inhibitory effects on platelet aggregation. Collagen (1 μg/mL) and U46619 (1 μM) stimulated about 85–98% aggregation in washed human platelets. Figure 2A–C shows the in vitro inhibitory effects (%) of various concentrations of Ir-1 (2, 5 and 10 μM), Ir-2 and Ir-4 (10, 20 and 50 μM) against collagen and Ir-1(50, 100 and 200), Ir-2 and Ir-4 (100, 200 and 500 μM) against U46619 induced aggregation in washed human platelets. Among the three compounds tested, Ir-1 had the most potent activity, inhibiting platelet aggregation induced by collagen (11.1 ± 3.7%) and U46619 (12.6 ± 6.3%) at a respective concentration of 10 and 200 μM (Figure 2C,D). Ir-2 and Ir-4 had effects on neither collagen nor U46619 induced platelets. Moreover, in plasma rich platelets (PRP), Ir-1 has almost 20% lower inhibitory effect against collagen-induced aggregation (32.5 ± 2.6%) than in the washed human platelets (11.1 ± 3.7%) data not shown. This result indicate that Ir-1 may slightly bind with plasma proteins and hence it exerts less effect in PRP.

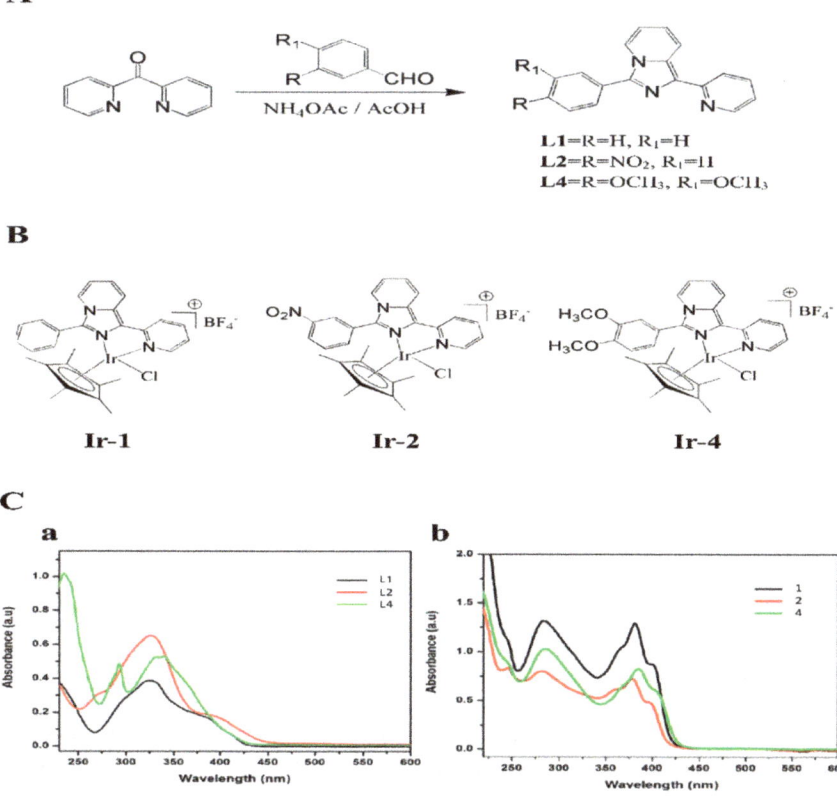

Figure 1. Synthesis of ligands and Ir-III complexes. (**A**) Scheme of synthesis of ligands 1-(2-pyridyl)-3-phenylimidazo[1,5-α]pyridine (L1), 1-(2-pyridyl)-3-(3-nitrophenyl)imidazo[1,5-α]pyridine (L2) and 9-[4-(1-pyridin-2-yl-imidazo[1,5-α]pyridin-3-yl)-phenyl-9H-carbazole (L4); (**B**) Scheme of synthesis of complexes [Ir(Cp*)(L1)Cl]BF$_4$ (Ir-1), [Ir(Cp*)(L2)Cl]BF$_4$ (Ir-2) and [Ir(Cp*)(L4)Cl]BF$_4$ (Ir-4); (**C**) Absorption spectra of ligands (**a**) and Ir-III complexes (**b**) in acetonitrile.

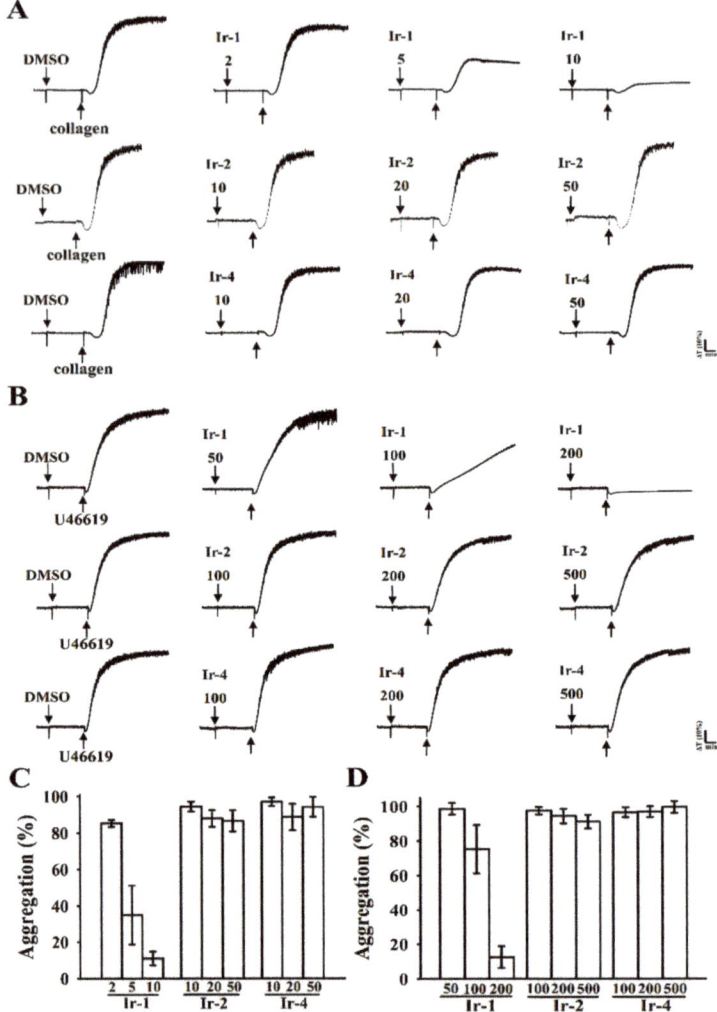

Figure 2. Anti-aggregation activity of iridium complexes (Ir1, Ir-2 and Ir-4) on collagen and U46619-induced platelet aggregation in washed human platelets. (**A**) Washed human platelets (3.6 × 10^8 cells/mL) were preincubated with the solvent control (0.1% DMSO) or Ir-1 (2–10 μM), Ir-2 and Ir-4 (10–50 μM) for 3 min and then treated with 1 μg/mL collagen for 6 min; (**B**) Washed human platelets were preincubated with the solvent control or Ir-1 (50–200 μM), Ir-2 and Ir-4 (100–500 μM) for 3 min and then treated with 1 μM U46619 for 6 min to stimulate platelet aggregation. Histograms of platelet aggregation in Ir-1, Ir-2 and Ir-4 treated platelets stimulated by collagen (**C**) and U46619 (**D**). Data are presented as means ± standard errors of the means (n = 4).

2.2. Ir-III Compounds on ATP Release and [Ca^{2+}]i Mobilization in Human Platelets

The release of dense granule content in platelets was assessed through ATP release analysis. Among the three tested compounds, only Ir-1 significantly prevented ATP release from activated platelets stimulated by collagen (Figure 3A). Activation of glycoprotein VI (GPVI), a collagen receptor, leads to quick intracellular calcium mobilization, which is crucial for provoking platelet secretion and aggregation [18]. To investigate the intracellular mobilization of free calcium stores, calcium levels were measured flurometrically using the calcium-sensitive dye, Fura-2 AM. Stimulation of platelets with collagen caused a marked increase of intracellular calcium concentration (Figure 3B). However, Ir-1 inhibited collagen-induced [Ca^{2+}]i mobilization on platelets in a manner similar to that observed with the inhibition of ATP release.

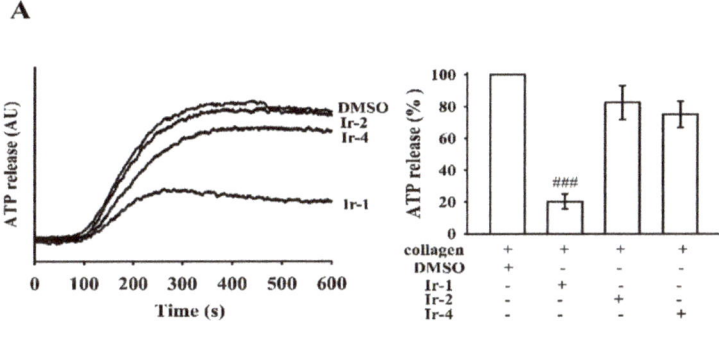

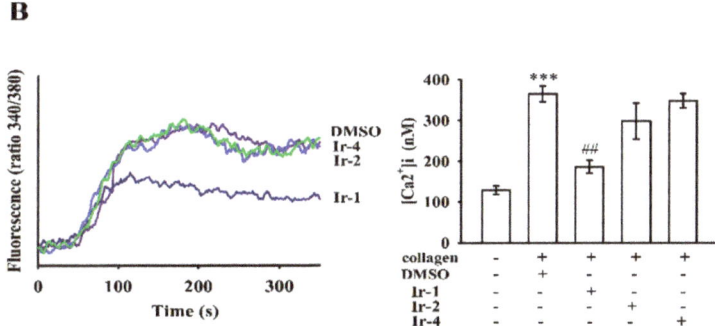

Figure 3. Effects of Ir-1, Ir-2 and Ir-4 on collagen induced ATP release and relative [Ca^{2+}]i mobilization in human platelets. Washed human platelets (3.6 × 10^8 cells/mL) were preincubated with 10 µM Ir-1, Ir-2 and Ir-4 or a solvent control (0.1% DMSO) and subsequently treated with 1 µg/mL of collagen to stimulate ATP release reaction (**A**), and to induce the cytoplasmic influx of Ca^{2+} from intracellular stores (**B**) as described in the Sections 4.3 and 4.4. Data are presented as the means ± S.E.M. ($n = 4$). *** $p < 0.001$ compared with the DMSO group. ### $p < 0.001$ compared with the collagen induced group. ## $p < 0.01$ compared with the DMSO group.

2.3. Ir-1 Attenuated Collagen Induced P-Selectin Expression without Causing Cytotoxicity

Platelet activation is associated with surface P-selectin expression from α-granules, thus triggering platelet aggregation. In normal platelets, surface P-selectin is positioned on the inner wall of α-granules. Platelet activation results in "membrane flipping", where the platelet releases α-granules, showing the inner walls of the granules on the outside of the cell [19]. In this study, Ir-2 and Ir-4 only slightly reduced P-selectin expression; however, Ir-1 had a significant effect on P-selectin expression stimulated by 1 µg/mL collagen (Figure 4A).

The aggregation curves of platelets preincubated with 100 µM of Ir-1, Ir-2 and Ir-4 for 10 min and then washed twice with Tyrode's solution showed no major differences from those of platelets preincubated with the solvent control (0.1% DMSO) (Figure 4B), demonstrating that the effects of Ir complexes on platelet aggregation are alterable and noncytotoxic. Additionally, the LDH study showed that the tested Ir complexes (100 µM) incubated with platelets for 20 min did not significantly increase LDH activity or exert cytotoxic effects on platelets (Figure 4C), demonstrating that Ir-compounds do not disturb platelet permeability or induce platelet cytolysis.

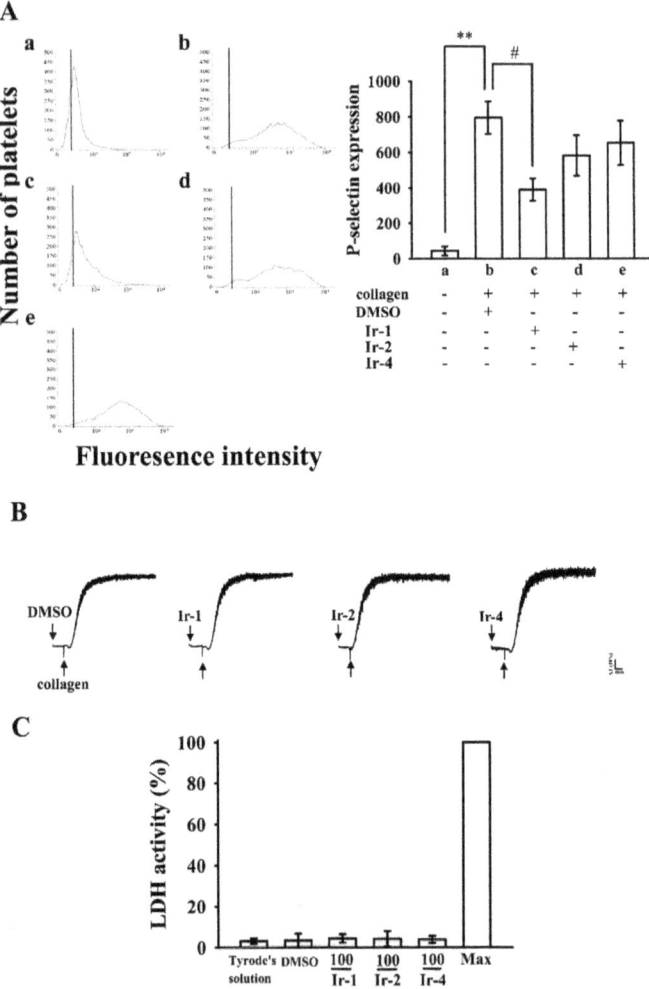

Figure 4. Effects of Ir-1, Ir-2 and Ir-4 on collagen-induced surface FITC-P-selectin expression and cytotoxicity in human platelets. (**A**) Washed human platelets (3.6 × 10^8 cells/mL) were preincubated with: (**a**) FITC only as a resting control; (**b**) the solvent control (0.1% DMSO); (**c**) Ir-1 (10 µM); (**d**) Ir-2 (10 µM); or (**e**) Ir-4 (10 µM) for 3 min and subsequently treated with 1 µg/mL of collagen to test the direct binding of FITC-P-selectin; (**B**) Washed platelets were preincubated with 0.1% DMSO or Ir-1, Ir-2 and Ir-4 (100 µM) for 10 min and subsequently washed two times with Tyrode's solution and collagen (1 µg/mL) was then added to trigger platelet aggregation; (**C**) Washed platelets (3.6 × 10^8/mL) were preincubated with 0.1% DMSO or with 100 µM of Ir-1, Ir-2 and Ir-4 for 20 min, and a 10-µL aliquot of the supernatant was deposited on a Fuji Dri-Chem slide LDH-PIII. Data are presented as the means ± S.E.M. (*n* = 4). ** *p* < 0.01 compared with the DMSO group. # *p* < 0.05 compared with the collagen induced group.

2.4. Ir-1 Tempered MAPK and Akt/PKC Phosphorylation

MAPKs, such as P38MAPK, JNK and ERK, are expressed in platelets and different agonists can activate them. Phosphorylation of these signaling molecules plays a central role in activating platelet granule secretion [20]. Consequently, to clarify the mechanism underlying the effects of tested Ir-complexes on agonist-induced platelets, we studied the Akt/PKC and MAPK pathway (Figure 5A–D). Among the tested compounds, only Ir-1 significantly attenuated the phosphorylation of Akt/PKC and MAPK molecules p38 and JNK (Figure 5). Ir-2 and Ir-4 had no effect on these molecules.

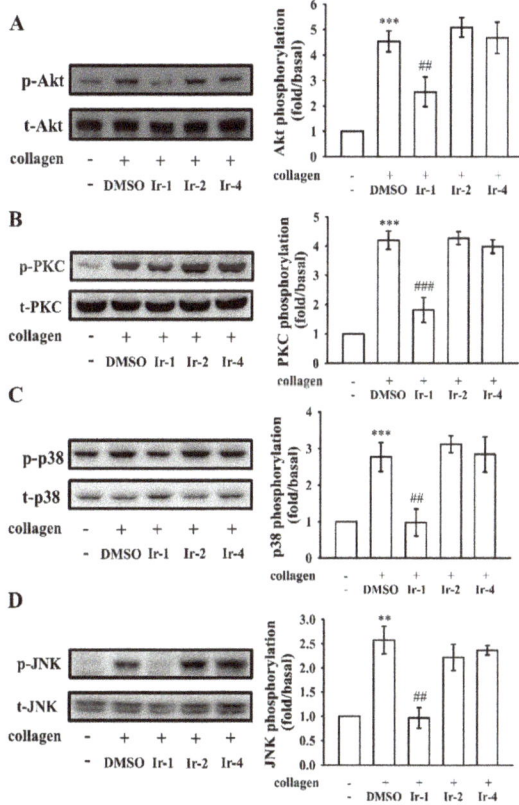

Figure 5. Effects of iridium-III complexes on the phosphorylation of Akt/PKC and MAPKs induced by collagen in human platelets. Washed platelets (1.2×10^9 cells/mL) were incubated with solvent control (0.1% DMSO) or 10 µM Ir-1, Ir-2 and Ir-4 and then treated with 1 µg/mL collagen to induce platelet activation. The subcellular extracts were analyzed by Western blotting for the phosphorylation of: Akt (**A**); PKC (**B**); p38MAPK (**C**); and JNK (**D**). Data are presented as the mean ± SEM ($n = 4$). ** $p < 0.01$ and *** $p < 0.001$ compared with the normal group, ## $p < 0.01$ and ### $p < 0.001$ compared with the collagen induced group.

2.5. Ir-1 Inhibits Platelet Aggregation via Interrupting the Association of JAQ-1 with GPVI

Integrin α2β1 and GPVI are major collagen receptors that mediate platelet adhesion and aggregation. To investigate whether Ir-1 inhibits platelet aggregation via GPVI, we used convulxin, a GPVI agonist, which is purified from the venom of *Crotalus durissus terrificus* to induce platelet aggregation. The results show that treatment with Ir-1 (5–20 µM) significantly inhibited platelet aggregation stimulated with 10 ng/mL of convulxin (Figure 6A,B).

The above result was further confirmed by flow cytometry analysis that Ir-1 inhibits platelet activation via interrupting the convulxin and GPVI interaction on the platelet membrane. The results revealed that the relative fluorescence intensity of FITC-JAQ1 (mAb raised against GPVI; 1 µg/mL) bound to the platelets was significantly higher than that of the resting counterparts (Figure 6C). This FITC-JAQ1 mAb binding significantly diminished in the presence of convulxin (10 ng/mL) or Ir-1 (20 µM). Overall, although these results may suggest that Ir-1 could interrupt the association between JAQ-1 and GPVI to its antiplatelet mechanism, however the possibility of other unidentified mechanisms involved in this reaction needs to be clarified in future studies.

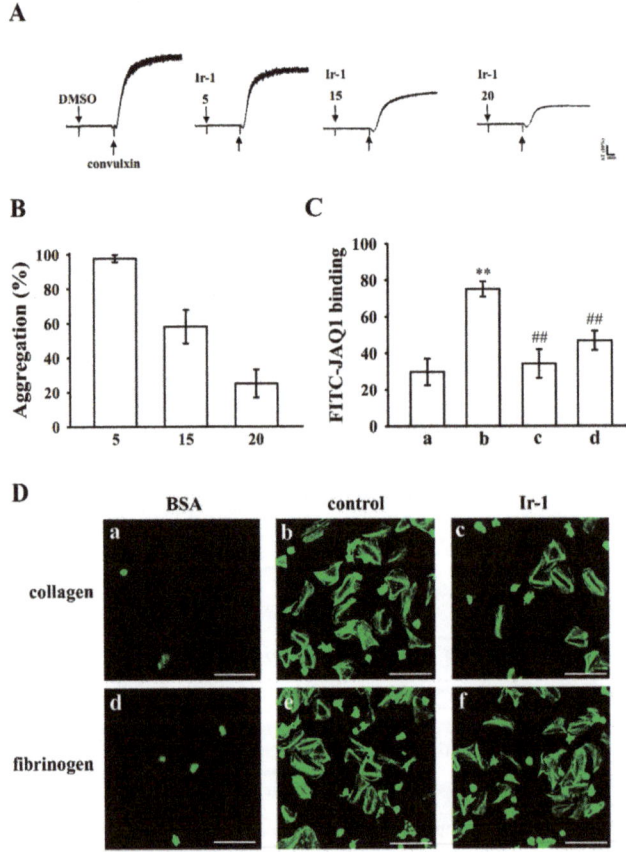

Figure 6. Effects of Ir-1 on convulxin-induced platelet aggregation, adhesion and spreading in human platelets. (**A**) Washed platelets (3.6 × 10^8 cells/mL) were preincubated with Ir-1 (5–20 µM) or the solvent control (0.1% DMSO), followed by the addition of 10 ng/ml of convulxin; (**B**) Concentration-response (%) histograms of Ir-1 in inhibition of convulxin-induced platelet aggregation; (**C**) Statistical graphs represent the platelets in the presence of: (a) FITC only (background); (b) FITC-JAQ1 mAb (1 µg/mL); (c) preincubated with convulxin (10 ng/mL); and (d) Ir-1 (20 µM), followed by the addition of FITC-JAQ1 mAb (1 µg/mL); (**D**) Washed human platelets were allowed to spread on: (**a,d**) bovine serum albumin (BSA); (**b,c**) collagen; and (**e,f**) fibrinogen-coated surfaces at 37 °C for 45 min in the presence of (**b,e**) the solvent control (0.1% DMSO) or (**c,f**) Ir-1 (10 µM, 5 min, at 37 °C) and then fixed with paraformaldehyde to stop spreading. Platelets were subsequently labeled with FITC-conjugated phalloidin and photographed under a confocal microscope (scale bar = 10 µm). Data are presented as means ± standard errors of the means (n = 3). ** $p < 0.01$, ## $p < 0.01$ compared with the control group.

2.6. Ir-1 Restricts Cell Adhesion and Spreading on Immobilized Collagen

As shown in Figure 6Da,b, platelets staining with FITC-conjugated phalloidin demonstrated that platelets adhered to immobilized collagen were significantly more than immobilized BSA. In addition, Ir-1-treated platelets had lower adhesion and spreading on immobilized collagen than did 0.1% DMSO-treated platelets (Figure 6Dc). Control platelets (0.1% DMSO, data not shown, $n = 3$) were fixed to immobilized collagen normally, whereas Ir-1-treated platelets showed less adhesion to the collagen-coated surface. Ir-1 inhibited platelet adhesion by approximately $49.7 \pm 1.1\%$. The percentage of spreading platelets treated with Ir-1 was approximately $34.3 \pm 3.2\%$. The platelet adhesion and spreading between 0.1% DMSO-treated platelets and Ir-1 on immobilized fibrinogen were no significant.

2.7. Ir-1 on Closure Time

Platelet aggregation in response to ADP and epinephrine (EPI) was recorded using a platelet function analyzer (PFA-100) with both collagen-ADP (C-ADP) and collagen epinephrine (C-EPI) cartridges. The closure time (CT) of the C-ADP-coated membrane in whole blood treated with 10 µM Ir-1 was significantly increased (279.6 ± 25.0 s) when compared to the solvent control DMSO (95.0 ± 30.6 s), however, the CT was not prolonged in C-EPI-coated membrane (Figure 7A). Ir-2 and Ir-4 did not prolong either C-ADP or C-EPI closure times as the levels remained within normal ranges as established by the PFA-100 test.

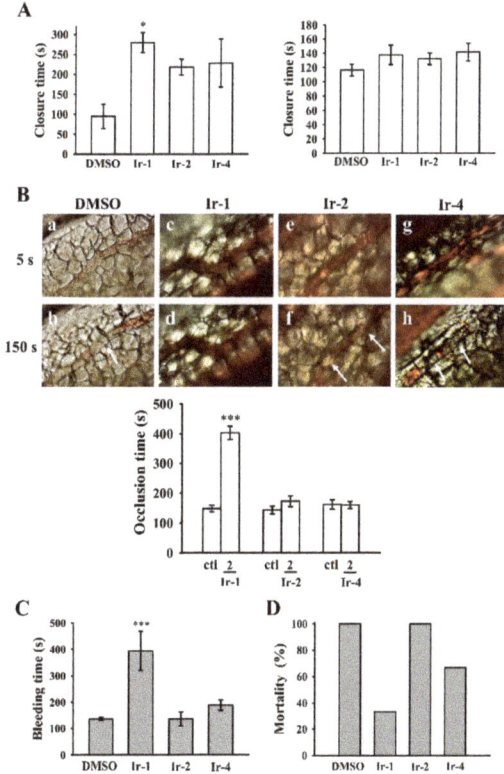

Figure 7. Effects of iridium complex on PFA-100 closure time and thrombotic platelet plug formation in the mesenteric venules, bleeding time and ADP induced pulmonary thrombosis in mice. (**A**) Shear-

induced platelet plug formation in human whole blood was determined by recording the closure time of C-ADP and C-EPI-coated membranes, as described in the Section 4.8; (**B**) Mice were administered an intravenous bolus of the solvent control (ctl; 0.1% DMSO) or Ir-1, Ir-2 and Ir-4 (2 mg/kg), and the mesenteric venules were irradiated to induce microthrombus formation (occlusion time). Microscopic images (400× magnification) of 0.1% DMSO-treated controls (a,b) and the 2 mg/kg Ir-1 (c,d), Ir-2 (e,f) and Ir-4 (g,h) treated groups were recorded at 5 s (a,c,e,g) and 150 s (b,d,f,h) after irradiation. The photographs are representative of six similar experiments. The arrow indicates platelet plug formation; (**C**) The bleeding time was measured through transection of the tail in mice after 30 min of administering 2 mg/kg Ir-1, Ir-2 and Ir-4 intraperitoneally; (**D**) Effects of Ir-1, Ir-2 and Ir-4 on ADP-induced pulmonary thrombosis in mice. ADP (700 mg/kg) was injected in the tail vein to induce acute pulmonary thrombosis. The survival rate was determined after ADP administration. The survival rate was evaluated using the Kaplan–Meier survival method (n = 8). Data are presented as the mean ± SEM (n = 8). * $p < 0.05$ and *** $p < 0.001$, compared with the 0.1% DMSO-treated group.

2.8. Effects of Ir Complexes on Occlusion Time and Bleeding Time

Platelet-rich thrombus formation in mesenteric venules was observed in fluorescein sodium and filtered light irradiated ICR mice. The time lapse for inducing occlusion in the irradiated vessel was 148.3 ± 11.2 s (n = 8). From the data shown in Figure 7B, among the tested Ir-III complexes, Ir-1 (2 mg/kg) expressively prolonged the occlusion time to 403.1 ± 22.3 s (n = 8). The thrombotic platelet plug formation was detected in mesenteric microvessels at 150 s, whereas it was noted at 5 s after irradiation in the solvent-treated group. Platelet plug formation was not observed at either 5 or 150 s after irradiation in mice that had been treated with Ir-1 (2 mg/kg). The rate of blood flow in the solvent-treated venule was slower than that of the Ir-1-treated venule, as the platelet plug converted at 150 s (Figure 7B).

The tail bleeding time of mice that were intraperitoneally injected with DMSO was measured as 135.8 ± 5.5 s (n = 8). A dose of 2 mg/kg Ir-1 treated mice showed a significant prolongation (394.0 ± 73.9 s) of the bleeding time 30 min after injection. Ir-2 or Ir-4 did not prolong the bleeding time, as their effects were similar to that in control mice (Figure 7C).

2.9. Ir-Complexes on ADP-Induced Acute Pulmonary Thromboembolism

An in vivo study was performed to test the effect of Ir-complexes on inhibiting acute pulmonary embolism mortality in mice. As shown in Figure 7D, a dose of 2 mg/kg Ir-1 prominently lowered the mortality rate in mice, from 100% to 33.3% in those that had been challenged with ADP (700 mg/kg) indicating that Ir-1 efficiently stops acute pulmonary thromboembolism in vivo.

3. Discussion

In this study, three iridium (III) complexes, [Ir(Cp*)(1-(2-pyridyl)-3-phenylimidazo[1,5-α]pyridine)Cl]BF$_4$ (Ir-1), [Ir(Cp*)(1-(2-pyridyl)-3-(3-nitrophenyl)imidazo [1,5-α]pyridine) Cl]BF$_4$ (Ir-2) and [Ir(Cp*)(9-[4-(1-pyridin-2-yl-imidazo[1,5-α]pyridin-3-yl)-phenyl]-9H-carbazole) Cl]BF$_4$ (Ir-4) with 1-(2-pyridyl)-3-phenylimidazo[1,5-α]pyridine, 1-(2-pyridyl)-3-(3-nitrophenyl)imidazo[1,5-α]pyridine and 9-[4-(1-pyridin-2-yl-imidazo[1,5-α]pyridin-3-yl)-phenyl]-9H-carbazole as ligands, respectively, were synthesized and evaluated for their antiplatelet activities. Among them, Ir-1 exhibited the most potent antiplatelet activity against collagen and U4661 induced human platelet aggregation, while Ir-2 and Ir-4 had no effect. Ir-1 also exhibited potent in vivo antithrombotic effects. Overall, these findings highlight the exciting potential of iridium (III) compounds to be developed as effective antiplatelet drugs for the treatment of thromboembolic diseases. In addition, Ir-1 may be considered as a leading compound to design a new class of antiplatelet drugs.

Ligand-gated Ca^{2+}-permeable ion channels are express on the platelet surface and provide a rapid route for Ca^{2+} entry to release ATP from damaged vascular cells or from activated platelets and other blood cells [21,22]. These channels shown to increase in vitro platelet $[Ca^{2+}]i$ responses following stimulation by several major hemostatic agonists, including ADP, collagen, thrombin and thromboxane A2, and also aggravate in vivo thrombosis [23]. Evaluation of platelet-surface P-selectin in activated platelets can be used as a substitute to measurement of platelet aggregation for analysis of platelet defects and in monitoring the effectiveness of drug treatments [24,25]. Therefore, inhibition of $[Ca^{2+}]i$ mobilization, ATP production and platelet-surface P-selectin is important for appraising the effectiveness of the antiplatelet drugs. Our previous studies found some newly synthesized Ir-III compounds, such as [Ir (Cp*) 1-(2-pyridyl)-3-(3-methoxyphenyl)imidazo[1,5-α]pyridine Cl]BF4 (Ir-3), [Ir(Cp*)1-(2-pyridyl)-3-(4-dimethylaminophenyl)imidazo[1,5-α]pyridine Cl]BF4 (Ir-6) and [Ir(Cp*)1-(2-pyridyl)-3-(2-hydroxyphenyl)imidazo[1,5-α]pyridine Cl]BF4 (Ir-11), potently inhibit collagen-activated $[Ca^{2+}]i$ mobilization, ATP production and platelet-surface P-selectin expression in washed human platelets. Consistent with these results, this work observed that, among the three tested Ir-III complexes (Ir-1, Ir-2 and Ir-4), Ir-1 effectively inhibited collagen stimulated $[Ca^{2+}]i$ mobilization, ATP production and P-selectin expression. These results indicate that inhibition of these granular substances may contribute to the important antiplatelet effects of Ir-1 compounds.

Due to the integrity of the cell membrane after the release of LDH, a decrease in LDH release from the cytoplasm and a supplement of enough oxygen for platelet metabolism are important factors for improving survival and quality of platelet concentrate during storage [26]. In this study, the LDH enzyme activity was expressively increased, as evidenced by a maximal value (MAX) of LDH in the sonicated platelets, which is used as a positive control as compared with the DMSO, Tyrode's solution and Ir-III complex treated groups. It seems that Ir-III complexes-treated platelets had no membrane damage and thus they could have beneficial effects on the platelets quality.

Akt pathway had reported in the activated platelets by GPVI via the modulation of the serine/threonine kinase, Akt [27]. This molecule was found to be phosphorylated by PKC and Ca^{2+}/calmodulin-dependent protein kinase [28]. Akt deficient mice showed impaired platelet activation induced by collagen [29]. MAPKs are reported to exist in platelets and be intricately involved in the action of numerous anti-platelet agents [30]. Studies with inhibitors have established that MAPKs contribute critically to platelet reactions in different agonists [31]. Several inflammatory cytokines and stress inducers activate JNK1/2 and p38 MAPK that lead to cellular apoptosis [32]. A study had also shown that JNK deficient platelets are directly correlated with increased bleeding time, decreased integrin $\alpha IIb\beta 3$ activation, and severe granule secretion [31]. Moreover, p38 MAPK is associated with thrombus formation, as demonstrated in $p38^{+/-}$ mice in a model of ferric chloride-induced carotid artery occlusion [21]; the removal of JNK1 also weakens in vitro collagen induced platelet aggregation and granule release and in vivo thrombus formation [31]. Consequently, the inhibition of Akt, PKC and JNK/p38 phosphorylation can be considered to be playing an important role in the antiplatelet action of drugs or compounds. This hypothesis is consistent with the current study that among the three tested Ir-III complexes, Ir-1 had potently suppressed collagen-induced Akt, PKC, p38 and JNK phosphorylation, while Ir-2 and Ir-4 did not affect these molecules. These findings support that Ir-1 could reduce collagen-induced platelet activation, including granule release, $[Ca^{2+}]i$ mobilization, and platelet aggregation, partly through the inhibition of Akt, PKC, p38 and JNK activation.

PFA-100, a new method of measuring the primary hemostasis induced by platelet adhesion and aggregation under shear stress conditions, has recently been familiarized. This test measures the time of platelet plug formation, called closure time [33]. The clinical effectiveness of PFA-100 has been confirmed in various platelet disorders, including the platelet dysfunction especially in uremic patients [34]. In addition, PFA-100 has evidenced to be useful in measuring surgical bleeding risk in patients who had oral surgery and other surgical procedures [33,35]. Further, some reports designate that the use of PFA-100 as perioperative screening test is connected with an increase in the use of desmopressin prophylaxis that still was not supportive in reducing the rate of bleeding complications [36]. In the present study, we analyzed the PFA-100 (C-EPI and C-ADP closure times) for the risk of bleeding complications after Ir-III complex treatment. Our results did show significant differences in the closure time values of the C-ADP cartridge of the PFA-100 test in Ir-1 treated platelets. In addition, we were not able to detect any significant changes in C-EPI cartridge of the PFA-100 closure time values.

Antiplatelet drugs are typically used in thrombogenic diseases, but acute intense thrombocytopenia is a documented complication of treatment with antiplatelet drug (e.g., GPIIb/IIIa inhibitors), and the reason is not yet fully identified. Thrombocytopenia may be related with a variety of conditions, and life-threatening bleeding is one of its worst side effects. Since GPVI expression scarcity is only associated with faintly prolonged bleeding times, it is worth developing novel GPVI antagonists for thrombogenic diseases. In this study, Ir-1 significantly tempered thrombus formation in two in vivo models of fluorescein sodium-induced platelet thrombus formation in the mesenteric microvessels and ADP-induced pulmonary thrombosis in mice. In addition, Ir-1 did not affect normal hemostasis without inducing mortality in mice. These results suggest that Ir-1 may recognize as safe antithrombotic agent. In this study, FITC-JAQ1 mAb bound to the platelets was significantly higher than that of the resting platelets. This FITC-JAQ1 binding significantly reduced by convulxin or Ir-1, indicating that Ir-1 may interrupt the association between the JAQ-1 and the collagen receptor GPVI on human platelets. As shown in Figure 6D, platelet spreading on fibrinogen-coated membrane seems visually to be attenuated after platelet pretreatment by Ir-1 (Figure 6D, compare e to f) although the difference is not significant. This result may clarify by a report that GPVI dimers represent a significant part of GPVI on the surface of resting platelets and are able to bind fibrinogen [37]. In mice naturally deficient in GPVI, the tail bleeding time is usually not prolonged, in contrast with the noticed in vivo effect of Ir-1. This phenomenon may suggest that Ir-1 has additional effects, besides the collagen-GPVI axis.

Generally, addition of polar substituents into the coordinated benzene ring lowers cytotoxicity or biological activity [38]. This hypothesis was confirmed from the IC_{50} values of monosubstituted benzenes: OPh < H (benzene) < CONH2, COOEt, COPh, COOMe, Br, CH2OH. Activities ranged from moderate (18 µM) to inactive (> 100 µM). In this study, based on the previous literature, these type of Ir-III (Ir-1, Ir-2 and Ir-4) compounds could interact with biological systems after hydrolysis, and the chloride ions in the complexes may be replaced by water molecule (as in cisplatin). The rate of hydrolysis may be tuned by the substituent on the ligand system. Mostly, the complexes hold increase in rate of hydrolysis display greater cytotoxicity than the compounds, which are inactive or weakly active with less hydrolyzing properties. A study showed that bovine, ovine, and caprine κ-casein and their hydrolysates exhibit platelet inhibitory activities due to their potent hydrolytic behaviors [39]. A previous important study also established that carbamoylpiperidine and nipecotoylpiperazine derivatives augment desired antithrombotic effects because of their increased levels of hydrophobicity [40]. Therefore, we postulated that the difference in the antiplatelet activities of complexes Ir-1, Ir-2, and Ir-4 is mainly dependent on the respective substitution on the phenyl (no substitution), nitrophenyl (electron withdrawing substitution) and dimethoxy (electron donating substitution) groups on the ring of the iridium ligands. Here, the absence of substitution on phenyl group in Ir-1 could increase the rate of hydrolysis on its ligand system and might play a role in its observed antiplatelet and antithrombotic effects.

4. Materials and Methods

4.1. Reagents

Thrombin, U46619, heparin, collagen, fibrinogen, FITC-phalloidin and bovine serum albumin (BSA) were purchased from Sigma (St. Louis, MO, USA). Fura-2AM was purchased from Molecular Probes (Eugene, OR, USA). An anti-phospho-p38 mitogen-activated protein kinase (MAPK) Ser^{182} monoclonal antibody (mAb) and convulxin were purchased from Santa Cruz Biotechnology (Santa Cruz, CA, USA). Anti-p38 MAPK, anti-phospho-c-Jun N-terminal kinase (JNK) (Thr^{183}/Tyr^{185}), anti-phospho-(Ser) protein kinase C (PKC) substrate (pleckstrin; p-p47), and anti-JNK polyclonal antibodies (pAbs) were purchased from Cell Signaling (Beverly, MA, USA). Anti-phospho-protein kinase B (Akt) (Ser^{473}) and anti-Akt mAbs were purchased from Biovision (Mountain View, CA, USA). Fluorescein isothiocyanate (FITC)-labeled anti-GPVI (JAQ1) mAb was obtained from Emfret Analytics (Würzburg, Germany). Hybond-P polyvinylidene fluoride (PVDF) membranes, an enhanced chemiluminescence Western blotting detection reagent, and antibodies, namely horseradish peroxidase (HRP)-conjugated donkey anti-rabbit immunoglobulin G (IgG), and sheep anti-mouse IgG, were purchased from Amersham (Buckinghamshire, UK). A fluorescein isothiocyanate (FITC) anti-human CD42P (P-selectin) mAb was obtained from BioLegend (San Diego, CA, USA).

4.2. Synthesis of Ligands and Ir-III Complexes

Synthesis and characterization of the ligands 3-phenyl-1-pyridin-2-yl-imidazo[1,5-*a*]pyridine(L1), 3-(3-nitrophenyl)-1-pyridin-2-yl-imidazo[1,5-*a*]pyridine (L2) and 3-(3,4-dimethoxyphenyl)-1-pyridin-2-yl-imidazo[1,5-*a*]pyridine (L4) are similar to that of the reported method by Wang et al. [41], as shown in Figure 1A. According to the method described [42], the iridium complexes were prepared by mixing the ligands with [Ir(Cp*)(Cl)$_2$]$_2$ (Figure 1B). A representative synthetic scheme for the metal complexation is illustrated below for TIr-1. The absorption spectra of ligands and complexes in acetonitrile is shown in Figure 1Ca,b.

[Ir (Cp*) (L1) Cl]BF$_4$ (Ir-1). To the suspension of 3-phenyl-1-pyridin-2-yl-imidazo[1,5-*a*]pyridine L1 (0.1 g, 0.36 mM) in methanol and dichloromethane solution, was added the methanolic solution of [Ir(Cp*)(Cl)$_2$]$_2$ (0.14 g, 0.184 mM) dropwise and the mixture was stirred at room temperature for 1 h. NH$_4$BF$_4$ (0.05 g, 0.54 mM) was then added and further stirred overnight. The volatile solvent was removed and the formed residue was washed with dichloromethane and filtered to remove excess salt. Finally, the solvent was reduced and the diethyl ether was added to induce precipitation yielding yellow solid. Yield 82%; ^{1}H NMR (400 MHz, DMSO-d_6) δ 8.84–8.82 (d, 1H J = 8Hz), 8.54–8.44 (m, 3H), 8.18–8.15 (t, 3H J = 6 Hz), 7.75 (s, 3H), 7.56–7.49 (m, 2H), 7.17–7.13 (t, 1H J = 8 Hz), 1.27 (s,15H); UV-Vis (λ_{abs}, nm) (ε, M^{-1}cm^{-1}): 401 (1739), 381 (2586), 365 (2043), 284 (2633), 245 (ESI-MS *m/z* 634 [M$^+$ + BF$_4^-$].

[Ir (Cp*) (L2) Cl]BF$_4$ (Ir-2). ^{1}H NMR (400 MHz, DMSO-d_6) δ 9.10 (s,1H), 8.86–8.85 (d, 1H J = 4 Hz), 8.63–8.51 (m, 6H), 8.20–8.17 (t, 1H J = 6 Hz), 8.07–8.03 (t, 1H J = 8 Hz), 7.57–7.53 (t, 2H J = 8 Hz), 7.21–7.18 (t, 1H J = 6 Hz), 1.27 (s, 15H). UV-Vis (λ_{abs}, nm) (ε, M^{-1}cm^{-1}): 400 (943), 378 (1449), 360 (1227), 280 (1601), 246 (1664) ESI-MS *m/z* 679 [M$^+$ + BF$_4^-$].

[Ir (Cp*) (L4) Cl]BF$_4$ (Ir-4). ^{1}H NMR (400 MHz, DMSO-d_6) δ 8.82 (s, 1H), 8.51 (s, 3H), 8.17–8.15 (t, 1H J = 4 Hz), 7.76–7.75 (d, 2H J = 4 Hz), 7.54–7.48 (m, 2H), 7.32–7.29 (m, 1H), 7.14–7.13 (d, 1H J = 4 Hz), 3.91 (s, 3H), 3.85 (s, 3H), 1.29 (s, 15H). UV-Vis (λ_{abs}, nm) (ε, M^{-1}cm^{-1}): 406 (1170), 385 (1651), 364 (1217), 285 (2051), 245 (1795) ESI-MS *m/z* 694 [M$^+$ + BF$_4^-$].

4.3. Platelet Aggregation and ATP Release Assay

Healthy men and women (20–35 years old) were engaged for the study. The subjects had no history of severe diseases, such as cardiovascular diseases (CVDs), hypertension, type 1 or type 2 diabetes, thyroid disorders, or hemostatic disorders. The subjects were educated to abstain from taking medication that is known to affect platelet function for a 14-day period before participating in the study. Written informed consent was gained from all subjects. The Institutional Review Board of Taipei Medical University, Taiwan (TMU-JIRB-N201612050; 20 January 2017) was approved this study, and it conformed to the directives of the Declaration of Helsinki.

According to the method described from our previous study, the human platelet suspensions were prepared. Briefly, human blood samples were collected from adult volunteers who abstained from the use of drugs or other substances that could affect with the experiment for at least 14 days before collection; the collected blood samples were mixed with an acid–citrate–dextrose solution. After centrifugation, the platelet-rich plasma was supplemented with 0.5 µM PGE1 and 6.4 IU/mL heparin. Tyrode's solution containing 3.5 mg/mL BSA was used to prepare the final suspension of washed human platelets. The final Ca^{2+} concentration in Tyrode's solution was 1 mM. The platelet aggregation study was conducted using a lumiaggregometer (Payton Associates, Scarborough, ON, Canada) [43]. An isovolumetric solvent control (0.1% DMSO) or Ir-1, Ir-2 and Ir-4 complexes were preincubated with platelet suspensions (3.6×10^8 cells/mL) for 3 min before the addition of collagen and U46619. The amount of platelet aggregation was measured as the percent compared with individual control (without Ir compounds) after the reaction proceeded for 6 min and is stated in light transmission units. During the measurement of the ATP release assay, 1 min before adding the collagen (1 µg/mL), 20 µL of luciferin–luciferase was added and the amount of ATP released was equated with that released by the control (without Ir compounds).

4.4. Measurement of Relative $[Ca^{2+}]i$ Mobilization

The concentration of $[Ca^{2+}]i$ was measured using Fura-2AM per the method described previously [42]. Concisely, citrated whole blood was centrifuged at $120\times g$ for 10 min, and the platelet rich plasma (PRP) was collected and subjected to 5 µM Fura-2AM for 1 h. As described in the above section, human platelets were prepared. The Fura-2AM-added platelets were pretreated with 10 µM Ir-1, Ir-2 and Ir-4 in the presence of 1 mM $CaCl_2$ and then stimulated with 1 µg/mL of collagen. Using a spectrofluorometer (Hitachi FL Spectrophotometer F-4500, Tokyo, Japan), the Fura-2 fluorescence was measured at excitation wavelengths of 340 and 380 nm and an emission wavelength of 510 nm.

4.5. Flow Cytometric Analysis

The platelet suspensions (3.6×10^8 cells/mL) were preincubated with 0.1% DMSO (solvent control) or 10 µM of each Ir-1, Ir-2 and Ir-4 and FITC-P-selectin (2 µg/mL) for 3 min, and 1 µg/mL collagen was added to trigger platelet activation. In other experiment, the FITC labeling of the anti-GPVI mAb (FITC-JAQ1 mAb) was done, in which the platelets (3.6×10^8 cells/mL) were preincubated with 10 ng/mL of convulxin or 20 µM Ir-1 for 3 min, followed by the addition of 1 µg/mL of FITC-JAQ1 mAb. For isotype controls, FITC-IgG antibody (Biolegend, Cat. No. 400108) was used. The suspensions were then assayed for fluorescein-labeled platelets by using a flow cytometer (FACScan System, Becton Dickinson, San Jose, CA, USA). Data were collected from 50,000 platelets per experimental group, and the platelets were identified with their characteristic forward and orthogonal light-scattering profiles. All experiments were repeated at least three times to confirm reproducibility.

4.6. Detection of Lactate Dehydrogenase (LDH)

Washed platelets (3.6×10^8 cells/mL) were preincubated with 0.1% DMSO or 100 µM each Ir-1, Ir-2 and Ir-4 for 20 min at 37 °C. A 10 µL of the supernatant was deposited on a Fuji Dri-Chem slide LDH-PIII (Fuji, Tokyo, Japan), and the optical density was read at 540 nm wavelength by using a UV-Vis spectrophotometer (UV-160; Shimadzu, Japan). "Max" is considered as maximal value of LDH recorded in the sonicated platelets.

4.7. Immunoblotting

Washed platelets (1.2×10^9 cells/mL) were pre-incubated with 10 µM Ir-1, Ir-2 and Ir-4 or 0.1 % DMSO for 3 min and then collagen was added to induce platelet activation. After the reaction stopped, the platelets were directly re-suspended in 200 µL of lysis buffer. Samples (60 µg protein) were resolved on a 12% sodium dodecylsulfate polyacrylamide gel electrophoresis (SDS-PAGE), and transferred to the PVDF membranes by using a Bio-Rad semidry transfer unit (Hercules, CA, USA). Membranes were blocked with TBST (10 mM Tris-base, 100 mM NaCl, and 0.01% Tween 20) containing 5% BSA for 1 h and probed with various primary antibodies. HRP-conjugated anti-mouse IgG or anti-rabbit IgG (diluted 1:3000 in TBST) antibodies were used and the bands were visualized using an enhanced chemiluminescence system.

4.8. Measurement of Closure Time Using PFA-100™ Platelet Function Analyzer

The platelet functions were analyzed using a Dade Behring PFA-100 system (Dade Behring, Marburg, Germany) according to a method described [44]. First, 0.8 mL of human whole blood was treated with Ir-1, Ir-2, Ir-4 (10 µM) or the solvent control (0.1% DMSO) for 2 min, and then poured onto the cartridges containing collagen-ADP (C-ADP) or collagen epinephrine (C-EPI)-coated membranes, and subjected to a high shear rate of 5000–6000/s. A platelet plug forms, then slowly occludes the aperture; subsequently, the blood flow gradually decreases and finally stops. The time required to obtain full occlusion of the aperture by the platelet clot is defined as the "closure time" and was recorded in the collagen membrane [44].

4.9. Confocal Microscopic Analysis of Platelet Adhesion and Spreading

Eight-chamber glass coverslides were coated with BSA (100 µg/mL), fibrinogen or collagen (100 µg/mL) at 4°C overnight. The coverslides were blocked with 1% BSA for 1 h after being washed twice with PBS. Washed platelets (3.6×10^8 cells/mL) preincubated with Ir-1 (10 µM) or the solvent control (0.1% DMSO) were allowed to spread on the protein-coated surfaces at 37 °C for 45 min. After removing the unbound platelets and two washes with PBS, the attached cells were fixed with 4% paraformaldehyde, permeabilized (0.1% Triton) and stained with FITC-labeled phalloidin (10 µM) for 1 h. The confocal study was done with a Leica TCS SP5 microscope furnished with a 100×, 1.40 NA oil immersion objective (Leica, Wetzlar, Germany).

4.10. Animals

ICR mice (20–25 g, male, 5–6 weeks old) were obtained from BioLasco (Taipei, Taiwan). All procedures were approved by the Affidavit of Approval of Animal Use Protocol-Taipei Medical University (LAC-2016-0395) and were in accordance with the Guide for the Care and Use of Laboratory Animals (8th edition, 2011). Since among the three tested Ir-III complexes, Ir-1 (10 µM) effectively inhibits platelet activation in vitro, this concentration was chosen and calculated accordingly into mouse dose 2 mg/kg [45].

4.11. Fluorescein Sodium-Induced Platelet Thrombi in Mesenteric Microvessels of Mice

This study conformed to the Guide for the Care and Use of Laboratory Animals (Approval No. LAC-2016-0395; 1 August 2017). As described previously [46], the jugular vein was exposed and cannulated using PE-10 tubing to administer the dye and compounds (by an i.v. bolus). Vessels (30–40 µm) were selected for irradiation (below 520 nm) to form a microthrombus. One minute after fluorescein sodium (15 µg/kg) given, Ir-1, Ir-2 and Ir-4 (2 mg/kg) were administered. The time lapse for inducing thrombus formation leading to cessation of blood flow was measured.

4.12. Measurement of Bleeding Time in Mouse Tail Vein

Experiments were performed through transection of the tails in male ICR mice. Briefly, after an intraperitoneal administration of 2.0 mg/kg Ir-1, Ir-2 and Ir-4 for 30 min, the mice tails were cut 3 mm from the tip. The tails were immersed in normal saline at 37 °C, and the time from incision to full cessation of bleeding was recorded.

4.13. Acute Pulmonary Thrombosis Induced by ADP in Mice

A dose of 2 mg/kg of Ir-1, Ir-2 and Ir-4 and vehicle solution (0.1 % DMSO, all in 20 µL) were injected into the tail vein of 20–25 g ICR mice for 30 min, followed by 700 mg/kg ADP injection into the contralateral vein [47]. The mortality rate was determined in mice of each group within 5 min after injection.

4.14. Statistical Analysis

The experimental data are produced as the mean ± standard error of the means (S.E.M.) and are presented by the number of observations (n). The unpaired Student t test was used to analyze the significance of variations between the control and experimental mice. The differences between multiple groups in other experiments were assessed through one-way analysis of variance (ANOVA). When ANOVA showed significant differences among the group means, the groups were compared using the Student Newman–Keuls method. In the analysis, p-values < 0.05 were considered statistically significant. Statistical evaluations were performed using SAS (version 9.2; SAS Inc., Cary, NC, USA).

5. Conclusions

In this work, we showed that, among the three newly synthesized organometallic iridium-III complexes, Ir-1, Ir-2 and Ir-4, Ir-1 has a promising in vitro antiplatelet and in vivo antithrombotic profiles. Ir-1 actively inhibits collagen-stimulated platelet activation by inhibiting the Akt/PKC pathways, and subsequently by suppressing activation of MAPKs. These alterations reduce the levels of surface P-selectin expression and $[Ca^{2+}]i$, and ultimately inhibit platelet aggregation. Our SAR study suggested that the inhibitory activity of Ir-1 is modulated by its increasing hydrolytic nature. Altogether, these results suggest that Ir-1 may be a leading novel Ir-III complex to design new antiplatelet drugs for the treatment of thromboembolic diseases.

Author Contributions: C.-H.Y., T.J., Y.C., and J.-R.S. conceived and designed the projects. C.-W.H., T.J., C.-H.H., T.K. and Y.-J.C. conducted the experiments. T.J. wrote the paper. T.K. contributed to the synthesis and analysis of the compounds. M.M. edited the English. All authors contributed clarifications and guidance on the manuscript. All authors were involved in editing the manuscript. All authors read and approved the final manuscript.

Funding: Shin Kong Wu Ho-Su Memorial Hospital (SKH-8302-104-DR-23 and SKH-8302-105-DR-21), Ministry of Science and Technology of Taiwan (MOST 104-2622-B-038-003, MOST 104-2320-B-038-045-MY2, MOST 106-2320-B-038-012, and MOST 106-2320-B-038-049-MY3), Shin Kong Wu Ho-Su Memorial Hospital–Taipei Medical University (SKH-TMU-104-05 and SKH-TMU-105-02), Taipei Medical University (DP2-107-21121-N-02), and the University Grants Commission, India (MRP-MAJOR-CHEM-2013-5144 and 69/2014 F. No. 10-11/12UGC) supported grants to this work.

Conflicts of Interest: The authors declare no conflict of interest.

References

1. Smith, J.N.; Negrelli, J.M.; Manek, M.B.; Hawes, E.M.; Viera, A.J. Diagnosis and management of acute coronary syndrome: An evidence-based update. *J. Am. Board Fam. Med.* **2015**, *28*, 283–293. [CrossRef] [PubMed]
2. Franchi, F.; Angiolillo, D.J. Novel antiplatelet agents in acute coronary syndrome. *Nat. Rev. Cardiol.* **2015**, *12*, 30–47. [CrossRef] [PubMed]
3. Zimmermann, N.; Hohlfeld, T. Clinical implications of aspirin resistance. *Thromb. Haemost.* **2008**, *100*, 379–390. [CrossRef] [PubMed]
4. Chen, W.H. Antiplatelet resistance with aspirin and clopidogrel: Is it real and does it matter? *Curr. Cardiol. Rep.* **2006**, *8*, 301–306. [CrossRef] [PubMed]
5. Algra, A.; De Schryver, E.L.; van Gijn, J.; Kappelle, L.J.; Koudstaal, P.J. Oral anticoagulants versus antiplatelet therapy for preventing further vascular events after transient ischaemic attack or minor stroke of presumed arterial origin. *Cochrane Database Syst. Rev.* **2006**, *3*, CD001342.
6. Belloc, C.; Lu, H.; Soria, C.; Fridman, R.; Legrand, Y.; Menashi, S. The effect of platelets on invasiveness and protease production of human mammary tumor cells. *Int. J. Cancer* **1995**, *60*, 413–417. [CrossRef] [PubMed]
7. Boucharaba, A.; Serre, C.M.; Gres, S.; Saulnier-Blache, J.S.; Bordet, J.C.; Guglielmi, J.; Clézardin, P.; Peyruchaud, O. Platelet-derived lysophosphatidic acid supports the progression of osteolytic bone metastases in breast cancer. *J. Clin. Investig.* **2004**, *114*, 1714–1725. [CrossRef] [PubMed]

8. Wenzel, J.; Zeisig, R.; Fichtner, I. Inhibition of metastasis in a murine 4T1 breast cancer model by liposomes preventing tumor cell-platelet interactions. *Clin. Exp. Metast.* **2010**, *27*, 25–34. [CrossRef] [PubMed]
9. Koo, M.H.; Nawarskas, J.J.; Frishman, W.H. Prasugrel: A new antiplatelet drug for the prevention and treatment of cardiovascular disease. *Cardiol. Rev.* **2008**, *16*, 314–318. [CrossRef] [PubMed]
10. Krötz, F.; Sohn, H.Y.; Klauss, V. Antiplatelet drugs in cardiological practice: Established strategies and new developments. *Vasc. Health Risk Manag.* **2008**, *4*, 637–645. [CrossRef] [PubMed]
11. Gasser, G.; Ott, I.; Metzler-Nolte, N. Organometallic anticancer compounds. *Med. Chem.* **2011**, *54*, 3–25. [CrossRef] [PubMed]
12. Ruiz, J.; Rodríguez, V.; Cutillas, N.; Samper, K.G.; Capdevila, M.; Palacios, O.; Espinosa, A. Novel C, N-chelate rhodium (III) and iridium (III) antitumor complexes incorporating a lipophilic steroidal conjugate and their interaction with DNA. *Dalton Trans.* **2012**, *41*, 12847–12856. [CrossRef] [PubMed]
13. Liu, Z.; Sadler, P.J. Organoiridium complexes: Anticancer agents and catalysts. *ACC Chem. Res.* **2014**, *47*, 1174–1185. [CrossRef] [PubMed]
14. Li, Y.; Tan, C.P.; Zhang, W.; He, L.; Ji, L.N.; Mao, Z.W. Phosphorescent iridium (III)-bis-N-heterocyclic carbene complexes as mitochondria-targeted theranostic and photodynamic anticancer agents. *Biomaterials* **2015**, *39*, 95–104. [CrossRef] [PubMed]
15. Hsia, C.W.; Velusamy, M.; Tsao, J.T.; Hsia, C.H.; Chou, D.S.; Jayakumar, T.; Lee, L.W.; Li, J.Y.; Sheu, J.R. New Therapeutic Agent against Arterial Thrombosis: An Iridium (III)-Derived Organometallic Compound. *Int. J. Mol. Sci.* **2017**, *18*, 2616. [CrossRef] [PubMed]
16. Shyu, K.G.; Velusamy, M.; Hsia, C.W.; Yang, C.H.; Hsia, C.H.; Chou, D.S.; Jayakumar, T.; Sheu, J.R.; Li, J.Y. Novel iridium (III) -derived organometallic compound for the inhibition of human platelet activation. *Int. J. Mol. Med.* **2018**, *41*, 2589–2600. [CrossRef] [PubMed]
17. Shyu, R.S.; Khamrang, T.; Sheu, J.R.; Hsia, C.W.; Velusamy, M.; Hsia, C.H.; Chou, D.S.; Chang, C.C. Ir-6: A Novel Iridium (III) Organometallic Derivative for Inhibition of Human Platelet Activation. *Bioinorg. Chem. Appl.* **2018**. [CrossRef] [PubMed]
18. Smith, J.B.; Selak, M.A.; Dangelmaier, C.; Daniel, J.L. Cytosolic calcium as a second messenger for collagen-induced platelet responses. *Biochem. J.* **1992**, *288*, 925–929. [CrossRef] [PubMed]
19. Borsig, L.; Wong, R.; Feramisco, J.; Nadeau, D.R.; Varki, N.M.; Varki, A. Heparin and cancer revisited: Mechanistic connections involving platelets, P-selectin, carcinoma mucins, and tumor metastasis. *Proc. Natl. Acad. Sci. USA* **2001**, *98*, 3352–3357. [CrossRef] [PubMed]
20. Adam, F.; Kauskot, A.; Rosa, J.P.; Bryckaert, M. Mitogen-activated protein kinases in hemostasis and thrombosis. *J. Thromb. Haemost.* **2008**, *6*, 2007–2016. [CrossRef] [PubMed]
21. Wang, L.; Ostberg, O.; Wihlborg, A.K.; Brogren, H.; Jern, S.; Erlinge, D. Quantification of ADP and ATP receptor expression in human platelets. *J. Thromb. Haemost.* **2003**, *1*, 330–336. [CrossRef] [PubMed]
22. Mahaut-Smith, M.P. The unique contribution of ion channels to platelet and megakaryocyte function. *J. Thromb. Haemost.* **2012**, *10*, 1722–1732. [CrossRef] [PubMed]
23. Fung, C.Y.; Jones, S.; Ntrakwah, A.; Naseem, K.M.; Farndale, R.W.; Mahaut-Smith, M.P. Platelet Ca^{2+} responses coupled to glycoprotein VI and Toll-like receptors persist in the presence of endothelial-derived inhibitors: Roles for secondary activation of P2X1 receptors and release from intracellular Ca^{2+} stores. *Blood* **2012**, *119*, 3613–3621. [CrossRef] [PubMed]
24. Ludwig, R.J.; Schön, M.P.; Boehncke, W.H. P-selectin: A common therapeutic target for cardiovascular disorders, inflammation and tumour metastasis. *Expert Opin. Ther. Targets* **2007**, *11*, 1103–1117. [CrossRef] [PubMed]
25. Alghatani, M.; Heptinstall, S. Novel strategies for assessing platelet reactivity. *Future Cardiol.* **2017**, *13*, 33–47. [CrossRef] [PubMed]
26. Tynngard, N. Preparation, storage and quality control of platelet concentrates. *Transfus. Apher. Sci.* **2009**, *41*, 97–104. [CrossRef] [PubMed]
27. Jackson, S.P.; Yap, C.L.; Anderson, K.E. Phosphoinositide 3-kinases and the regulation of platelet function. *Biochem. Soc. Trans.* **2014**, *32*, 387–392. [CrossRef]
28. Deb, T.B.; Coticchia, C.M.; Dickson, R.B. Calmodulin-mediated activation of Akt regulates survival of c-Myc-overexpressing mouse mammary carcinoma cells. *J. Biol. Chem.* **2004**, *279*, 38903–38911. [CrossRef] [PubMed]

29. Chen, J.; De, S.; Damron, D.S.; Chen, W.S.; Hay, N.; Byzova, T.V. Impaired platelet responses to thrombin and collagen in AKT-1-deficient mice. *Blood* **2004**, *104*, 1703–1710. [CrossRef] [PubMed]
30. Mazharian, A.; Roger, S.; Berrou, E.; Adam, F.; Kauskot, A.; Nurden, P.; Jandrot-Perrus, M.; Bryckaert, M. Protease-activating receptor-4 induces full platelet spreading on a fibrinogen matrix: Involvement of ERK2 and p38 and Ca^{2+} mobilization. *J. Biol. Chem.* **2007**, *282*, 5478–5487. [CrossRef] [PubMed]
31. Adam, F.; Kauskot, A.; Nurden, P.; Sulpice, E.; Hoylaerts, M.F.; Davis, R.J.; Rosa, J.P.; Bryckaert, M. Platelet JNK1 is involved in secretion and thrombus formation. *Blood* **2010**, *115*, 4083–4092. [CrossRef] [PubMed]
32. Chang, L.; Karin, M. Mammalian MAP kinase signalling cascades. *Nature* **2001**, *410*, 37–40. [CrossRef] [PubMed]
33. Favaloro, E.J. Clinical utility of the PFA-100. *Semin. Thromb. Hemost.* **2008**, *34*, 709–733. [CrossRef] [PubMed]
34. Ho, S.J.; Gemmell, R.; Brighton, T.A. Platelet function testing in uraemic patients. *Hematology* **2008**, *13*, 49–58. [CrossRef] [PubMed]
35. Arrieta-Blanco, J.J.; Bartolomé-Villar, B.; Juzgado, A.; Mourelle Martinez, R. Assessment of PFA-100 system for the measurement of bleeding time in oral surgery. *Med. Oral Patol. Oral Cir. Bucal.* **2006**, *11*, E514. [PubMed]
36. Karger, R.; Reuter, K.; Rohlfs, J.; Nimsky, C.; Sure, U.; Kretschmer, V. The Platelet function analyzer (PFA-100) as a screening tool in neurosurgery. *ISRN Hematol.* **2012**, *2012*, 1–7. [CrossRef] [PubMed]
37. Induruwa, I.; Moroi, M.; Bonna, A.; Malcor, J.D.; Howes, J.M.; Warburton, E.A.; Farndale, R.W.; Jung, S.M. Platelet collagen receptor Glycoprotein VI-dimer recognizes fibrinogen and fibrin through their D-domains, contributing to platelet adhesion and activation during thrombus formation. *J. Thromb. Haemost.* **2018**, *16*, 389–404. [CrossRef] [PubMed]
38. Habtemariam, A.; Melchart, M.; Ferna´ndez, R.; Parsons, S.; Oswald, I.D.H.; Parkin, A.; Fabbiani, F.P.; Davidson, J.E.; Dawson, A.; Aird, R.E.; et al. Structure-Activity Relationships for cytotoxic ruthenium(II) arene complexes containing N,N-, N,O-, and O,O-chelating ligands. *J. Med. Chem.* **2006**, *49*, 6858–6868. [CrossRef] [PubMed]
39. Manso, A.; Escudero, C.; Alijo, M.; López-Fandiño, R. Platelet aggregation inhibitory activity of bovine, ovine, and caprine κ-casein macropeptides and their tryptic hydrolysates. *J. Food. Prot.* **2002**, *65*, 1992–1996. [CrossRef] [PubMed]
40. Alevriadou, B.R.; McIntire, L.V.; Lasslo, A. Inhibition of platelet adhesion and thrombus formation on a collagen-coated surface by novel carbamoylpiperidine antiplatelet agents. *Biochim. Biophys. Acta* **1992**, *1137*, 279–286. [CrossRef]
41. Wang, J.; Dyers, L.; Mason, R.; Amoyaw, P.; Bu, X.R. Highly efficient and direct heterocyclization of dipyridyl ketone to N, N-bidentate ligands. *J. Org. Chem.* **2005**, *70*, 2353–2356. [CrossRef] [PubMed]
42. Bennett, M.A.; Huang, T.N.; Matheson, T.W.; Smith, A.K. (η6-Hexa methylbenzene) ruthenium complexes. *Inorg. Synth.* **1982**, *21*, 74–78.
43. Sheu, J.R.; Lee, C.R.; Lin, C.H.; Hsiao, G.; Ko, W.C.; Chen, Y.C.; Yen, M.H. Mechanisms involved in the antiplatelet activity of Staphylococcus aureus lipoteichoic acid in human plalets. *Thromb. Haemost.* **2000**, *83*, 777–784. [PubMed]
44. Jilma, B. Platelet function analyzer (PFA100): A tool to quantify congenital or acquired platelet dysfunction. *J. Lab. Clin. Med.* **2001**, *138*, 152–163. [CrossRef] [PubMed]
45. Reagan-Shaw, S.; Nihal, M.; Ahmad, N. Dose translation from animal to human studies revisited. *FASEB J.* **2008**, *22*, 659–661. [CrossRef] [PubMed]
46. Lin, K.H.; Kuo, J.R.; Lu, W.J.; Chung, C.L.; Chou, D.S.; Huang, S.Y.; Lee, H.C.; Sheu, J.R. Hinokitiol inhibits platelet activation ex vivo and thrombus formation in vivo. *Biochem. Pharmacol.* **2013**, *85*, 1478–1485. [CrossRef] [PubMed]
47. Lu, W.J.; Lee, J.J.; Chou, D.S.; Jayakumar, T.; Fong, T.H.; Hsiao, G.; Sheu, J.R. Anovelroleofandrographolide, an NF-κB inhibitor, on inhibition of platelet activation: The pivotal mechanisms of endothelial nitric oxide synthase/cyclic GMP. *J. Mol. Med.* **2011**, *89*, 1261–1273. [CrossRef] [PubMed]

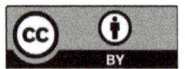

© 2018 by the authors. Licensee MDPI, Basel, Switzerland. This article is an open access article distributed under the terms and conditions of the Creative Commons Attribution (CC BY) license (http://creativecommons.org/licenses/by/4.0/).

MDPI
St. Alban-Anlage 66
4052 Basel
Switzerland
Tel. +41 61 683 77 34
Fax +41 61 302 89 18
www.mdpi.com

International Journal of Molecular Sciences Editorial Office
E-mail: ijms@mdpi.com
www.mdpi.com/journal/ijms